The Neuropsychology of Asian Americans

STUDIES ON NEUROPSYCHOLOGY, NEUROLOGY, AND COGNITION

Series Editor:
LINAS BIELIAUSKAS, University of Michigan

Studies on Neuropsychology, Neurology and Cognition provides state-of-the-art overviews of key areas of interest to a range of clinicians, professionals, researchers, instructors, and students working in clinical neuropsychology, neurology, rehabilitation, and related fields.

Topics cover a broad spectrum of core issues related to theory and practice concerning brain and behavior, including: practical and professional issues (e.g. diagnosis, treatment, rehabilitation); cognitive development over the lifespan (e.g. child, geriatric); domain-specific cognitive issues (e.g. sport, toxicology); methodology related to brain and behavior (e.g. functional brain imaging, statistics and research methods); as well as relevant allied issues (e.g. ethics, minorities and culture, forensics)

The authors, editors, and contributors to each title are internationally recognized professionals and scholars in their field. Each volume provides an essential resource for clinicians, researchers, and students wanting to update and advance their knowledge in their specific field of interest.

PUBLISHED

Fujii — *Neuropsychology of Asian Americans*
Anderson, Jacobs, & Anderson – *Executive Functions and the Frontal Lobes*
Crowe — *The Behavioral and Emotional Complications of Traumatic Brain Injury*
Morgan & Ricker — *Textbook of Clinical Neuropsychology*
Kalechstein & van Gorp — *Neuropsychology of Substance Use*
DeLuca & Kalmar — *Information Processing Speed in Clinical Populations*
Stern — *Cognitive Reserve*
Tuokko & Hultsch — *Mild Cognitive Impairment*
Poreh — *Quantified Process Approach to Neuropsychological Development*
Leon-Carrion, von Wilde, & Zitnay — *Brain Injury Treatment*
Bush & Martin — *Geriatric Neuropsychology*
Berent & Albers — *Neurobehavioral Toxicology, Vols. I, II, and III*
Bush — *A Casebook of Ethical Challenges in Neuropsychology*
Ciccetti & Rourke — *Methodological and Biostatistical Foundations of Clinical Neuropsychology and Medical and Health Disciplines, 2nd Edition*
Lovell et al. — *Traumatic Brain Injury in Sports*
Wilson — *Neuropsychological Rehabilitation*
Lamberty, Courtney, & Heilbronner — *The Practice of Clinical Neuropsychology*
Ferraro — *Minority and Cross-cultural Aspects of Neuropsychological Assessment*
Rourke, Rourke, & van der Vlugt — *Practice of Child-clinical Neuropsychology*
Sweet — *Forensic Neuropsychology*

For continually updated information about published and forthcoming titles in the Neuropsychology, Neurology, and Cognition series, please visit: ***www.psypress.com/nnc***

The Neuropsychology of Asian Americans

Edited by

Daryl E. M. Fujii

Psychology Press
Taylor & Francis Group
NEW YORK AND LONDON

Psychology Press
Taylor & Francis Group
711 Third Avenue,
New York, NY 10017

Psychology Press
Taylor & Francis Group
27 Church Road
Hove, East Sussex BN3 2FA

First issued in paperback 2015

Psychology Press is an imprint of the Taylor and Francis Group, an informa business

International Standard Book Number: 978-1-138-88296-6 (pbk)
International Standard Book Number: 978-1-84169-784-0 (Hardback)

Library of Congress Cataloging-in-Publication Data

The neuropsychology of Asian-Americans / editor, Daryl Fujii.
p. ; cm. -- (Studies on neuropsychology, neurology and cognition)
Includes bibliographical references and index.
ISBN 978-1-84169-784-0 (hardcover : alk. paper)
1. Neuropsychology--United States. 2. Neuropsychology--Asia. 3. Asian Americans--Psychology. 4. Cultural psychiatry--United States. I. Fujii, Daryl, 1961- II. Series: Studies on neuropsychology, neurology, and cognition.
[DNLM: 1. Neuropsychology--methods--United States. 2. Asian Americans--ethnology--United States. 3. Asian Americans--psychology--United States. 4. Cultural Competency--United States. 5. Mental Disorders--ethnology--United States. 6. Professional-Patient Relations--United States. WL 103.5 N94963 2011]

QP360.N4947 2011
612.8--dc22 2010019933

Visit the Taylor & Francis Web site at
http://www.taylorandfrancis.com

and the Psychology Press Web site at
http://www.psypress.com

Contents

Series preface

One of the major goals of our book series *Neuropsychology, Neurology and Cognition* is to facilitate the application of neuropsychological knowledge to clinical populations. In editing *The Neuropsychology of Asian Americans*, Dr. Daryl Fujii provides the basis for application of neuropsychological principles and practices to the fastest-growing major racial/ethnic group in the United States in terms of percentage growth. According to the 2000 U.S. census, Asian Americans made up 4.3% of the U.S. population, showing a 63% increase from data gathered in the 1990 census. Asian Americans thus constitute a significant and increasing base of need for clinical services.

In this volume, multiple authors address optimal parameters for providing clinical services to subgroups of Asian Americans in terms of clinical interaction, parameters of the testing context, and suggestions for providing the results of neuropsychological assessment in ways which are culturally competent and sensitive. Even more importantly, the chapters provide a central repository of listing of available resources for each subgroup ranging from Cambodian Americans, to Laotian Americans, to Hmong Americans. Each group, of course has a rich and unique cultural history and context which must be taken into account for competent and ethical clinical practice. The second part of this ground-breaking text addresses the state of knowledge and practice of neuropsychology within the various Asian countries and cultures, leading the reader toward an informed journey of understanding and further exploration of issues and possibilities in expanding their experience with Asian American Neuropsychology.

I welcome this valuable contribution our series and highly recommend *The Neuropsychology of Asian Americans* to anyone who is privileged to interact with the Asian American community in a clinical, research, or scholarly context. It will be an interaction which increases in richness and frequency with each passing decade.

Linas A. Bieliauskas
Ann Arbor
May, 2010

Acknowledgments

It is with great pride that I present to you this book. It has truly been a labor of love as well as an enlightening experience. It is dedicated to all the industrious Asian Americans and their ancestors living in the homeland. I thank all the contributing authors for their expertise and willingness to allow me to revise (or butcher) their writing. I also thank the following clinicians, who have contributed their personal knowledge and experiences to enrich our understanding of Asian Americans: Suwitda Cholitkul, Shin Shin Tang, Suryadutt Venkat, Hoa Vo, and Koichiro Yamasaki. Special thanks to my loving wife, Sam Yoon Fujii, who had the patience to put up with me for the past 3 years that I spent on this project, as well as the past 18 years. Thanks to my eggies, Dylan, Cody, and furry son Norbert; brother, Jay, and family, Naomi and Jarin; parents, Earl and Judy Fujii; and Grandpa Ito Doomo Arigato Gozaimasu. I also wish to acknowledge my in-laws, Chon You Soon, Sam Sil, and Glen Cannon; Sam Su Yoon and Chung Hee Lee; and Jae Song Lee. Kamsahamnida.

Daryl Fujii

Contributors

Agnes S. Chan, PhD
Department of Psychology
Chinese University of Hong Kong
Hong Kong

Mei-Chun Cheung, PhD
Institute of Textiles and Clothing
Hong Kong Polytechnic University
Hong Kong

Jeanyung Chey, PhD
Department of Psychology
Seoul National University
Seoul, South Korea

Simon L. Collinson, DPhil
Department of Psychology
National University of Singapore
Singapore

Lauren Kwon Dawson, PhD, ABPP
Rehabilitation Hospital of the Pacific
Honolulu, Hawaii

Normah Che Din, MA
Health Psychology Unit
Universiti Kebangsaan
Kuala Lumpur Federal Territory, Malaysia

Sopagna Eap, PhD
Department of Psychology
Pacific University
Forest Grove, Oregon

Daryl Fujii, PhD, ABPP
Veterans Affairs Community Living Center
Honolulu, Hawaii

Angelica Isomura-Motoki, PhD
Department of Neuropsychiatry
Showa University School of Medicine
Tokyo, Japan

Mi-Yeoung Jo, PsyD, ABPP
Los Angeles, California

Vidyulata Kamath, PhD
Department of Psychiatry
University of Pennsylvania Medical Center
Philadelphia Pennsylvania

J. Keshav Kumar, PhD
Department of Clinical Psychology
Neuropsychology Unit
National Institute of Mental Health and Neurosciences
Bangalore, India

Theanvy Kuoch, MA, LPC
Khmer Health Associates, Inc.
West Hartford, Connecticut

Minh-Thu Le, PhD
Beverly Hills, California

Phuoc Dinh Le, PhD
Los Angeles, California

Lourdes Ledesma, PhD
Manila, Philippines

Winnie W. Leung, MPhil
Neuropsychology Laboratory
Department of Psychology
Chinese University of Hong Kong
Hong Kong

Maria Raquel Lopa-Ramos, PhD
Neurodevelopmental Center
St. Luke's Medical Center
Quezon City, Philippines

Masaru Mimura, MD, PhD
Department of Neuropsychiatry
Showa University School of Medicine
Tokyo, Japan

Jennifer Monzones, MA
Department of Psychology
Fordham University
New York, New York

Kevin L. Nadal, PhD
John Jay College of Criminal Justice
City University of New York
New York, New York

Dung Ngo, PhD
Department of Psychology
University Wisconsin–Lacrosse
Lacrosse, Wisconsin

Heyeon Park
Department of Psychology
Seoul National University
Seoul, South Korea

Vaishali S. Phatak, PhD, ABPP
Regional Epilepsy Center
University of Washington
Seattle, Washington

Kattiya Ratanadilok, PsyD
Kampangsan, Thailand

Mary Scully, RN, CS
Khmer Health Advocates, Inc.
West Hartford, Connecticut

Vincent G. Tsushima, PhD, JD
Hawaii Pacific University
Honolulu, Hawaii

William T. Tsushima, PhD
Straub Clinic and Hospital
Honolulu, Hawaii

Alyssa Kaying Vang, PsyD
Children's Hospitals and Clinics of Minnesota
St. Paul, Minnesota

Tony M. Wong, PhD, ABPP
Brain Injury Rehab Program
Unity Health System
Rochester, New York

Tony Wu, PhD
Los Angeles Guidance Clinic
Los Angeles, California

Barbara W.K. Yee, PhD
Department of Family and Consumer Sciences
University of Hawaii at Manoa
Honolulu, Hawaii

Donald Yeo, PsyD
Department of Neurology
Singapore General Hospital
Singapore

1 Introduction

Daryl Fujii

Introduction

Although relatively small in number compared to the total American population, Asians are the fastest-growing ethnic minority in the United States. According to the 2000 U.S. Census Bureau, there were 10,171,820 Asians living in the United States, which is about 3.6% of population. The figure rises to 11,859,446, or 4.2% of the total population, if persons of part-Asian ancestry are included. These numbers reflect a 48% to 72% increase for various subgroups from 1990 to 2000 in comparison to 13% of the general population (Barnes & Bennett, 2002). The growth in the Asian population will not only continue but exponentially increase, as by 2050 it is projected that the number of Asian Americans will increase 213% to 33.4 million, or 8% of U.S. population (U.S. Census Bureau, 2004).

Given the growing number of Asians, it is likely that a clinical neuropsychologist will at some point in time be referred a client of Asian heritage. An Asian client may pose a special challenge for Western neuropsychologists, as many are not familiar with Asian culture, and most standard tests and procedures may have questionable validity and reliability with this population (Fujii & Wong, 2005; Wong & Fujii, 2004). Salient issues in working with Asians include ethnic diversity, language barriers, acculturation, and different value systems and communication styles.

Asian Americans are a highly diverse group. The 2000 U.S. Census Bureau lists 24 different ethnicities under the Asian category. The 11 largest Asian ethnicities in the United States are as follows (Barnes & Bennett, 2002):

1. Chinese (2,422,970, 23.8%)
2. Filipinos (1,864,120, 18.3%)
3. Asian Indians (1,645,510, 16.2%)
4. Vietnamese (1,110,201, 10.9%)
5. Korean (1,072,682, 10.5%)
6. Japanese (795,051, 7.8%)
7. Cambodian (178,043, 1.8%)
8. Hmong (170,049, 1.7%)
9. Laotian (167,792, 1.6%)

10. Pakistani (155,909, 1.5%)
11. Thai (110,851, 1.1%)

Not only are Asians ethnically diverse, but they are demographically diverse as well. For example, although known as the "model minority" due to high academic and occupational achievement, persons with a bachelor's degree or higher range from a high of 63.9% for Asian Indians to 7.7% and 7.5% for Laotian and Hmong, respectively. Similarly, although the median family income of all Asians was $9,000 higher than the median for all American families ($59,300 vs. $50,000), median incomes of subgroups vary from a high of $70,849 for Japanese to a low of $32,384 for Hmong. These differences illustrate that "one size does not fit all" when understanding Asian ethnic groups, as characteristics of one ethnicity do not necessarily apply to another. This diversity increases the knowledge base required for working with Asian Americans, thereby making it more difficult to work with this population.

Language barriers are another issue. It is estimated that 69% of the Asian Americans are foreign born. Asian Indians, Vietnamese, Koreans, and Thais are the subgroups with the highest percentage of foreign-born persons, ranging from 75% to 78% (Reeves & Bennett, 2004). By contrast, the Asian ethnic group with the lowest percentage of foreign born is the Japanese, at 39% (Reeves & Bennett, 2004). An implication of this demographic is that a large number of Asian Americans are not proficient in English. Data from the 2000 U.S. Census Bureau indicate that 79% of Asian households speak a language other than English at home, with percentages ranging from 47% for Japanese households to over 90% for Cambodians, Laotians, and Vietnamese, and 96% for Hmong (Reeves & Bennett, 2004). Forty percent of Asians are reported to speak English less than "very well," with the highest percentage being the Vietnamese, 62%. The Japanese were the only subgroup with over 50% of the households speaking only English at home (Reeves & Bennett, 2004).

An issue related to immigration is acculturation. In addition to language spoken at home and whether one was foreign born, years living in the United States is another contributor to level of acculturation. Data from the 2000 census indicate varying patterns of immigration for each Asian subgroup. For example, the numbers of Asian Indian immigrants have steadily increased over the past decades, with 18.2% immigrating before 1980, 27.8% immigrating in the 1980s, and 54% during the 1990s. Immigration patterns for Filipinos have been relatively steady across the three decades, with 31.3%, 33%, and 35.6% immigrating to the United States before 1980, during the 1980s, and the 1990s, respectively. By contrast, immigration patterns of Southeast Asians, including Cambodians, Hmong, and Laotians, resemble a bell-shaped curve, with significantly large numbers of persons immigrating in the 1980s, and much fewer immigrating before 1980 and after 1989 (Reeves & Bennett, 2004). The different patterns in longitudinal immigration would suggest different levels of acculturation both between and within specific Asian ethnicities.

Acculturation issues are particularly salient in Asian populations. Unlike many Western societies, which are heavily influenced by Judeo-Christian religions and beliefs, Asian values are influenced by Eastern religions such as Buddhism and Hinduism, which emphasize selflessness and a harmony with nature and others. The different foundational influence is a double-edged sword, as it affects both a foreign-born individual's adjustment to Western society and a neuropsychologist's ability to understand behaviors and develop rapport, the latter essential for data gathering. In addition, typical Asian behaviors associated with illness, such as routinely agreeing with authority figures, including health care professionals, to show respect even if one disagrees, and a tendency to somaticize emotional problems, may confuse Western clinicians who may be unfamiliar with these behaviors (Wong & Fujii, 2004).

Despite the growing numbers of Asian Americans, there are very few Asian neuropsychologists practicing in America. Preliminary data indicate the numbers of Asian American neuropsychologists in comparison to the total number of neuropsychologists are lower than the percentage of the population in America. A rough estimate of Asian American neuropsychologists based upon identifying Asian surnames on the International Neuropsychological Society's (INS) membership directory for U.S. citizens resulted in roughly 115 names, or about 3% of the total number of American neuropsychologists (n = 3855). Numbers are very similar (3.1%) when Canadian neuropsychologists are included (130/4211). These percentages are about 20% or 28.5% lower than the percentage of Asians or part-Asians in America, respectively.

Not only are there too few neuropsychologists, but the ethnic distribution of neuropsychologists does not coincide with that of Asian Americans. As mentioned previously, the largest Asian ethnicities in descending order are Chinese, Filipinos, Asian Indians, Vietnamese, Koreans, and Japanese. By contrast, the Asian ethnicities with the most neuropsychologists in order are Chinese, Asian Indian, Korean, and Japanese. Thus, among the Asian ethnic groups with the highest populations, both Filipinos and Vietnamese have very few practicing neuropsychologists.

Using a similar methodology with the American Academy of Clinical Neuropsychology (AACN) directory, 11 board-certified Asian neuropsychologists were identified: Japanese, 4; Chinese, 3; Korean, 2; and Asian Indians, 2; which is roughly 1.7% of all neuropsychologists certified by the American Board of Professional Psychology (ABPP). Again, the ethnic distribution does not coincide with the ethnic distribution of Asian Americans. Another interesting statistic is the distribution across states: Hawaii, 3; California, 3; Ohio, 2; New York, 2; and Washington, DC, 2. These numbers indicate that board-certified Asian neuropsychologists are primarily located on the coasts and in Hawaii, leaving 46 states without an ABPP-credentialed Asian neuropsychologist.

Numbers are even smaller for neuropsychologists reporting proficiency in Asian languages. The following are the number of neuropsychologists speaking Asian languages listed on the National Academy of Neuropsychology (NAN) directory: Chinese, 4 (Chinese, Cantonese, Mandarin unique clinicians combined); Vietnamese, 4; Asian Indian, 3 (Gurajati, Hindi, Urdu unique clinicians combined); Filipino, 3; Japanese, 2; Korean, 1; and Malay, 1. Although numbers are small, the distribution of speakers is generally consistent with the Asian population broken down by ethnic groups. The following is the distribution of clinicians across the states (including Canada): Washington, 5; California, 4; Utah, 2; Oregon, 1; Texas, 1; Ohio, 1; Indiana, 1; Virginia, 1; Massachusetts, 1; and Alberta, 1. These numbers indicate a strong West Coast bias followed by the Midwest and East Coast.

It should be emphasized that the methodology for procuring these data is crude. First, the population estimates are based upon 2000 census data, while the clinician numbers are based upon 2008 data. Differences in data sources would suggest that population numbers underestimate the actual numbers of Asian Americans. Similarly, our number likely underestimated the numbers for both Asian neuropsychologists and neuropsychologists proficient in Asian languages. Our data do not account for Asians who have non-Asian surnames due to marriage or adoption, those who do not belong to one of the major neuropsychological associations, or those who did not list their foreign language ability. Also, some Asian surnames are identical to Western names, for example, Lee, Young, Alvarez, and Martinez; thus, some clinicians may have been mistaken for European or Hispanic and not included as Asian. Given this caveat, it should be mentioned that the author did experience significant difficulty in finding potential contributors to this book for many of the ethnic subgroups, particularly the ones with few numbers as reported by this methodology, thereby lending credence to these results.

The relatively small numbers of Asian neuropsychologists, particularly for many of the specific ethnicities, such as Filipino and Vietnamese, are alarming for Asian clients seeking neuropsychological services, as it is assumed that a neuropsychologist who shares the same ethnic background and speaks the same language as the client would be more likely to produce a culturally informed evaluation due to familiarity with the culture, ability to develop rapport, and better communication. It should also be emphasized that just because a neuropsychologist is of a related Asian heritage as a client (e.g., Chinese clinician, Hmong client), this does not guarantee culturally informed services, as there is much diversity within specific Asian ethnicities, and an Asian clinician may be just as naïve about a specific culture than a non-Asian one. In any case, an implication of the shortage of Asian neuropsychologists is that non-Asian neuropsychologists will have ample opportunity to provide services to Asian clients.

In summary, Asians are the fastest-growing ethnic minority in the United States. Asians are diverse with the U.S. Census, listing 24 distinct ethnicities in the Asian category. There are few Asian neuropsychologists who can provide services to this population, particularly in ethnic subgroups such as Filipinos, Vietnamese, Cambodian, Laotians, Hmong, and Thai. Thus, many Asian clients in need of neuropsychological services would likely have to seek services from a non-Asian clinician or Asian clinician who may not be entirely familiar with the client's culture. Asian clients can pose special challenges to neuropsychologists due to issues of ethnic diversity, language barriers, acculturation, and differences in values and communication style. Given the number of pertinent issues that require attention for a clinician to perform a culturally informed evaluation, a neuropsychologist, particularly non-Asian, may be reluctant to work with an Asian client.

Purpose of this book

The purpose of this book is twofold. The first purpose, associated with the section on neuropsychology of Asian Americans, is to provide clinical neuropsychologists with a knowledge base of the demographic, cultural, and neuropsychological literatures, and practical recommendations for working with the major Asian ethnic groups to facilitate culturally informed neuropsychological evaluations. The overall goal is to increase the resource pool of neuropsychologists who are competent in delivering services to Asian Americans.

A second, but related purpose, associated with the second part of this book, is to educate researchers and clinicians on neuropsychological practices and scientific literature in several Asian countries. For clinicians, these chapters may identify neuropsychological resources that would be useful for evaluating or treating a person from that Asian country. This information could also assist clinicians performing court evaluations in meeting *Daubert* level standards of evidence by incorporating tests used by clinicians, or citing rationales for test selection based upon neuropsychological practices in an Asian person's native country. Another area of interest for clinicians would be learning about professional issues such as educational and training procedures and requirements, licensure, and professional organizations in different Asian countries.

For researchers, a peek into the neuropsychological literature can hopefully lead to a cross-fertilization of research ideas, or cross-cultural validation or refutation of neuropsychological findings or assumptions based upon Western research. This exposure to new ideas can hopefully inspire new directions for research or developing new technologies.

The remainder of the chapter will describe a framework for clinicians on how to use the information in this book to perform culturally informed neuropsychological evaluations with Asians.

How to use information from the book

Each Asian American chapter is organized similarly, covering topics such as immigration history, reason for immigration, educational system in home country, educational achievement and occupational attainment in America, cultural values, family structure, attitudes toward illness, neuropsychological testing, recommendations for testing, and an illustrative case sample. Information from these chapters should be used in the following manner:

1. Provide a knowledge base for understanding and developing rapport with persons from a specific Asian ethnic group
2. Assist in determining testing strategy or test selection
3. Assist in test interpretation
4. Assist in making recommendations

Due to lack of norms and shared clinical issues for several Asian American ethnicities (Cambodian, Hmong, Laotian), recommendations for these groups are very similar. Although repetitive, the same recommendations are repeated in these chapters for easy reference.

Provide a knowledge base

Before selecting a test strategy, clinicians require a knowledge base for understanding a person with a different cultural background. In many ways, this lack of understanding would be like trying to watch a 3D movie without the special glasses. Perceptions are blurry and it is difficult to appreciate the movie. However, once the glasses are worn, it is amazing how crystal clear the images become. Knowledge from each chapter can assist the clinicians in the following ways:

1. Provide a conceptual framework for understanding a person who was born and raised in another country. Some important factors include primary reasons for immigration, immigration patterns, acculturation, values, belief system, and general experiences in the country of origin and America that may shape values and behaviors.
2. Provide a context for evaluation. For example, many Asians do not typically see psychologists or mental health professionals unless a condition is serious due to shame, stigma, or attribution to karma, the latter because the person cannot do anything about his fate, which is deserved.
3. Help to understand the dynamics of the clinician-client relationship as perceived by the Asian client. For example, an Asian client may perceive the psychologist as an authority figure who is all-knowing or someone who is respected and with whom you should not disagree.
4. Help provide a strategy for interviewing the client and developing rapport. Many Asians may have trust issues and can be passive in providing information. Thus, encouraging clients to talk about their country, experience with immigration, or their name, or allowing family to participate in the interview process may be useful.
5. Provide guidance for working with interpreters. With a general knowledge base, clinicians can better inform interpreters of goals, clarify uncertainties, and map out strategies for interviewing or possibly translating tests.
6. Provide clues for understanding specific behaviors. For example, saying yes or head nodding may not mean agreement, but instead be polite gestures to an authority figure.
7. Provide a framework for understanding the client. Given the person's cultural background, presentation, and personal history, what can you surmise about this individual? What is his or her level of acculturation given his or her generation? How is he or she functioning socially, academically, or occupationally in comparison to his or her peers? What are some hypotheses for cognitive functioning? In this regards it should be emphasized that there is marked diversity within each Asian ethnic group, and thus rigid stereotyping should be avoided.

Testing strategy and test selection

Next, information can be used to assist the clinician in determining testing strategy or test selection: In performing neuropsychological evaluations with Asian clients,

Fujii and Wong (2005) recommend either a norm-based testing or hypothesis testing strategy. The authors argue that both methodologies are sound and would meet *Daubert* standards for admissibility of scientific evidence in a court of law if the report is used for forensic purposes. The criteria for determining relevance and reliability of scientific evidence include (1) whether a technique can be tested, (2) whether a technique has been subject to peer review, (3) whether the error rate for the technique is known, and (4) whether the technique has general acceptance in the scientific community (for a review see Fujii & Wong, 2005).

The norm-based testing approach is the standard procedure of neuropsychological assessment whereby the clinician uses tests such as the Wechsler Adult Intelligence Scale–IV or Wisconsin Card Sort that have been standardized, normed, and validated. In this method, the science is based in the empirically validated tests and their psychometric properties. Evaluations based upon this strategy should meet *Daubert* criteria 1, 2, and 4. The strategy could meet criteria 3 for specific populations if there are empirical studies reporting sensitivities and specificities for diagnoses or a clinical criterion.

In the hypothesis testing approach, the clinician develops a hypothesis of normal functioning or a pattern of deficits based upon what is known about a specific neurological disorder, and then supports or refutes the hypothesis based upon data obtained through interviews, observations, neuroimaging data or other labs, and test scores. Although this methodology is not new and is often implicit in clinical decision making, it is recommended that this decision-making process be made explicit in the report with articulated hypotheses.

In this approach, it is recommended that clinicians use consensus statement criteria or the literature on neurobehavioral syndromes for developing hypotheses. For example, if a diagnosis of frontotemporal dementia is suspected, a clinician may use the Neary et al. (1998) consensus statement as criteria to base his or her hypotheses for the presence of this disorder. The clinicians would then look for data from different sources to determine if the client's cognitive, behavioral, and emotional symptoms, onset and progression of illness, neuroimaging data, and available test data are consistent with each consensus statement criteria for a frontotemporal dementia. If the person meets criteria, hypotheses about prognosis and future functioning can be made as well as clinical recommendations. Similarly, if an individual sustained a right frontal stroke, the clinician would hypothesize cognitive, behavioral, or emotional syndromes associated with lesions to this area. Thus, clinicians should be familiar with the cognitive-behavioral neurology literature. *Principles of Behavioral and Cognitive Neurology* (Mesulam, 2000), *Neuropsychiatry and Behavioral Neuroscience* (Cummings & Mega, 2003), and *Clinical Neuropsychology* (Heilman & Valenstein, 2003) are recommended resources. It is argued that the hypothesis testing strategy should meet *Daubert* criteria 1, 2, and 4.

The hypothesis testing approach is more useful for diagnostic purposes versus specific measurement of cognitive deficits, but can be useful for prediction or providing rough estimates or educated guesses of cognitive functioning, as well as making recommendations. Although this type of evaluation can be conducted by other disciplines, such as neurology or psychiatry, it is argued that psychologists generally tend to be more thorough and systematic in their data gathering and development of behavioral or practical recommendations.

For Asian clients, a norm-based testing approach with Western-based tests is recommended if the client meets any of the following criteria: (1) the client received a college-level education with courses that are generally taught in English, (2) the client has lived in the United States for many years from a young age and is competent in English, (3) English is the primary language spoken at home, or (4) the client has performed at the average level or higher on national standardized tests (e.g., Stanford Achievement Test). Depending on observation of English fluency and background history, test selection may emphasize nonverbal tests, and any interpretation of verbal tests should be made with caution. A norm-based test strategy is also recommended if normed and validated tests are available for a person's ethnic group and demographic profile. In these cases, however, the clinician would have to procure the tests and may need an interpreter if he or she does not speak the language.

A hypothesis testing approach is recommended when (1) a client does not match American demographics for neuropsychological test samples due to low level of education or quality of education, and poor command of English, (2) there is no supportive literature suggesting equivalent performances on similar neuropsychological tests, and (3) there are no normed tests developed in the client's language or country. Information on education and English skills, the neuropsychological literature in the client's native country, and neuropsychological or academic performances in the United States would be particularly relevant to determine testing strategy.

If norm-based tests are not available for a particular ethnic group, and the clinician would like some neuropsychological measurement data for a ballpark estimate of functioning, it is recommended that the clinician translate tests with the most cross-cultural validation or validation in a country similar in education, location, and socioeconomic status. An example of a cross-culturally validated instrument would be the World Health Organization (WHO) neuropsychological battery, which has normative samples in Germany, Brazil, Zaire, Kenya, and Thailand (Maj et al., 1994). Words for the 15-item auditory verbal learning test can be found in Mitrushina, Boone, Razani, and D'Elia (2005). When translating materials, the clinician should be aware of issues in translation and equivalence, and back-translate items if possible (for a review, see Fouad & Chan, 1999). Caveats for interpreting findings from these translations are discussed in the next section.

Assist in test interpretation

Information from each chapter would be useful for providing a context for understanding test scores. Gross estimates of premorbid and general functioning can be made based upon amount and quality of education, English skills and exposure, acculturation, occupational and academic history, and neuropsychological literature. If deemed appropriate, clinicians could make interpretive adjustments when reviewing scores. For a norm-based test strategy, interpretive adjustments could be made if norms from an ethnic group are low. For example, if an ethnic group has been found to perform significantly lower than Americans on the Trailmaking Test, a low score on this test should not be interpreted as impaired functioning. For a hypothesis testing strategy, interpretive adjustments could be made if there is evidence that the amount and quality of education is low for an ethnic group and the clinician decides to use some Western tests. For example, if an ethnic group scores a mean of 90 on Raven's Progressive Matrices (RPM), the clinical implication of a 79 score should not be the same as it would for Western norms.

There are several caveats when attempting to make interpretive adjustments. First, just because an ethnic group produces lower scores on Western tests, the clinician should not automatically perceive these people to be less intelligent than Westerners, as other factors, such as education, quality of education, English skills, and acculturation, can significantly affect test scores. A perfect example is the significantly low scores of many European immigrants who entered America through Ellis Island and whose progeny became successful in the new land. Second, when making interpretive adjustments with a hypothesis testing strategy, clinicians should use broad strokes when making interpretations. Thus, much less confidence can be placed in smaller differences between scores. More confidence can be placed with larger discrepancies, consistency of poor scores within a domain, or deficit patterns that are consistent with expectations for a specific neurological disorder or findings on neuroimaging. Third, when attempting to make adjustments, clinicians need to consider the education and occupational levels of the samples that produced the available test scores. Dates of studies are also important, as for many third-world countries or those with emerging economies, the educational systems can make significant improvements in a few decades. In addition, exposure to and teaching of English can also change over a relatively short period of time. Thus, test norms collected on urban 15-years-olds in 1975 would apply to 49-year-old immigrants who lived in urban areas in their native country, but less so for a 15-year-old who immigrated from a rural area in 2006.

When writing reports, it is imperative that clinicians describe limitations in validity and provide rationales for interpretive adjustments. As mentioned previously, for hypothesis testing approaches, hypotheses should be stated, and then supported or refuted based upon the evidence from interviews, observation, history, and medical data. As a rule, clinicians should emphasize caution in interpretation of test scores as well as functional implications. Caution is especially imperative when interpreting translated tests, although normal performances can be more confidently interpreted to rule out impaired functioning. It is recommend that clinicians indicate a confidence level of interpretation (e.g., high, medium, low). This confidence level can be specific to tests, diagnosis, or functional implications. Clinicians should also list additional information needed to support or refute hypotheses, as well as alternative hypotheses.

Assist in making recommendations

Finally, information from each chapter would be useful for making recommendations congruent with the values of the individual and family members. Clinicians should be aware of how values, spiritual beliefs, and beliefs about mental and medical illness can influence how individuals and families react to neuropsychological findings and recommendations. Some considerations include: How do findings fit in the individual's belief system or values? What are individual and family strengths that would facilitate understanding of findings and support follow-through on recommendations? How can these strengths be mobilized? What beliefs or values can hinder appreciation of findings and follow-through on recommendations? How can these challenges be overcome?

Once recommendations are conceptualized, the next step is to determine the most effective manner of communicating neuropsychological findings and recommendations to individual and families in order to maximize understanding and follow through. Knowledge of values and beliefs, as well as dynamics with clinicians, and communication styles, will be useful for determining strategies.

References

Barnes, J., & Bennett, C. (2002). *The Asian population: 2000*. Washington, DC: U.S. Bureau of the Census.

Cummings, J. L., & Mega, M. S. (2003). *Neuropsychiatry and behavioral neuroscience*. New York, NY: Oxford University Press.

Fouad, N. A., & Chan, P. M. (1999). Gender and ethnicity: Influence on test interpretation and reception. In J. Lichtenberg & R. Goodyear (Eds.), *Scientist-practitioner perspective on test interpretation* (pp. 31–57). Boston, MA: Allyn & Bacon.

Fujii, D. E., & Wong, T. M. (2005). Neuropsychological assessment with Asian-Americans immigrants: Recommendations for meeting *Daubert* standards. *Journal of Forensic Neuropsychology*, *4*(4), 3–31.

Heilman, K. M., & Valenstein, E. (2003). *Clinical neuropsychology* (4th ed.). New York, NY: Oxford University Press.

Maj, M., Satz, P., Janssen, R., Zaudig, M., Starace, F., D'Elia, et al. (1994). WHO neuropsychiatric AIDS study, cross-sectional phase II: Neuropsychological and neurological findings. *Archives of General Psychiatry*, *51*, 51–61.

Mesulam, M. M. (Ed.). (2000). *Principles of behavioral and cognitive neurology* (2nd ed.). New York, NY: Oxford University Press.

Mitrushina, M., Boone, K., Razani, J., & D'Elia, L. (2005). *Handbook of normative data for neuropsychological assessment* (2nd ed.). New York, NY: Oxford University Press.

Neary, D., Snowden, J., Gustafson, L., Passant, U., Stuss, D., Black, et al. (1998). Frontotemporal lobar degeneration: A consensus on clinical diagnostic criteria. *American Academy of Neurology*, *51*, 1546–1554.

Reeves, T. J., & Bennett, C. E. (2004). *We the people: Asians in the United States*. Washington, DC: U.S. Census Bureau.

U.S. Census Bureau. (2004). *Census Bureau projects tripling of Hispanic and Asian populations in 50 years: Non-Hispanic Whites may drop to half of total population*. Retrieved April 2009 from http://www.census.gov/Press-Release/www/releases/archives/population/001720.html

Wong, T. M., & Fujii, D. E. (2004). Neuropsychological assessment of Asian Americans: Demographic factors, culture diversity, and practical guidelines. *Applied Neuropsychology*, *11*, 23–36.

2 Neuropsychology of Cambodian Americans

Daryl Fujii, Barbara W.K. Yee, Sopagna Eap, Theanvy Kuoch, and Mary Scully

Brief history

Cambodia is located in Southeast Asia and was once the kingdom of Angkor (802–1431). The country was inhabited for about 2000 years by the Khmer, whose culture was strongly influenced by Indian civilization and Hinduism (see Chan, 2004, for detailed Cambodian history). Cambodia was raided by Thailand and Vietnam from the fourteenth to mid-nineteenth centuries. The French colonized Cambodia in 1863. Not considered to be a strategic colony like Vietnam, the French did little to develop infrastructure, such as roads, hospitals, schools, or industries, in the mostly agrarian society. In fact, the Vietnamese were assigned by the French to be administrators in Cambodia (Kim, 2002). Cambodia was granted independence in 1953 and was governed by King Sihanouk and his political party members until 1970.

Cambodia's peaceful independence was disrupted in the late 1960s by the fallout of the Vietnam War, as Americans dropped 2.7 million tons of bombs on the border area between Cambodia and Vietnam. Civil war broke out in 1970 between the Communist-backed Khmer Rouge and Lon Nol's Khmer Republic, causing millions of refugees to flood the major urban areas, seeking safety, only to endure the disease, malnutrition, and starvation caused by overcrowded camps.

The Khmer Rouge, under the leadership of Pol Pot, proved victorious in 1975. In an attempt to reeducate the population, this regime was responsible for one of the worst reigns of genocide in history. An estimated 1.5 million Cambodians, or approximately 20% of the total Cambodian population, were killed by execution, disease, or starvation in brutal labor camps. The educated and wealthy were the primary targets, as approximately 90% of Cambodia's doctors, lawyers, teachers, clergy, and businesspersons were exterminated. The regime also targeted minority groups such as the Cham for total extermination. According to numerous sources, the Khmer Rouge government relocated 2.5 million city dwellers to rural Cambodia, separating children from parents and spouses from one another. Such policies resulted in rapid disruption of long-standing traditional Cambodian culture, society, and governance. Cambodians who fled their country during this period experienced extreme losses:

of family members, of their culture and way of life, and of their social support systems. Many who attempted to escape to Thailand fell victim to land mines or witnessed people dying from these mines, or were victims of rape, capture, and torture by Communist soldiers.

Pol Pot's reign of terror ended in 1979 when the Vietnamese took over the country. Still, many Cambodian refugees continued to experience difficulties in Thai refugee camps, which were so overcrowded that some people were actually turned away. The camps were dangerous places where fires, bandit attacks, and rape were a constant threat. In the dry season families lived on one bucket of water per person per day for drinking, washing, and laundry. In the rainy season cholera, dengue, and malaria were a threat that equaled the violence and deadly boredom of living behind barbed wire. Malnutrition was also a problem in these refugee camps, as food was heavily rationed. Most Cambodians spent between 1 and 12 years in refugee camps before immigrating to the United States between 1980 and 1989 (McKenzie-Pollock, 1993). Refugees and immigrants from Cambodia are the Khmer (the most populous ethnic Cambodian group), the Cham (a Muslim minority group), and the Khmer Loeu (or highlander Khmer).

Cambodian population demographics in the United States

The 2000 U.S. census counted 206,052 Cambodian Americans in the United States (see demographic review for more detailed statistics cited in Niedzwiecki & Duong, 2004, from the 2000 U.S. census). However, this number is estimated to be at least a 30% undercount of Cambodians based on admission rates of 195,752 Cambodians, of whom 145,172 arrived as refugees and 50,582 as immigrants, and a rate of Cambodians born in the United States of about 33% of the 2000 census.

States with the largest number of Cambodian residents in the 2000 census were California (84,559), Massachusetts (22,886), Washington (16,630), Pennsylvania (10,207), Texas (8,225), Minnesota (6,533), Rhode Island (5,290), and Virginia (5,180). States with Cambodian residents of 1,000 to 4,999 according to the 2000 Census (from highest to lowest) include New York, Illinois, Oregon, Ohio, Georgia, Florida, Connecticut, North Carolina, Maryland, Colorado, Utah, Arizona, Tennessee, and Maine. Like other Asian American ethnic groups, Cambodians are located in urban areas (97.9%) and have a larger average household size, of 4.39 persons, in comparison to the U.S. total of 2.59, or when compared to Asians overall (3.07).

The Cambodian American population living in the United States is a more youthful one than the general population. The median age of the Cambodian population in the United States is 22.8 years of age, compared to the median age of 35.4 years for the total U.S. population (Niedzwiecki & Duong, 2004, from the 2000 U.S. census). In the 2000 census, approximately 46% were 0–19 years of age, 28.8% were 20–39, 19.8% were 40–59, and 5.5% were 60 and older.

Cambodian Americans are poorly educated. Twenty-six percent have no formal schooling, while only 28% are literate in English (Ngo, 2006). Cambodian Americans residing in Portland, Oregon, averaged 2 years of formal education (Kinzie & Leung,

1996), while those living in California averaged between 3.1 and 10.5 years (Gong-Guy, 1987).

In 2000, Southeast Asians were among the poorest groups of Americans (Niedzwiecki & Duong, 2004, from the 2000 U.S. census). In the 2000 census, Cambodians averaged $10,215 per capita income in 1999, as compared to the U.S. overall of $21,587, Asians overall at $20,719, African Americans at $14,222, and Hispanics at $12,111. The median family income of Cambodians was $35,434 compared to $50,046 for the U.S. total median families. The 2000 U.S. census also revealed that Cambodian Americans had higher poverty rates than the average American, with 30.7 of Cambodians in poverty in 1999. Across selected communities, 22% of Cambodians received public assistance income. The only ethnic populations in California to have per capita incomes below $10,000 were Hmong Americans, Cambodian Americans, and Laotian Americans. In California, 40% of Cambodian immigrants, 32.2% of Laotians, and more than half of all Hmong live in poverty.

Cambodian American children have not fared well academically. They have lower standardized tests scores, lower grade point averages, and dropped out at a higher rate than Vietnamese and Hmong Americans (Ngo, 2006). In a 1997 study examining GPAs in six different immigrant and refugee children in Southern California, Cambodians had the lowest GPAs in comparison to Vietnamese, Mexican, Filipino, Laotian, and other immigrants from Asian and Latin America, and were also most likely to be categorized as "limited English proficient" (Rumbaut & Cornelius, 1995; Rumbaut & Ima, 1988). Kim (2002) reported that Cambodian students had a mean reading score of 14%, while their mean math score was 35%. Academic achievement in Cambodian American students has been associated with socioeconomic class, as children of middle-class families do better academically than those of working-class families and those below the poverty line (Hopkins, 1992).

Several reasons have been proposed to explain the poor academic achievement of Cambodian American children. Environmentally, Cambodian American families are more likely to attend inner city schools, with 5% of Cambodian youths involved in gangs (Kim, 2002). In fact, it is not uncommon for poor Cambodians to move from school district to school district to search for cheaper housing, better jobs, or safer neighborhoods (Smith-Hefner, 1999). Another problem is the lack of educational support. For example, despite the high number of children with limited English proficiency, one study found that in 1997, California had only 5 certified Khmer teachers for 20,645 Khmer-speaking students, a miniscule ratio of 1:4,129 (Chu, 1997).

Poor academic achievement has also been attributed to cultural beliefs and characteristics. Most parents have a poor command of English (Lee, 2006) and little formal education, and thus either cannot help their children or are unaware of specific roles teachers play (Yang, 2004). Due to Buddhist belief in destiny, Cambodian American parents may have the attitude that their children will either do well academically or not, and they cannot influence their performance (Um, 1997). They may also be reluctant to question authority figures, such as teachers, and thus may appear uninvolved (Um, 1997).

Testing issues

History of education in Cambodia

Education in Cambodia was traditionally provided by Buddhist monks for young males. In 1917, the French initiated a government-run education system for the elite, which primarily included many children of Vietnamese administrators overseeing the county. Universal education was only established after Cambodia gained independence in 1953 (Cambodia Cultural Profile, 2005). Consistent with previous educational systems, males outnumbered females due to cultural values. The Cambodian educational system operated under the French model, divided into primary and secondary educational systems. The primary education curriculum consisted of arithmetic, history, ethics, drafting, geography, hygiene, language, and science. Subjects were taught in Khmer for the first year, and in French from the second year. Vocational colleges soon followed, with the first public college, the Khmer Royal University, established in 1965. Six more universities were developed within the next few years. Prior to the outbreak of civil war in 1970, approximately 9,000 students attended college in Cambodia, while others went abroad in France, the United States, Canada, China, the Soviet Union, and Germany (Wikipedia, 2008).

Cambodia's educational system was decimated during the 1970s, initially from civil war, and then abolished by the Khmer Rouge, which systemically destroyed teaching materials and executed teachers. By the end of the Khmer reign in 1979, illiteracy climbed to 40% as most young people under the age of 14 had no formal education. Compulsory education until the ninth grade was reinstated in 1979, when the Khmer Rouge was overthrown with the assistance of the Vietnamese. Still, attendance was limited, especially in rural areas, due to a shortage of qualified teachers, lack of classrooms, and the expectation that children assist families on the farms. In addition, schools required an enrollment fee of 25 to 150 riels per month, which not every family could afford (Cambodia Cultural Profile, 2005; Wikipedia, 2008). With the reinstatement of the educational system, the literacy rates of Cambodians have steadily increased. For example, the youth literacy rate (literacy defined as "with understanding, both read and write a short simple statement on everyday life") has increased from 66.8% in 1980 to 80.3% in 2004. Literacy for adult Cambodian women has increased from 33.2% in 1980 to 60.2% in 2003, while for males it has increased from 74.4% in 1980 to 81.1% in 2003 (Globalis, n.d.).

Mental health issues

As mentioned previously, the Cambodian genocide during the reign of Pol Pot was one of the greatest human rights catastrophes of the twentieth century. Individuals who remained in Cambodia from 1970 through 1980 are estimated to have experienced 8 to 16 major traumatic events that may have included torture, rape, death of family members, or witnessing torture and death. Due to the widespread and prolonged experiences of trauma by most, Cambodian refugees have been found to demonstrate the highest rates of psychiatric disorders among Southeast Asian immigrants. Marshall, Schell, Elliott, Berthold, and Chun (2005) found that 62% presented with posttraumatic stress disorder (PTSD), while 42% met criteria for major depression. Refugees demonstrated a strong dose-response relationship to trauma exposure, but low rates of alcohol abuse. Interestingly, these symptoms were present even after two decades of living in the United States. Dose-response relationships and longevity of PTSD have also been found in Cambodian refugees settling in New Zealand (Cheung, 1994). Although lower in numbers, Gong-Guy (1987) reported 48% of Cambodian Americans needed psychiatric services, while 16% met the criteria for PTSD. Specific symptoms of PTSD include reexperiencing, avoidance, emotional numbing, and hyperarousal (Palmieri, Marshall, & Schell, 2007). Traumatic brain injury is also common, with one study reporting 567 incidents among 967 Cambodian adults who resided in a Thailand refugee camp (Mollica, Henderson, & Tor, 2002). Psychiatric problems are not only found in adults, as Cambodian American adolescents have also demonstrated significant mental health needs. In a study with 40 adolescents, Kinzie et al. (1986) reported 50% met criteria for PTSD, 53% for a depressive disorder, while 67% met criteria for at least one *Diagnostic and Statistical Manual of Mental Disorders*, third edition (DSM-III) diagnosis.

Treatment outcomes for traumatized Cambodian refugees are mixed. In a sample of 23 severely traumatized Cambodian refugee patients with posttraumatic stress disorder under continuous treatment for 10 years, 13 had good outcomes, but 10 had relatively poor treatment outcomes (Boehnlein et al., 2004). The complexity of explanatory factors related to treatment outcomes for these severely traumatized Cambodian refugee patients puzzled these authors. Even after examining differences in education, type of trauma, current stresses, marital support, treatment approaches, and physical health, unknown risk factors that were not included in this study accounted for the differential effectiveness of treatment.

Although reportedly infrequent in Cambodia prior to its civil war, alcohol and drug abuse, particularly of crack cocaine and methamphetamine, have been identified as significant problems for Cambodian Americans (Bromley & Chhem Sip, 2003; Sasao, 1991). This change in behavior has been attributed to the need to cope with traumas from the war as well adjusting to a new country (Hatanaka, Morales, & Kaseyama, 1991). Low-income families are particularly at high risk (Kuramoto, 1995).

Health issues

There is some evidence indicating that Cambodian Americans experience poorer health than other Asian Americans and the general U.S. population. In a study examining the health status of 1,026 Cambodian Americans living in Lowell, Massachusetts, Cambodians were found to be three times more likely to report not visiting a doctor because of high costs (Centers for Disease Control and Prevention, 2004). Over half of the Cambodian American men smoked (50.4%), and the Cambodian American women smoked (10.9%) more than other Asian American women. The Cambodians were less likely than the white population to eat five servings of fruits and vegetables daily (16.4%) and less likely to have been screened for serum cholesterol (47.7%). The Cambodian American women were less likely to have had a Pap test (64.2%).

Rates of uptake for pneumococcal vaccine (18.8%) and screening mammography rates were also lower than in the white population. In addition, the Asian Americans in Lowell who were 45 years and older (the majority of whom were Cambodian in this sample) were dying from diabetes at rates six times that of the general population in Massachusetts. Cambodians in California have been found to have four times the rate of stroke of the white population (107 vs. 28 per 100,000) and higher cardiovascular mortality. Prevalence of chronic hepatitis B infection is high among Cambodian Americans born in Cambodia, and as a result, incidence rates of liver cancer are higher for Cambodian American men than for the general population. Chewing betel nut among Cambodian middle-aged and elderly women increases the risk of their developing cancers of the mouth.

Pertinent cultural variables

Family structure

Family structure in Cambodia is characterized by clearly defined roles that are strictly adhered to. The father is the head of the family and the head decision maker, particularly for issues outside of the family. However, in the United States, children may be granted greater responsibilities as language proficiency may limit the abilities of parents to navigate through American systems and culture. This role shift can be culturally disruptive and result in family conflict. The mother's role is to manage the family finances, take care of the household, and maintain family values. Publicly, wives defer to male authority and are tolerant of male privilege. Still, they have more equality in their relationship when compared to surrounding Asian countries. Many Cambodian women lost their husbands during the Khmer Rouge era because men were more vulnerable to starvation, the leading cause of death at that time. Thus, females have adopted a more prominent role in most Cambodian families. Children are subservient to parents and the eldest son is generally favored. Siblings refer to each other by their gender and birth order, for example, older sister or younger brother (McKenzie-Pollock, 1993). Indeed, individuals are often referred to by titles that designate their place in the family, irrespective of whether they are actually related by blood; for example, younger uncle or older uncle. Referring to individuals by their first name is discouraged and only occurs when the other person is younger. A younger person using the formal name of someone older is a sign of disrespect. Cambodians are very respectful of their elderly, and the elders in the family are treated with kindness and deference. The extended family is very important to Cambodian Americans, and despite general low-income levels, many families still send back money to relatives living in Cambodia.

Religious values

Theravada Buddhism is the predominant religion among Cambodians (97%); the remaining are either Muslim or Christian. All Buddhists equate life to suffering caused by one's desires, and that suffering in one's current life results from misdeeds in previous lives. Core values are harmony and balance, and conflicts are to be avoided at all costs. Theravada Buddhism, however, has a more individualistic philosophy, stressing personal development and individual good behavior to attain enlightenment before helping others (Kim, 2002). It has been speculated that this belief system may result in Cambodian communities being less cohesive than other Southeast Asian communities (Kim, 2002). Although some Cambodians may not adhere strictly to Buddhist tenets, Cambodian culture is very much tied to their identity as Buddhist. As such, they may perceive Cambodians of other religions to be outsiders.

Illness beliefs and traditional healing practices

Traditionally, Cambodians believed that illness is caused by spirit possession, evil spells cast by other people, mistakes in performance of rituals over the life cycle, or neglect of rituals (see review in Graham & Chitnarong, 1997). Cambodians have traditionally treated their own illnesses and illnesses of family members on their own, without the intervention of outside parties. This behavior developed in response to the scarcity of physicians and hospitals in Cambodia, and the high costs of Western medical care. In traditional Cambodian practices, illness is conceived as an imbalance of hot and cold elements in the body. Herbal remedies, dermal techniques (e.g., coin rubbing or pinching), special foods, and rituals are all used to restore the balance of these elements and thereby to restore health. If the illness does not respond to the home remedies, then a *khru khmer* (traditional healer) or health practitioner is seen.

A common complaint among Cambodians is wind illness (*khyol*), having wind (*kerd khyol*), or catching the wind (*khyol chab*), which is comparable to feeling ill or having a sickness or fever. The wind illness is believed to be caused by imbalance in the body that is caused by (1) overwork, lack of food or sleep, and exposure to diverse weather (hot to cold to rain); (2) illness from a common cold, diabetes mellitus, or hypertension; or (3) imbalance specifically of the four human elements (wind, water, earth, and fire). Such traditional Cambodian health beliefs are based upon Chinese medicine (Yee & Keo, 2006).

When seeking Western medical treatment, older Cambodian Americans are likely to expect to receive medications to treat the illness; if medications are not forthcoming, the Cambodian elder may "doctor shop" until medications are finally prescribed. Traditionally, medications are taken until an individual feels better and then are discontinued. In addition, older Cambodian Americans may expect medications to take effect quickly, and they may also adjust medication doses downward in the belief that Western remedies are "too strong." The skillful clinician working with older Cambodian patients may wish to take extra care in explaining medication regimens and negotiating a therapeutic plan where drugs are involved.

Similar to physical illness, serious emotional disturbance such as mania and psychosis would be attributed to possession by malicious spirits, but also to inherent factors such as bad karma acquired through misdeeds in past lives, or to bad luck in familial lineage. Those experiencing mental problems would be treated by the Khru or by a monk and might be kept out of public view because of shame. Rarely would they receive Western treatment (Yee, 2005).

Following the Khmer Rouge regime, survivors often describe having "hot head," a condition they associate with their suffering during the war and the Khmer Rouge. Survivors have an awareness of physical and psychological distress and seek traditional and Western approaches to treatment. Due to Buddhist beliefs and stigma, families, however, generally do not seek help for mental illness until a relative's behavior is impossible to ignore or manage (Kinzie & Leung, 1996), or associated with a crisis such as domestic violence, child abuse or neglect, legal difficulties, or financial emergencies (Bromley & Chhem Sip, 2003). For many Cambodian Americans, typical symptoms of PTSD, such as nightmares, startle reactions, irritability, and reexperiencing traumas, are not worth mentioning to physicians. In addition, Cambodians, like other Asian cultures, tend to hold in negative feelings such as depression and anxiety, sublimating negative feelings into physical illness such as headache, backache, or stomach disorder (Bromley & Chhem Sip, 2003). Thus, persons with emotional disorders will typically seek treatment from physicians for medical symptoms.

Recommendations for neuropsychological assessment

Literature searches uncovered no neuropsychological norms on an exclusively Cambodian sample; thus, Western tests would most likely not be valid to estimate actual cognitive functioning. This would indicate that for a majority of adult cases, a formal neuropsychological evaluation may not be possible. Still, a conceptual impression from a multimodal assessment based upon social and functional history from client and collateral sources, behavioral observations, medical records, including neuroimaging if available, and history of progression of cognitive and behavioral changes, in comparison to expectations from neurological disorder, can still be useful for making diagnoses and recommendations for improving functioning.

This type of assessment based on history and presentation would be insufficient to determine subtle cognitive changes from mild brain injuries. However, given Cambodian culture in which behavioral or emotional problems are not brought to the attention of professionals until it is very disturbing to family or significantly affecting finances, it is highly likely this type of evaluation can be useful because for many Cambodian Americans, their deficits would be noticeable by the time of referral. Although ideally a Cambodian American neuropsychologist would perform the evaluation, due to the paucity of these professionals in combination with the pressing need for such an evaluation when a referral is finally made, it is likely a non-Cambodian American would be asked to perform a neuropsychological evaluation on a Cambodian American. The following are conceptual issues to consider when providing neuropsychological consultation to Cambodian Americans.

Children

1. Western tests are most relevant for Cambodians born and educated in the United States and for whom English is their primary language. However, many Cambodian American children are bilingual, as Cambodian is spoken

in over 90% of households (Reeves & Bennett, 2004). If English is not the child's primary language, then verbal tests would underestimate verbal abilities. Thus, the examiner would have to determine the exposure to and skill level of English. The following are questions to determine English exposure history:

a. Is Cambodian the primary language spoken at home? If so when did the child learn English? Is Cambodian the primary language spoken with friends? In which language is the child most comfortable conversing?
b. Is the child enrolled in English as a Secondary Language (ESL) classes? What is the child's academic achievement in reading and language? Is there a significant discrepancy in English versus math skills?
c. If Cambodian is preferred, consider an interpreter. However, since most Cambodian American children are bilingual, you should qualitatively assess their English skills through conversation. This evaluation could be supplemented with school records or talking with the child's teachers. Keep in mind that comprehension is generally more advanced than expression; thus, it may be that an interpreter would be most useful for facilitating maximal verbal responses or obtaining history versus basic understanding.

2. Evaluate for level of acculturation that is useful for interpretation, particularly to determine if cultural variables could contribute to discrepancies in test performances (Ponton & Corona-LoMonaco, 2007). Lim, Heiby, Brislin, and Griffin (2002) have developed a Khmer acculturation scale (KAS) that may be used with Cambodians living in the United States. The KAS incorporates a bidimensional measure of acculturation that independently assesses for both Khmer and Anglo orientation. Additionally, there are several acculturation measures that are often utilized for Asian ethnic groups (Phinney, 1992; Suinn, Rickard-Figueroa, Lew, & Vigil, 1987). If the clinician does not have access to these scales, aside from language spoken (see 1a), other indicators of culture include (a) ethnicity of friends, (b) foods eaten or preferred foods, (c) preferred music, (d) religion, (e) reading preferences, (f) cultural values, and (g) age when immigrated to the United States.
3. School records are a good resource to assist in determining premorbid functioning. However, when evaluating grades it would be important to review attendance, enrollment in mainstream classes, and enrollment in remedial English. Be sure to explore reasons for poor attendance, for example, gang involvement, assisting parents, frequent moves, or chaotic home life.
4. Given that most parents have low levels of education and work at menial jobs due to poor English skills, parents' education and occupation may not be helpful to estimate premorbid abilities, particularly if both are low. More significant would be parents who have a relatively high level of education in Cambodia, for example, high school. Similarly, low socioeconomic class would not be as significant as if the family were middle class.

5. In understanding the behavior or emotional state of Cambodian American children, it would be important to evaluate the emotional state of the parents. Many parents may have PTSD or depression, which could significantly affect the home environment or ability to carry out recommendations.

Adults

1. Given that most Cambodians who immigrated to America have poor command of English, it is highly likely that an interpreter will be required. Comprehensive recommendations on how to select and work with interpreters are beyond the scope of this chapter. Some basic considerations include meeting the interpreter beforehand to familiarize him or her with the purpose and requirements of the evaluations as well as provide guidelines for interaction (for a review see Ponton & Corona-LoMonaco, 2007). Clinicians should avoid using family, particularly children, as interpreters due to potential biases and difficulties that it can cause in Cambodian American family dynamics. In addition, interpreters should be used as cultural guides for both putting behaviors into context and giving recommendations. Given the small size of the Cambodian community, however, clinicians should inform the client and an English-speaking family member beforehand of the identity of the interpreter. It is possible that the interpreter and the client are familiar with one another in some capacity. Thus, the client may prefer a family member over a close acquaintance as the interpreter in order to keep family business within the family.
2. Traditionally, Cambodians who receive Western medical treatment would see a generalist due to lack of resources, with only the most severe cases referred to a specialist (Kinzie & Leung, 1996). Thus, to ease possible worries, the clinician may have to thoroughly explain the reason for referral and purpose of evaluation.
3. To obtain a thorough pertinent history and to assist in developing rapport, encourage the client to provide a detailed account of his or her life in Cambodia, the impact of the war, and the traumas that he or she experienced prior to immigrating to the United States. If not spontaneously revealed, clients can be prompted for experiences of head injuries, traumatic events, malnutrition, and loss of loved ones.
4. Evaluate for acculturation. Of particular importance is age at time of immigration (see children recommendation 2).
5. Evaluate for specific symptoms of PTSD, depression, anxiety, and substance abuse and dependence. If present, inquire about the client's explanation for the symptoms. Many Asian cultural groups somatasize mental health problems (Lin & Cheung, 1999). A denial of mental health symptoms does not necessarily suggest a lack of distress. However, clinicians should not assume that somatization is due to stigma against mental illness, but rather to a lack of awareness that emotional problems can manifest as physical problems. Thus, psychoeducation regarding these phenomena may

be very therapeutic for Cambodians, whose understanding of psychology is relatively less developed than it is in the Western world.

6. Due to lack of neuropsychological norms for Cambodians, for diagnostic referrals, we recommend a hypothesis testing approach based upon expectations of presentation for a specific neurological disorder (Fujii & Wong, 2005). Hypotheses should be developed from consensus statements or other widely accepted expert-based diagnostic guidelines. Data collected with a multimethod approach utilize client and collateral interviews describing the onset of, quality, severity, and progression of cognitive, behavioral, and emotional symptoms of the presenting problem, as well as any medical and imaging data. This information would be compared to different diagnostic criteria for goodness of fit.
7. For referrals requesting a functionality evaluation after a known neurological disorder, it is recommended that clinicians utilize the literature and consensus statements to guide exploration of associated cognitive, behavioral, or emotional problems. Of particular importance are changes since the onset of a disorder. Inquire about the impact that these symptoms are having on the client and family.
8. As mentioned previously, because there are no known norms with Cambodians, comprehensive neuropsychological testing is not recommended. However, clinicians may perform limited testing with homemade translated tests, keeping in mind that these are gross measurements at best, and would only be significant if performances are highly discrepant from expectations of the most similar normative group.
9. Due to low levels of education, there is a high level of illiteracy among adult Cambodian immigrants. Thus, clinicians should be knowledgeable of the literature on how illiteracy affects brain functioning (for reviews see Ardila & Rosselli, 2007; Castro-Caldas, 2007). For example, illiterates were less likely to develop aphasia and more likely to produce semantic versus phonemic paraphasias after left hemisphere lesions than literates (Castro-Caldas, 2007). On testing, illiterates' scores were not significantly different than those of literates of similar socioeconomic status on naming and identification of real versus pictures of objects, verbal fluency of familiar objects such as items in a supermarket, verbal memory recognition, and orientation. Cognitive areas most affected by education and literacy include digit span, verbal abstractions, calculations, and long-term semantic memory (Reis, Guerreiro, & Petersson, 2003). Clinicians should keep in mind that although an adult Cambodian is illiterate in English, he or she may be literate in a different language, for instance, Khmer. Other possibilities include French or Chinese.
10. Given this study, it would be most prudent to evaluate Cambodian adults on tests or evaluations that are least affected by literacy. When testing for verbal memory, although there are no Cambodian norms, we recommend using the World Health Organization (WHO) UCLA Auditory Verbal Learning Test (AVLT) (Maj et al., 1994) as the stimulus, with careful translation

into Cambodian (word list can be found in Mitrushina, Boone, Razani, & D'Elia, 2005). Words for this list were selected for their commonality across cultures, and the test was validated with samples from several countries, including Thailand.

11. We also recommend measures that estimate severity of impairment based on functionality, such as the Clinical Dementia Rating (Hughes, Berg, Danziger, Coben, & Martin, 1982).
12. General estimates of premorbid functioning can be based upon several factors: (a) education in Cambodia, with quality of education based upon hours in the classroom, subjects learned, availability of school materials, and student-to-teacher ratios; (b) children's academic achievement; and (c) current socioeconomic status. For these indicators, because the expectations would be low for both categories a and c, information would be most significant if education and socioeconomic status are average or higher. It is important to note that many Cambodians had to start a new life when they immigrated to the United States. Thus, it is possible that the individual enjoyed higher socioeconomic status in Cambodia than in the United States. The reverse is true as well.
13. The following are recommendations for writing the report: (a) make the implicit explicit by describing the thinking behind your conclusions, (b) don't forget to incorporate the potential contribution of psychological disorders such as PTSD in the formulation and recommendations, (c) indicate your level of certainty given the type of data that you have collected, and (d) describe all nonstandardized test administrations.
14. The following are suggestions for making recommendations and providing feedback: (a) focus on crisis resolution; (b) emphasize community strengths, such as reliance on family, ethnic community, and strong individual and group survival skills; (c) describe the rationale for recommendations; (d) avoid interactions that result in a loss of face; (e) be sure that the family is present and the father is involved in decision making; and (f) be respectful of family decisions if nontraditional forms of treatment are selected (Bromley & Chhem Sip, 2003).
15. Be cognizant of traditional Cambodian values of harmony and balance and the avoidance of conflict. It is possible that a Cambodian American client may become angry or upset if he or she perceives the clinician to be too confrontational. In this case, the client may politely tell the clinician that he or she will not return due to lack of transportation or work responsibilities, or just not show up at all for a follow-up appointment (McKenzie-Pollock, 1993).

Illustrative case sample

VY is a 40-year-old male, born in Cambodia, who immigrated to the United States in 1987. He is married and has three children, ages 17, 16, and 12. VY was working two jobs, as a groundskeeper at a public park and a busboy in a Chinese restaurant. About a month ago, VY was riding his bike to his busboy job when he witnessed a seven-year-old girl dart across the street from the restaurant while chasing a ball. She was immediately hit by an automobile. Distracted, VY ran into the curb and hit his forehead on the sidewalk. He lost consciousness for about a minute. He was taken to the emergency room and then sent home. After the accident, VY was absent from work for two weeks due to headaches, difficulty with concentration, mood changes, and problems with doing everyday home routines. The family relied heavily on VY's income, and thus took him to see a physician. He believed that these symptoms were due to VY's head injury and referred VY for neuropsychological testing.

Before seeing VY, Dr. G arranged to meet a Cambodian interpreter to go over the purpose and ground rules of the interview process and neuropsychological testing. VY's English-speaking son was informed of who his interpreter was beforehand so that his father could request a different interpreter if he knew the interpreter and felt uncomfortable having his information shared with a member of his community. The family approved of the interpreter. Dr. G asked the interpreter about how best to approach VY to demonstrate respect and make him feel comfortable. The WHO UCLA AVLT was also translated into Cambodian. When VY arrived to the interview with his family, he looked very anxious. Through the interpreter Dr. G explained that his physician referred him to evaluate whether his accident has affected his ability to work, and particularly if it has resulted in problems with thinking and behaviors. Dr. G wanted to help him to return to work. VY and his family accepted this explanation and were relieved that VY symptoms were not life threatening.

Dr. G began the interview by asking VY about his life in Cambodia and how he immigrated to the United States. VY reported that his parents were rice farmers. He was the middle of five children and attended rural schools for two years from ages 6 to 8. When the Khmer Rouge took over in 1975, VY was separated from his parents and siblings and placed in a labor camp where he had to till the soil from morning to night and often was fed only one cup of rice per day. This went on for four years until the Khmer Rouge was overthrown. VY later heard through word of mouth that his parents had died from starvation in another labor camp. While escaping to a refugee camp in Thailand, he witnessed several children explode after running on a mine. VY spent eight years in the refugee camp. He met his wife there and they married in 1986, a year before immigrating to the United States. VY admitted to smoking a pack of cigarettes per day and drinking two or three beers once or twice a week since immigrating to the United States.

In inquiring about reasons for his inability to return to work, VY reported headaches and stomachaches, caused by a bad case of *khyol*, or wind illness. Upon further questioning, Dr. G discovered that VY had been experiencing daily flashbacks and nightmares about his family and children dying in the Cambodian war. He was having sleep problems and could not concentrate or have the energy to go to work. He did not want to return to his busboy job, as thoughts of returning made him very nervous. The park where he worked as a groundskeeper also reminded him of mine fields in Cambodia. VY denied experiencing symptoms of depression.

According to his oldest son, PY, VY's behavior changed immediately after the accident. He had episodes of screaming in the middle of the night. VY initially did not want to see a physician, partially due to shame, but decided that he had to seek help as he could not support the family. PY also reported that his father drank a six-pack several times a week. PY reported that his father was illiterate. He did not notice a significant memory problem in his father, although his father would deny experiencing bad symptoms.

Dr. G performed a brief cognitive battery based on tests that were found to be least affected by illiteracy. VY was oriented to person, place, date, and time. He was able to generate 13 words on a fluency test requiring him to identify items in a supermarket, which was in the low average range for samples of comparable educational level. VY appeared to utilize a strategy in which he would name fruits, then vegetables, then meats. On the AVLT, VY was able to recall 5 words on the first trial, 10 on the fifth trial, 9 after an immediate delay, 8 after 15 minutes, and identified 12/15 on a recognition trial. Again, these scores were about low average for a cohort with comparable educational levels. VY was also administered Raven's Progressive Matrices, earning a score of 82.

Dr. G diagnosed VY with PTSD and recommended treatment from a psychologist specializing in this disorder. Given his adequate scores on a brief battery within the context of VY's education level and illiteracy, the mildness of his head injury, and the fact that family did not notice changes in memory or other cognitive functions, Dr. G did not believe that VY suffered significant cognitive problems from the injury. Still, he recommended follow-up testing and evaluation, if VY did not improve and return to work after PTSD treatment.

After three months of PTSD treatment, VY was able to return to this groundskeeper job, but quit his busboy job, as the location was a trigger to his flashbacks. He did find another job as a custodian in a supermarket. Dr. G decided that VY was functioning adequately, and thus did not require a return appointment.

References

Ardila, A., & Rosselli, M. (2007). Illiterates and cognition: The impact of education. In B. Uzzell, M. Ponton, & A. Ardila (Eds.), *International handbook of cross-cultural neuropsychology* (pp. 181–198). Mahwah, NJ: Lawrence Erlbaum Associates.

Boehnlein, J. K., Kinzie, J. D., Sekiya, U., Riley, C., Pou, K., & Rosborough, B. (2004). A ten-year treatment outcome study of traumatized Cambodian refugees. *The Journal of Nervous & Mental Disease, 192,* 658–663.

Bromley, M. A., & Chhem Sip, S. K. (2003). Substance abuse treatment issues with Cambodian Americans. In S. L. Ashenberg Straussner (Ed.), *Ethnocultural factors in substance abuse treatment* (pp. 321–343). New York, NY: Guilford Press.

Cambodia Cultural Profile (2005). *Introduction to Cambodia: Education.* Retrieved August 9, 2008 from http://www.culturalprofiles.net/Cambodia/Directories/Cambodia_Cultural_Profile/-36.html

Castro-Caldas, A. (2007). Relationship between functional brain organization and education. In B. Uzzell, M. Ponton, & A. Ardila (Eds.), *International handbook of cross-cultural neuropsychology* (pp. 199–214). Mahwah, NJ: Lawrence Erlbaum Associates.

Centers for Disease Control and Prevention. (2004). Health status of Cambodians and Vietnamese—Selected communities, United States, 2001–2002. *Morbidity and Mortality Weekly Report, 53,* 760–765.

Chan, S. (2004). *Survivors: Cambodian refugees in the United States*. Urbana, IL: University of Illinois Press.

Cheung, P. (1994). Posttraumatic stress disorder among Cambodian refugees in New Zealand. *International Journal of Social Psychiatry, 40,* 17–26.

Chu, N. V. (1997). Re-examining the model minority myth: A look at Southeast Asian youth. *McNair Journal, 5.* http://www-mcnair.berkeley.edu/97Journal/Chu.html

Fujii, D., & Wong, T. (2005). Neuropsychological assessment with Asian-American immigrants: Recommendations for meeting *Daubert* standards. *Journal of Forensic Neuropsychology, 4*(4), 3–31.

Globalis. (n.d.). *Cambodia.* Retrieved March 3, 2008 from http://globalis.gvu.unu.edu/indicator_detail.cfm?Country=KH&IndicatorID=124

Gong-Guy, E. (1987). *The California Southeast Asian mental health needs assessment.* California State Department Mental Health Contract 85-7682-2A-2.

Graham, E. A., & Chitnarong, J. (1997). *Ethnographic study among Seattle Cambodians: Wind illness*. Retrieved January 1, 2008, from http://ethnomed.org/ethnomed/clin_topics/cambodian/ethno_wind.html

Hatanaka, H., Morales, R., & Kaseyama, N. (1991). *Asian Pacific alcohol peer consultation and training project.* Los Angeles, CA: Special Services for Groups.

Hopkins, M. (1992). Becoming bicultural: Preserving culture through adaptation. In P. A. Devoe (Ed.), *Selected papers on refugee issues* (pp. 71–80). Arlington, VA: American Anthropological Association.

Hughes, C., Berg, L., Danziger, W., Coben, L., & Martin, R. (1982). A new clinical scale for the staging of dementia. *British Journal of Psychiatry, 140*, 566–572.

Kim, R. Y. (2002). Ethnic differences in academic achievement between Vietnamese and Cambodian children: Cultural and structural explanations. *Sociological Quarterly*, *43*, 213–235.

Kinzie, J. D., & Leung, P. K. (1996). Psychiatric care of Indochinese Americans. In A. Gaw (Ed.), *Culture, ethnicity, and mental illness* (pp. 281–304). Washington, DC: American Psychiatric Press.

Kinzie, J. D., Scak, W., Angell, R., et al. (1986). The psychiatric effects of massive trauma on Cambodian children: I. The children. *Journal of the American Academy of Child and Adolescent Psychiatry*, *25*, 370–376.

Kuramoto, F. (1995). Asian Americans. In J. Philleo, F. Brisbaine, & L. G. Epstein (Eds.), *Cultural competence for social workers: A guide for alcohol and other drug abuse prevention professionals working with ethnic/racial communities* (pp. 105–155). Rockville, MD: U.S. Department of Health and Human Services, Public Health Service, Substance Abuse and Mental Health Services Administration, Center for Substance Abuse Prevention.

Lee, S. J. (2006). Additional complexities: social class, ethnicity, generation, and gender in Asian American student experiences. *Race, Ethnicity and Education, 9*, 17-28.

Lim, K. V., Heiby, E., Brislin, R., & Griffin, B. (2002). The development of the Khmer acculturation scale. *International Journal of Intercultural Relations, 26,* 653–678.

Lin, K. M., & Cheung, F. (1999). Mental health issues for Asian Americans. *Psychiatric Services, 50,* 774–780.

Maj, M., Satz, P., Janssen, R., Zaudig, M., et al. (1994). WHO neuropsychiatric AIDS study, cross-sectional phase II: Neuropsychological and neurological findings. *Archives of General Psychiatry, 51*, 51–61.

Marshall, G., Schell, T. L., Elliott, M. N., Berthold, S. M., & Chun, C. A. (2005). Mental health of Cambodian refugees 2 decades after resettlement in the United States. *Journal of the American Medical Association, 294,* 571–579.

McKenzie-Pollock, L. (1993). Cambodian families. In M. McGoldrick, J. Giordano, & J. K. Pearce (Eds.), *Ethnicity and family therapy* (pp. 307–315). New York, NY: Guilford Press.

Mitrushina, M., Boone, K., Razani, J., & D'Elia, L (2005). *Handbook of normative data for neuropsychological assessment* (2nd ed., pp. 618–622). New York, NY: Oxford University Press.

Mollica, R. F., Henderson, D. C., & Tor, S. (2002). Psychiatric effects of traumatic brain injury events in Cambodian survivors of mass violence. *British Journal of Psychiatry, 181*, 339–347.

Ngo, B. (2006). Learning from the margins: The education of Southeast and South Asian Americans in context. *Race Ethnicity and Education, 9*, 51–65.

Niedzwiecki, M., & Duong, T. C. (2004). *Southeast Asian American statistical profile.* Washington, DC: Southeast Asian Resource Action Center (SERAC). Retrieved January 7, 2008, from http://www.searac.org/seastatprofilemay04.pdf

Niedzwiecki, M., Yang, K. Y., & Earm, S. (2003). *Southeast Asian American elders in California: Demographics and service priorities revealed by the 2000 census and a survey of mutual assistance associations (MAAs) and faith-based organizations (FBOs).* Washington, DC: Southeast Asia Resource Action Center (SEARAC). Retrieved January 7, 2008, from http://www.searac.org/sea-eldersrpt-fin.pdf

Pachuta, D. M. (1989). Chinese medicine: The law of five elements. In A. A. Sheikh & K. S. Sheikh (Eds.), *Eastern and Western approaches to healing: Ancient wisdom and modern knowledge* (pp. 64–90). New York, NY: John Wiley & Sons.

Palmieri, P. A., Marshall, G. N., & Schell, T. L. (2007). Confirmatory factor analysis of posttraumatic stress symptoms in Cambodian refugees. *Journal of Traumatic Stress, 20,* 207–216.

Phinney, J. S. (1992). The multigroup ethnic identity measure. *Journal of Adolescent Research, 7,* 156–176.

Ponton, M., & Corona-LoMonaco, M. E. (2007). Cross-cultural issues in neuropsychology: Assessment of the Hispanic patient. In B. Uzzell, M. Ponton, & A. Ardila (Eds.), *International handbook of cross-cultural neuropsychology* (pp. 265–282). Mahwah, NJ: Lawrence Erlbaum Associates.

Reeves, T., & Bennett, C. (2004). *We the people: Asians in the United States. Census 2000 special reports.* Washington, DC: U.S. Census Bureau.

Reis, A., Guerreiro, M., & Petersson, K. M. (2003). A sociodemographic and neuropsychological characterization of an illiterate population. *Applied Neuropsychology, 10*, 191–204.

Rumbaut, R. G., & Cornelius, W. A. (1995). *California's immigrant children.* La Jolla, CA: Center for U.S.-Mexican Studies, University of California, San Diego.

Rumbaut, R. G., & Ima, K. (1988). *The adaptation of Southeast Asian refugee youth.* San Diego, CA: Southeast Asian Refugee Youth Study, Department of Sociology, San Diego State University.

Sasao, T. (1991). *Statewide Asian drug service needs assessment: A multimethod approach.* Sacramento, CA: California Department of Alcohol and Drug Programs.

Smith-Hefner, N. J. (1999). *Khmer American: Identity and moral education in a diasporic community.* Berkeley, CA: University of California Press.

Suinn, R. M., Rickard-Figueroa, K., Lew, S., & Vigil, P. (1987). The Suinn-Lew Asian self-identity acculturation scale: An initial report. *Educational and Psychological Measurement, 47,* 401–407.

Um, K. (1997). Resettlement into limbo: Implications for the schooling and education of Cambodian children. In B. Te, M. Cordova, W. Walker-Moffat, & J. First (Eds.), *Unfamiliar partners: Asian parents and U.S. public schools* (pp. 29–35). Boston, MA: National Coalition of Advocates for Students.

Yang, K. Y. (2004). Southeast Asian American children: Not the "model minority." *The Future of Children, 14*, 127–133.

Yee, B. W. K. (2005). *Health and health care of Southeast Asian elders: Vietnamese, Cambodian, Hmong and Laotian elders* (Ethnic Specific Modules). Retrieved September 9, 2005, from http://www.stanford.edu/group/ethnoger

Yee, B. W. K., & Keo, Y. R. (2006). Cambodian elders. In *Doorway thoughts: Cross-cultural health care for older adults* (Vol. 2, pp. 36–55). New York, NY: The American Geriatrics Society.

3 Neuropsychology of Chinese Americans

Tony M. Wong

The term *Chinese American* will be used here in reference to those of Chinese descent who are currently residing in the United States, whether they are born in America or have immigrated to this country from other lands. To describe or characterize a group of people based on shared ethnic, racial, or cultural factors, especially in a volume that is addressed to clinical practitioners, can be risky. Although such attempts might be helpful in providing important contextual information and guidance to clinical neuropsychologists who are providing services to individuals from a group with whom they are not entirely familiar, it would at the same time be easy to misapply this information by rigidly stereotyping an individual from a particular ethnic group based on characteristics that may be common to that group. Just as the use of the term *Asian* or *Asian American* could be somewhat misleading and obscure the underlying heterogeneity of this group (Wong & Fujii, 2004; Wong, 2000), classifying an individual as *Chinese* or *Chinese American* can mask the marked diversity behind this relatively large subgroup. Therefore, in order to provide information that might be helpful to clinical neuropsychologists who evaluate or treat patients of Chinese descent, the goal of this chapter is as much to describe factors that account for the differences within this Asian American subgroup as it is to portray characteristics that might be common among this group.

Population demographics in the United States

The Chinese have been the largest Asian subgroup in America since such comparative statistics have been officially documented in 1990 (U.S. Census Bureau, 1991). In 2000, they accounted for 23.7% of the total Asian population in the United States (U.S. Bureau of the Census, 2000), and 0.9% of the total U.S. population. Moreover, significant and substantial growth was seen in this subgroup in the decade from 1990 to 2000, as their numbers in this country increased by over 40% to 2,432,585. Immigration appears to have played a large role in these significant numbers, as an estimated 1.5 million of the Chinese in the United States, or approximately 62%, are foreign born, according to the 2000 census (U.S. Bureau of the Census, 2001). In contrast to the historically and overwhelmingly high ratio of men to women among the Chinese in America, which was due to earlier restrictive immigration policies that limited the influx of Chinese women, the census data since 1990 show that

Chinese women now slightly outnumber Chinese men, with a sex ratio of 92.9 in the United States in 2000.

With respect to geographic distribution, the 2000 U.S. census data show that the highest numbers of Chinese reside in California, New York, and Texas, with Hawaii, Massachusetts, and New Jersey added to this list when states with the highest percentages of Chinese American residents are considered. The fewest people of Chinese descent, in numbers and percentages, live in Mississippi, Montana, North Dakota, South Dakota, West Virginia, and Wyoming.

As a whole, Chinese Americans are relatively well educated. In 2006, it was estimated that 51.7% of this group who were 25 years of age or older possessed a bachelor's degree or higher (U.S. Census Bureau, 2007), compared to 27.0% of the total population. The contrast in educational attainment is even greater when looking at those who had graduate or professional degrees, as this described 26.3% of Chinese Americans, compared to 9.9% of the entire U.S. population. Interestingly, however, 18.4% of the adults of this racial subgroup did not graduate from high school, compared to 15.9% of the total population, and 16.0% had a high school diploma as their highest level of formal education achieved, compared to 30.2% of the entire American population, suggesting a bimodal distribution of educational attainment for Chinese Americans. According to the same census data, Chinese Americans also appear to fare well on other major socioeconomic indicators. For example, 53.4% of this subgroup were employed in management or professional occupations, compared to 34% of the overall U.S. population, indicating that, at least in recent years, the Chinese in America compare favorably with their non–Chinese American peers, with respect to both educational attainment and occupational status. Chinese Americans also have a higher per capita income than the overall U.S. population ($29,189 vs. $25,267, respectively).

Immigration history

As is the case when working with individuals from any ethnic/cultural subgroup in America, and in order to minimize overgeneralizations, stereotyping, and misunderstanding, it is helpful to appreciate the historical context underlying the current demography of Chinese Americans in the United States. Descendants of one of the oldest and longest continuous civilizations in history, Chinese Americans initially emigrated from a vast land that "embodies complexities in language, religion, customs, political system, legal heritage and physical landscape" (Tong, 2003, p. 2). As such, there exists a marked diversity within the group designated as Chinese American, which may include, depending on an individual's specific family and immigration history, distinct differences in language/dialect and in sociocultural background.

Although there has been evidence of Chinese exposure to North America from the early fifteenth century via maritime exploration and trading junkets, the first record of Chinese presence in the mainland United States was in 1785, when three Chinese sailors arrived in Baltimore as part of an abandoned interracial shipping crew (Tong, 2003; Tsai, 1986). However, it was not until the mid–nineteenth century, after the discovery of gold in California in 1848, when the first wave of large-scale immigration of Chinese to the United States occurred. Large numbers of Chinese men immigrated to the Western United States to pursue gold mining opportunities, or in response to recruitment efforts by the Central Pacific Railroad Company, which was building the western portion of the first transcontinental railroad (Chan, 1991). A majority of these early immigrants were Cantonese- or Taishanese-speaking villagers from Guangdong's Pearl River Delta (Lai, 2004).

This large-scale emigration of Chinese to America and other countries, particularly from this southern coastal province of China, was prompted by a number of factors present at that time in their native country. This included discontent due to heavy taxation, corruption, and oppression (Tsai, 1986), and a dramatic increase in the population in Guangdong, as the populace grew 79.5% during the period from 1787 to 1850, compared to a 47% increase in the total population (Tong, 2003).

The political and economic uncertainty, coupled with the significant struggle for limited cultivable land due to the enormous population increase in the region, naturally led to the diaspora to other lands to pursue economic viability. Thus, Chinese men of largely peasant/unskilled background came to America to pursue the hope and opportunity of the "Gam Saan," or "Gold Mountain," with the intent of returning with or sending their fortunes back to their families in China. However, the growing presence of Chinese immigrants, competition with Caucasian laborers, and prevailing nativist sentiment resulted in palpable and openly hostile anti-Chinese sentiment and the enactment of a series of exclusion laws, beginning with the Exclusion Act of 1882, the only U.S. law ever to limit immigration and naturalization based on race. These and various other anti-Chinese laws had significant impact upon the quality of life of these early Chinese immigrants and laborers, preventing them from bringing over their wives and families, severely limiting their rights (e.g., citizenship, land ownership), and facilitating financial and social hardship. The exclusion laws also had the net effect of decreasing the flow of Chinese immigration (from a high of 107,488 Chinese residents in 1890 to 61,639 in 1920; Gaw, 1993; Qin, 2005) and creating a society of bachelors in the Chinese American community.

Beginning around the time of World War II, a combination of social, political, legal, and other factors led to a series of changes in immigration policy in the United States that resulted ultimately in a shift in the pattern and volume of Chinese immigration into America. The Magnuson Act, or the Chinese Exclusion Repeal Act of 1943, was passed by the U.S. Congress, repealing the series of exclusion acts that began in 1882, and allowing Chinese residents to become naturalized citizens. As Tong (2003) notes, this law was more symbolic than substantive, as it also set an admission quota of 105 Chinese per year, and entry into the United States continued to be regulated on the basis of race rather than national origin. Nevertheless, the passage of this act did herald a new era, and set the stage for further liberalization of immigration policy. This and subsequent acts allowed for more Chinese women to immigrate into America, and for further reunification and establishment of families of Chinese heritage in the United States (Wong & Fujii, 2004).

In 1962, the Refugee Act provided 25,000 nonquota visas to Chinese, and in 1965, the Immigration and Nationality Act amendments were passed, abolishing the national origin quotas that have existed since 1924. These acts were significant factors contributing to what is considered the second wave of large-scale Chinese immigration. Beginning during the postwar years and especially since 1965, the pattern of Chinese immigration into the United States changed. Whereas, prior to 1945, most Chinese Americans originated from Guangdong Province, ethnic Chinese from more diverse areas of China and the world were immigrating to America. These would include China, Hong Kong, Taiwan, and areas of Southeast Asia (e.g., Vietnam, Laos, and Cambodia). In addition, "overseas Chinese" from such countries as Japan, Korea, Philippines, Singapore, and Malaysia, as well as countries in South America and Europe, joined the rapid influx of Chinese immigrants (Lee, 1996). In addition to a shift with respect to region or country of origin of Chinese immigrants, there has also been a concomitant change in where these immigrants tended to settle in America. For example, the earlier immigrants, particularly those during the nineteenth century and the earlier portion of the twentieth century, tended to reside in the Western states and especially in California. This was ostensibly due to the economic promises of the Gold Rush and the construction of the Transcontinental Railroad. Even up to 1980, over half of all Chinese living in the United States were in the Pacific states (Tsai, 1986). Also, the early Chinese immigrants, due in large part to racial hostility by the majority culture, retreated to urban ethnic enclaves (Tong, 2003). These "Chinatowns" originally developed in San Francisco, Los Angeles, and other California cities, but as the Chinese migrated toward the east and south, they also emerged in such places as New York City, Philadelphia, Baltimore, Boston, Washington, D.C., Prescott (Arizona), and El Paso. More recent Chinese immigrants, though still tending to reside in major metropolitan areas, have largely dissociated themselves from the traditional Chinatowns, and have become more suburbanized.

The sociological composition of Chinese living in America has been influenced significantly by the above immigration policies and patterns (Wong, 2000; Wong & Fujii, 2004), as well as other extant factors during the various epochs in which Chinese immigration occurred (e.g., the People's Republic of China began to allow emigration in 1977, leading to an increase of professionals from that country immigrating to America). Although, in addition to what has already been discussed, there are several other dimensions in which the composition of Chinese Americans have changed over the years in response to changes in immigration-related factors, what is clear is that the Chinese in America are as diverse as Americans of European descent (Tsai, 1986). Therefore, as a group, persons of Chinese descent living in America today are quite heterogeneous with respect to region/country of origin, native or ancestral language/dialect, current English proficiency, immigration status, socioeconomic background, level of education, social norms, and other factors that can also contribute to one's acculturation in this country. Neuropsychologists who are providing services to Americans of Chinese descent, then, need to be aware of the diversity inherent in this group, and consider carefully the level of acculturation for their particular client or patient in trying to make appropriate adjustments in their approach to neuropsychological assessment.

In addition to the relative level of acculturation between individuals within a particular age cohort, another important consideration is the differences in socioeconomic attainment due to generational differences. Until the 1940s, when the exclusion acts were repealed and other factors led to an increase in the volume and diversity of Chinese immigration into the United States, most Chinese Americans emigrated from the rural regions in Guangdong Province, and worked primarily as laborers or merchants. Although with exceptions, most during this period also did not have much formal education, and English language facility was relatively limited. These factors, along with prevailing nativist sentiment, largely limited the social mobility and approval of these immigrants. Since the postwar period, both the socioeconomic profile and the social acceptance of Chinese Americans began to change.

Qin (2005) found that the educational attainment of Chinese in the United States was well below the norm in 1940. He noted that the census reported that only 2.8% of Chinese males aged 25 and over had completed four or more years of college, compared to 5.8% of white males. Moreover, 78.2% of Chinese males had not gone beyond grade school levels, ranking second only to black males (84.6%). Overall, the Chinese compared unfavorably with their white counterparts at all levels of educational attainment during that period. However, the educational attainment of Chinese in America improved in the decades following, such that by 1950, their educational achievement, reflected in median years of schooling completed, was at about the same level of the rest of the U.S. population. Tong (2003) notes that when the Communist victory in China occurred in 1949, some Chinese students were stranded in America and were subsequently allowed to obtain permanent residence status. Also, beginning in the late 1950s, significant numbers of students from Taiwan and Hong Kong arrived to pursue higher education. These and other events contributed not only to an increase in the median years of educational attainment for Chinese Americans as a group, but also diversified the community with respect to country/region of origin and language.

Wong (1980) found that by 1970 both foreign-born and native-born Chinese males had equaled or surpassed white males in median years of schooling completed, percentage with four years of high school or more, and percentage with four or more years of college. From 1970 to the present, educational achievement of Chinese Americans has continued to advance, and is reflected in the most recent census data, which show that over 50% of this group have earned at least a bachelor's degree, and over 25% have earned graduate or professional degrees. It has been surmised that the marked educational achievement of Chinese Americans in the past decades has been due, in part, to the rapid influx into this country, especially since 1960, of highly educated professionals of Chinese origin and of students pursuing college and professional degrees. A historic cultural preference for education as a means of status attainment has also been a popular explanation for the educational progress of Chinese in this country.

As with educational attainment, occupational diversity for Chinese Americans became more pronounced following World War II. Prior to that time, the initial Chinese immigrants largely worked in the mines and railroads in the western United States, and, in the period following that, worked as laundry and restaurant workers in various Chinatowns around the country. In the 1940s and 1950s, Chinese males aged 14 and over were found to cluster occupationally in the low-paying census categories "service" and "laborer/operator," but also in the "managers/official" category. But as Qin (2005) noted, this latter category is somewhat misleading, as many of the Chinese who were classified as "managers" were owners of small ethnic businesses operating in the racially homogenous enclaves, as opposed to being large employers in the more mainstream sectors of society. A more telling reflection of Chinese Americans' occupational status at that time was the fact that the proportions of Chinese in the "professional/technical" category were very low in 1940 (2.4% and 7.4%, respectively, for men and women) and 1950 (6.3% and 11.0%, respectively, for men and women), although there was a noteworthy increase within that decade. The presence of the stranded students and scholars due to the Communist takeover of China mentioned during the discussion of educational attainment contributed to this increase in the number of Chinese employed in professional and technical jobs. Over the ensuing decades, the occupational achievement of Chinese Americans continued to make impressive gains, as their representations in professional/technical jobs rose dramatically, along with a concomitant decline in the "manual labor," "service," and "clerical" categories.

In addition to educational and occupational attainment as indicators of socioeconomic status or progress, trends in earnings or income of Chinese Americans can also be examined. Such analyses have tended to suggest that earnings attainment for Chinese Americans have improved significantly over the years. In addition, the data might suggest that Chinese Americans might have achieved economic parity even with the Euro-American population. For example, by 1970, the median family income for Chinese Americans exceeded the median family income of their white counterparts by about $1000. However, as Chan (1991) suggested, this figure is deceiving, as a higher proportion of Chinese American families than white families had more than one person in the household working, which accounts for the higher family income. Thus, if per capita rather than per family income data were used, then it might be observed that Chinese Americans were earning less income than the national average during that period. Similarly, Qin's (2005) analysis showed that from 1980 to 2000, when per capita income is used as the measure, while there was a clear and significant increase in income over that period, earnings for Chinese Americans continued to lag behind those of their white counterparts. Despite these caveats, the aggregate income data for Chinese Americans show remarkable improvement in earnings over the decades following World War II.

Testing issues

There are several challenges associated with the neuropsychological assessment of Asian American immigrants, but the primary issue is one of test validity (Fujii & Wong, 2005). Because most neuropsychological tests used in the United States have been developed and normed on individuals of Euro-American background for whom English is the first language, when these procedures are used with immigrants whose primary language is different, potential threats to validity are introduced. In addition to language, level of acculturation, level and quality of education, and cultural factors also need be considered when conducting neuropsychological evaluations with Asian Americans, including Chinese Americans, particularly those who have immigrated to America. Careful consideration of these factors would help determine whether any adjustments in test selection or evaluation approach need to be made for a particular Chinese American client. It might be reasonably assumed that patients who are well educated and assimilated into American society with good English skills can be assessed in a manner similar to that used with Euro-American patients; i.e., the science of neuropsychological testing can be primarily based on empirically validated American norm-based testing (Fujii & Wong, 2005). Second-generation (and beyond) Chinese Americans will often fall within this category. Conversely, Chinese patients who are poorly educated, do not have strong English skills, and are not well acculturated are likely to present a greater challenge to the clinical neuropsychologist attempting to perform a valid examination.

As discussed elsewhere in this chapter, Chinese Americans are relatively well educated, with the most recent census data showing that over half of this group possess a bachelor's degree or higher. However, there is individual variation underlying this group statistic, and the specific educational history of the patient or client being evaluated needs to be considered. For overseas-born Chinese immigrants who were educated in their country of origin before arriving in America, the quality of education in that country may be important to consider, especially because they have emigrated from various countries and regions of the world, with differing educational systems and legacies. For example, although Mainland China (People's Republic of China), the Hong Kong SAR (Special Administrative Region), and Taiwan (Republic of China) are some of the primary regions from which Chinese in America have emigrated, and are all considered "China" with respect to their majority ethnic, cultural, and language identities, their educational systems are different.

In Mainland China, great strides in public education have been made since the 1940s, when it was estimated that about 80% of the population was illiterate. However, although it was estimated recently that more than 93% of the population area of the country has achieved universal nine-year basic education, and a literacy rate above 96% in the young and middle-aged populations, only 40% of Chinese students go to upper secondary schools (Asia Society, 2005). Moreover, the Asia Society's report noted that a significant gap between rural and urban schools exists, in that the rural schools lag behind the urban with respect to teacher qualifications, facilities, and quality. Thus, it appears that, overall, the quality of education in Mainland China still lags behind that of the United States at this time.

Hong Kong and Taiwan, however, present a different picture. Due to greater economic resources, a much smaller population base to address, and historical factors, the quality of education in these regions is overall higher than that in the People's Republic of China, and is more similar to that of the United States.

Beyond quality of education, there are also differences with respect to the role of English in these educational systems and, consequently, English language ability of students/immigrants emerging from these systems. Although the educational systems in all three regions currently have English as a compulsory second language, until the 1997 transfer of Hong Kong from British rule to China, English was the primary medium of instruction there. In addition, some schools there continue to use English as the primary language of instruction, and English also continues to be used widely in Hong Kong due to its prior history as a British Crown Colony. The educational system in Hong Kong also has more of a Western style than to those in the People's Republic of China and in Taiwan.

In summary, then, depending on the region of China in which an immigrant received his or her public education, both the quality of that education and English language facility have to be accounted for when preparing a neuropsychological evaluation of that individual. Similar analyses or considerations need to take place for Chinese who have emigrated from other regions of the world. For example, many Chinese have immigrated to America from Singapore, where education quality and English usage are relatively high, or from Vietnam, where the education and English skills are not as advanced. Some practitioners might find the Bilingual Verbal Ability Tests (Munoz-Sandoval, Cummins, Alvarado, & Ruef, 1998), which include a measure of overall verbal ability as well as a measure of English proficiency, useful in their assessments of Chinese patients who are bilingual. This test was translated into 17 languages, including Chinese, plus English. However, reliability and concurrent validity studies during the construction of this test were only conducted on the Spanish-English samples. So, until this instrument's psychometric properties are more solidly established with Chinese bilingual individuals, it should be used with caution with this group.

In addition to educational history/background and English familiarity, the level of acculturation and other culturally related issues need to be considered in the neuropsychological evaluation of a Chinese American. Acculturation refers to the level to which an individual participates in the values, language, and practices of the majority culture versus those of his or her own community (Manly et al., 1998). Chinese Americans who are less acculturated or familiar with the Euro-American culture may respond differently to the standard neuropsychological tests based on Western norms than those who are more acculturated. Manly et al. (1998) found that level of acculturation in an African American sample accounted for a significant proportion of the variance on several neuropsychological measures. This and other similar findings suggest that acculturation is an important moderator variable to consider in the evaluation of individuals from a dissimilar culture (Wong, Strickland, Fletcher-Janzen, Ardila, and Reynolds, 2000), including Chinese immigrants.

From a practical perspective, assessing an individual's level of acculturation involves determining not only the degree to which he or she is familiar with American culture, but also the extent to which he or she is comfortable with and participates in the American culture, irrespective of how long that individual may have lived in the United States. Therefore, asking about things such as the individual's primary peer group, his or her recreational/community interests or involvement, and other related information might be helpful in determining one's general acculturation level.

After taking into consideration the specific sociocultural profile of a Chinese American patient, test selection itself is important in conducting a valid neuropsychological evaluation. Fujii and Wong (2005) argued that, for Asian Americans who are poorly educated and have limited English skills, it is best to administer tests that have been developed and validated for the patient's specific ethnic group.

However, while this may be a sound approach conceptually, this may still be a challenge practically. Although Chan, Shum, and Cheung (2003) found that there was a marked increase of published articles regarding cognitive or neuropsychological assessment in Asia from 1981 to 2001, including 40% of which covered test development or adaptation, only eight neuropsychological tests were ultimately determined to be clinically validated according to their criteria, with five of these tests normed on Chinese.

While there may be, in the future, an increase in the number of clinically validated tests available for use with Chinese patients, due to the heterogeneity of the Chinese/Chinese American population, even the selection, use, and interpretation of these instruments must be conducted judiciously. For example, one of the clinically validated instruments listed in the Chan, Shum, and Cheung (2003) study is the Hong Kong List Learning Test (Chan & Kwok, 1999), a verbal list learning test developed specifically for use with Chinese patients and found, in multiple studies, to have good discrimination between normal controls and various neurologic patient groups. However, this test was normed in and developed in Hong Kong with Cantonese-speaking subjects. Therefore, its properties with Mandarin-speaking or other Chinese language/dialect groups are currently unknown.

Despite this caveat, however, it is still preferable to use neuropsychological tests that are normed on a group that is closer in linguistic and cultural background to the patient's, as this would likely obtain a more reasonable approximation of one's cognitive status. In the absence of appropriate tests that are normed on Chinese, the neuropsychologist may have to rely on the use of neuropsychological tests that are normed and standardized on American subjects. Although the temptation may be to use tests that are less language dependent or ostensibly nonverbal, such as the Wechsler Performance scales; motor tests such as Grip Strength, Fingertapping, or pegboard tests; Rey-Osterrieth figure; or other similar procedures, it should also be understood that these instruments are not "culture free" or "culture fair," especially when using with those who have low educational levels (Fujii & Wong, 2005; Wong, 2000).

Until the amount of quality neuropsychological instrumentation available for use with Chinese (or other Asian) patients increases, consideration might be given to the multimethod hypothesis testing approach recommended by Fujii and Wong (2005), which integrates data from different sources (e.g., behavioral observations, history, medical reports, collateral reports) in addition to neuropsychological test results. Also, a current compilation of Asian neuropsychological references, including those for Chinese, can be found in Fujii, Artiola i Fortuny, and Norman (2007), and can be a helpful resource to guide test analysis and selection.

Despite the historical shortage of neuropsychological procedures properly validated for use with Chinese and Chinese-speaking patients, there has been an increasing presence in the neuropsychological and psychological literature of investigations into the psychometric and normative properties of certain measures when applied to Chinese populations. These findings may be useful under certain circumstances in guiding test selection and interpretation for those providing neuropsychological services to Chinese patients. For example, Hsieh and Tori (2007) report normative data on a battery of eight neuropsychological procedures that were administered to 324

Mandarin-speaking adults in Beijing, China. Due to practical limitations, the procedures they used, which consisted of Animal Naming, Color Trails, Five-Digit Test, Fuld Object Memory Test, Raven's Standard Progressive Matrices, Symbol Digit Modalities Test, Trailmaking Test A, and the Digit Span Test, may not represent an ideal battery to some, especially within a clinical context where a more comprehensive set of procedures might be needed. Also, the applicability of these norms beyond Mandarin-speaking individuals from Mainland China might an issue.

Despite these limitations, however, this represents an improvement over what has been previously available, and potentially provides clinicians and researchers with at least a partial repertoire of ethnic-specific norms to use with certain Chinese patients. Normative data have also been obtained and described on the Trailmaking Test A and the Chinese version of the Trailmaking Test B (Lu & Bigler, 2002), the Chinese version of the Mattis Dementia Rating Scale (Chan, Choi, Chiu, & Lam, 2003), the Chinese version of the Category Fluency Test (Chan & Poon, 1999), and the Wisconsin Card Sorting Test for children and adolescents in Taiwan (Lin, Chen, Yang, Hsiao, & Tien, 2000; Shu, Tien, Lung, & Chang, 2000). As with the Hsieh and Tori norms discussed previously, the external validity of these latter sets of norms need to be considered before using them on a wider Chinese population, as these data were obtained on specific Chinese groups in different locales (e.g., Taiwan, Hong Kong, United States).

Apart from these test-specific norms for Chinese populations, there have also been some reports, albeit controversial, asserting that IQs among Chinese compare very favorably to those of Western groups (e.g., Chan & Lynn, 1989; Lynn, 1991). Beyond norms per se, a number of studies describe the cross-cultural applicability to Chinese samples of certain neuropsychological procedures previously developed for use with Western populations. For example, Chan and his colleagues demonstrated that the results from the Test of Everyday Attention, when administered to both a nonclinical Chinese sample and a traumatic brain injury sample from Hong Kong, yielded a factor structure that was consistent with a three-factor model of attention. Cheung, Cheung, and Chan (2004) provided evidence that a modified version of the Boston Naming Test is applicable to the Chinese population, yielding a sensitivity of 73.1% and a specificity of 75.3% in differentiating normal from brain-damaged participants in a Hong Kong sample.

Lee and Chan (2000b) found that Chinese orthography did not generate a greater Stroop effect than English orthography in evaluating 85 participants belonging to Chinese-English bilingual and English monolingual groups. Finally, Lee, Cheung, Chan, and Chan (2000) showed that the Trailmaking Test and the Color Trails Test were generally fair across two language samples, but that the two instruments were highly correlated for the English sample, rather than the Chinese sample. Also, Lee and Chan (2000a) found in their Hong Kong sample that these two instruments represented equivalent constructs only when the participants were older and had higher levels of education.

In addition to current test results and other contemporary data collected in a neuropsychological examination, an estimate of premorbid cognitive/intellectual status is often obtained by a neuropsychologist so that change, or lack thereof, can be inferred. Wong and Fujii (2004) noted that conventional methods of obtaining this estimate, such as the use of a reading/vocabulary test, or asking about the patient's current occupation, may not be valid for immigrant populations. They suggested instead that information that would be useful in arriving at a reasonable premorbid estimate of abilities includes the region of the native country in which the individual was born and raised, the reason and timing of when immigration took place, occupation and educational level in the native country, parent's occupation and education history in the native country, and education and occupation in America.

An approach that might be considered, which incorporates these suggestions in a structured manner, is to use one of the demographically based indices, such as the Barona equation (Barona, Reynolds, & Chastain, 1984), to estimate baseline intellectual level, but using information from the native country for the variables. Because this equation was not originally derived with data obtained from Chinese individuals, only a gross, tentative estimate of premorbid intellectual level would be appropriate using this method. Despite this limitation, the distinct advantage of using an algorithm over a more subjective estimation method is in its objective consistency.

Finally, an adaptation of the "best performance(s)" method to estimating baseline cognitive level described by Lezak, Howieson, and Loring (2004) may also be a reasonable alternative. This method, in its original form, uses the best performance, whether it might be the highest test score or set of scores, nonscorable behavior, or evidence of premorbid achievement, as the best estimate of premorbid ability. In a slight adaptation this approach, the focus is on a test score or set of scores, and it can be inferred that the patient's premorbid level of performance would not be below that of his/her best performance normatively on any individual neuropsychological test or subset of tests in a given battery, even if it was on a test that was normed on an American population. This is based on the assumption that test bias typically occurs in the adverse direction, leading to an underestimate of the immigrant's abilities. Therefore, it can be reasonably assumed that the patient's abilities are "at least" at the level of his/her highest level of performance during a neuropsychological examination, if not higher. Even with this consideration, however, Lezak et al.'s admonition against using test scores in isolation is still applicable. Therefore, corroboration for this estimate of baseline level of abilities should be obtained from collateral information, such as occupational and/or educational history, and a thorough overall history.

Another test issue of relevance, particularly in forensic contexts, that deserves brief mention is that of symptom validity testing, which refers to methods used to detect poor effort or malingering. Although there are not currently symptom validity measures specifically designed for and normed on Chinese individuals, it might be reasonably assumed that some of the available forced choice–based procedures, such as the Hiscock and Hiscock (1989) method and the Test of Memory Malingering (Tombaugh, 1996), can be used with Chinese examinees to detect the more acute instances of malingering. That is, because both procedures use a forced, two-choice methodology, and are ostensibly not highly dependent on language for understanding and performing the tasks, significantly below-chance performance can be reasonably interpreted as indicative of malingering. Interestingly, the subject in question in the Hiscock and Hiscock study was of Chinese descent, although the purpose of the investigation and report was not cross-cultural in nature. The limitation of using these instruments with Chinese individuals, especially those who are less acculturated and/or whose English proficiency is not high, is that they are less sensitive to more subtle forms of malingering or compromised effort. The Word Memory Test (Green, 2003), a more sophisticated measure of malingering and effort, and which has a Mandarin translated version, might be considered where appropriate.

Other dementia screens translated into Chinese include the Montreal Cognitive Assessment (MoCA), which has several dialects including those spoken in Beijing, Cantonese, Hong Kong, and Taiwan, (Nasreddine et al., 2005, translations can be found online at http://www.mocastest.org/), Cognistat, which is translated into Cantonese and Mandarin (Kiernan, Mueller, Langston, & van Dyke, 2009), and the Informant Questionnaire on Cognitive Decline in the Elderly (IQCODE) (Jorm, 2004), a nonneuropsychological measure of dementia based upon informant report. Although potentially useful, these dementia screens should be used with caution as specific Chinese norms are not reported.

Other recommendations

The following are some additional recommendations to consider when delivering neuropsychological services to Chinese American patients:

Consider the socioeconomic status, context, and history of Chinese patients. As discussed earlier in this chapter, the generational cohort to which a Chinese American patient or client belongs may make a significant difference with respect to the socioeconomic context of that individual. For example, earlier immigrants from China are likely to be less formally educated and have a lower occupational status than the more recent immigrants, and are consequently less acculturated. Conversely, later generations of Chinese Americans are likely to be much more acculturated, having been born in this country, and with high levels of educational attainment and occupational status. Of course, beyond the general trends, obtaining the specific history/profile of the individual is crucial, as ultimately this information will be helpful for the neuropsychologist in determining what cross-cultural adjustments need to be made in order to obtain a valid neuropsychological evaluation for that person.

Wong (2000) and Wong and Fujii (2004) illustrated how the specific history of Chinese immigrants from disparate times and regions might lead to differing sociocultural presentations. They used as an example those who are descended from the early immigrants of the nineteenth century, who primarily had their origins from the rural villages outside of Guangzhou in Guangdong Province, and were primarily speakers of Cantonese or Taishanese. The more elderly among these, despite their relatively lengthy tenure in the United States, have little formal education, retain many of their native cultural traditions, and are poor speakers of English. These were contrasted against more recent Chinese immigrants, who tend to be more diverse socioeconomically and educationally, and likely speak Mandarin, the national language of China, and also have some basic proficiency in English, especially if they are well educated. Country of origin was also illustrated by these authors as an important factor of consideration. For example, Chinese immigrants from Singapore may be more likely to assimilate to American than those from China, due to Singapore's relatively more Westernized culture (Lee, 1996).

Consider the primary language/dialect background of Chinese patients. The ideal situation, when assessing patients who do not have good English skills, is to have a competent neuropsychologist conduct an evaluation with a patient in his or her primary language. However, this can be particularly complicated with Chinese patients, as there are traditionally seven major language or dialect groups in China. The two most commonly known in America are Mandarin, which is the official language of China, and Cantonese. In addition to the other five major Chinese language groups, there are several additional language groups and dialects or subdialects. Therefore, there may not always be a neuropsychologist available who can perform the evaluation in an individual's native language or dialect. Although an interpreter with the proper language/dialect background can be engaged to assist with the evaluation, there are potential problems with this approach (Artiola i Fortuny & Mullaney, 1998; Wong, 2000; Wong et al., 2000). If the use of an interpreter cannot be avoided, it is recommended that suggestions offered by Wong et al. (2000) regarding this approach be considered.

Be aware of cultural factors that might affect or influence neuropsychological testing of a Chinese patient. Obtaining a valid neuropsychological evaluation is more than merely selecting the appropriate tests and administering them in mechanistic fashion. Although a neuropsychological evaluation at its best provides information on brain functioning, it is still fundamentally a behavior sample, and neuropsychological test performance can be affected by the interaction between the examiner and the patient. Therefore, as Fujii and Wong (2005) suggested, if a neuropsychologist is not culturally sensitive, the client may be approached in a manner that damages rapport or prevents the optimal collection of information. Wong (2000) offered suggestions regarding facilitative behaviors with Asian American clients that can be applied with Chinese Americans. These include being aware of and respecting cultural nuances, being sensitive to cultural taboos, establishing rapport in a culturally appropriate manner, respecting cultural preferences that are not harmful, and reassuring confidentiality.

Be sensitive to how the Chinese sociocultural worldview might differ from that of the American neuropsychologist. Beyond the neuropsychological testing situation itself, there are important cultural considerations that might impact the entire neuropsychological consultation process. For example, the Chinese culture, as is true for most Asian cultures, views the family or extended family as the fundamental unit, as opposed to Western culture, which sees the individual as the most fundamental unit (Wong, 2000). As such, the Chinese patients or clients may have differing expectations, compared to their Western counterparts, with respect to such issues as family access to information, involvement and input in the assessment and intervention, and caretaking role of the family. Conceptualization of neuropsychological symptoms and syndromes may also be an issue. For example, geriatric memory problems may be viewed by Chinese clients as normal consequences of growing old (Elliott, Di Minno, Lam, & Tu, 1996; Wong & Fujii, 2004).

Case sample

Mr. C. is a 53-year-old, right-handed man of Chinese descent. He was referred for a neuropsychological examination by his primary care physician in order to determine his current neurocognitive status, as he sustained a traumatic brain injury with bilateral frontal hemorrhages secondary to a motor vehicle accident about five years ago. He spent about 13 days in the acute hospital unit following his accident and a little over a month in a brain injury rehabilitation program before being discharged home, with outpatient services. A native of Beijing, China, Mr. C. earned a bachelor's degree in chemical engineering in China, and had worked as a chemical engineer in Beijing for about 12 years before immigrating to the United States in 1998 to pursue further studies. He attended a university in Texas, where he earned a master's degree in chemical engineering in 2000. He had just finished this degree and was in the process of seeking a job when his accident occurred.

Since his discharge home, Mr. C. has complained of persisting memory problems. His wife and their 17-year-old daughter have noticed increased irritability. Mr. C. is currently physically and medically stable, and has no problems with his activities of daily living (ADLs). His family, however, is concerned that he has a limited daily routine, consisting primarily of surfing the Internet, and occasionally making unnecessary purchases online. His primary care physician feels that his patient has clearly made progress cognitively over the last five years, but is uncertain as to the extent of his current cognitive limitations, due to language/cultural issues.

Because Mr. C.'s primary language is Chinese (Mandarin), and his conversational English is limited, it was decided that his neuropsychological examination would be conducted in Mandarin. In order to minimize or account for, as much as reasonably possible, the effects of language or culture upon this examination:

1. A professional interpreter, who had no prior relationship to either the examiner or the examinee, was used. The interpreter was carefully instructed to translate in a verbatim, but culturally compatible, fashion, so that no unnecessary or unanticipated cues or embellishments might be provided to the patient.
2. When practically feasible, tests or procedures for which instructions or items rely heavily on English were translated and conducted in Chinese. For example, the Digit Span subtest was administered in Mandarin by the

interpreter (with prior preparation and instruction). Also, the depression and symptom inventories were carefully translated into and printed in Chinese prior to the patient's examination.

3. One of the very few tests/procedures reported in the scientific literature that assesses attention and is normed with Chinese subjects was utilized during this evaluation: the Random Chinese Word Cancellation Test (Chen-Sea, Cermak, & Henderson, 1993).
4. Overall, due to the constraints of language, culture, and the accompanying problems they introduce into achieving a valid examination, an emphasis was placed on utilizing tests and procedures that assess nonverbal cognitive functions that are ostensibly less likely to be affected by language or cultural background. However, it should also be noted that it is the common understanding of professionals familiar with cross-cultural assessment that even these nonverbal procedures are not necessarily culture free.

In order to obtain a broad estimate of the patient's premorbid or preaccident baseline intellectual functioning level, the Barona index (Barona et al., 1984) was used. The Barona equation is an empirically or mathematically derived index that is demographically based, and takes into account age, gender, ethnicity, education, occupation, urban versus rural residence, and region of residence. Although the index was designed and derived for individuals residing in the United States, in order to obtain the most generous estimate of the patient's intellectual level, it was decided to use "Northeast" instead of "South" as the patient's region of residence. Although Mr. C. currently lives in the South (Texas), he is a native of Beijing, and it can be reasonably asserted for the purposes of this index that it would be more appropriate to use the Northeast variable, which is higher, and results in a higher index/score. All other variables did not require any adjustment, as it is assumed that the valence of the variables of age, gender, ethnicity, education, and urban versus rural residence would be in a similar direction even when applied cross-culturally (e.g., there is a positive correlation between level of education and intellectual level regardless of cultural/ethnic identity). This resulted in the following scores:

Estimated Verbal Intellectual Quotient:	115 (high average)
Estimated Performance Intellectual Quotient:	111 (average)
Estimated Full-Scale Intellectual Quotient:	115 (high average)

It should be noted that these obtained scores should be viewed only as broad estimates of the patient's intellectual baseline, both because they are derived, and not actual scores, and because these are estimates of what might be theoretically obtained with the Wechsler Adult Intelligence Scale–Revised, an intellectual battery that is normed on English-speaking U.S. residents.

Despite the largely nonstandard administration of the neuropsychological battery (i.e., use of an interpreter and use of primarily Western-normed procedures), the results showed residual strengths in attention, memory, language, arithmetic skills, and nonverbal/visual reasoning. Although a precise measurement of underlying capacity cannot be assumed due to the inherent limitations of a cross-cultural neuropsychological examination, at least broad estimates of the domains mentioned were obtained, and suggest that they are at or near premorbid levels, with some mild decrement possible. Impaired areas of functioning suggested by the test results included concept formation, mental flexibility, reduced cognitive efficiency, and information processing speed. Overall, these results suggest that most of his cognitive functions, including episodic memory, appear to be relatively intact, whereas aspects of his executive functioning are below normal expectation. This profile of findings is consistent with the patient's history of anterior brain injury as well as his current behavioral repertoire.

References

Artiola i Fortuny, L., & Mullaney, H. (1998). Assessing patients whose language you do not know: Can the absurd be ethical? *The Clinical Neuropsychologist, 12*, 113–126.

Asia Society. (2005). *Education in China: Lessons for U.S. educators*. Retrieved October 26, 2007, from http://www.asiasociety.org

Barona, A., Reynolds, C. R., & Chastain, R. (1984). A demographically based index of premorbid intelligence for the WAIS-R. *Journal of Consulting and Clinical Psychology, 52*, 885–887.

Chan, A. S., Choi, A., Chiu, H., & Lam, L. (2003). Clinical validity of the Chinese version of Mattis Dementia Rating Scale in differentiating dementia of Alzheimer's type in Hong Kong. *Journal of the International Neuropsychological Society, 9*, 45–55.

Chan, A. S., & Kwok, I. (1999). *Hong Kong List Learning Test*. Hong Kong: Department of Psychology and Clinical Psychology Centre, The Chinese University of Hong Kong.

Chan, A. S., & Poon, M. W. (1999). Performance of 7- to 95-year-old individuals in a Chinese version of the category fluency test. *Journal of the International Neuropsychological Society, 5*, 525–533.

Chan, A. S., Shum, D., & Cheung, R. W. Y. (2003). Recent development of cognitive and neuropsychological assessment in Asian countries. *Psychological Assessment, 15*, 257–267.

Chan, J., & Lynn, R. (1989). The intelligence of six-year-olds in Hong Kong. *Journal of Biological Science, 21*, 461–464.

Chan, R. C. K., & Lai, M. K. (2006). Latent structure of the Test of Everyday Attention: Convergent evidence from patients with traumatic brain injury. *Brain Injury, 20*, 653–659.

Chan, S. (1991). *Asian Americans: An interpretive history*. Boston, MA: Twayne.

Chen-Sea, M., Cermak, S. A., & Henderson, A. (1993). Performance of normal Chinese adults and right CVA patients on the Random Chinese Word Cancellation Test. *Clinical Neuropsychologist, 7*, 239–249.

Cheung, R. W., Cheung, M. C., & Chan, A. S. (2004). Confrontation naming in Chinese patients with left, right or bilateral brain damage. *Journal of the International Neuropsychological Society, 10*, 46–53.

Elliott, K. S., Di Minno, M., Lam, D., & Tu, A. M. (1996). Working with Chinese families in the context of dementia. In G. Yeo & D. Gallagher-Thompson (Eds.), *Ethnicity and the dementias* (pp. 89–108). Washington, DC: Taylor & Francis.

Fujii, D., Artiola i Fortuny, L., & Norman, M. (2007). *Multicultural references*. Retrieved October 29, 2007, from the American Academy of Clinical Neuropsychology Web site: http://www.theAACN.org

Fujii, D. E., & Wong, T. M. (2005). Neuropsychological assessment with Asian-American immigrants: Recommendations for meeting *Daubert* standards. *Journal of Forensic Neuropsychology, 4*, 3–31.

Gaw, A. C. (1993). Psychiatric care of Chinese Americans. In A. Gaw (Ed.), *Culture, ethnicity, and mental illness* (pp. 245–280). Washington, DC: American Psychiatric Association.

Green, P. (2003). *Green's Word Memory Test for Microsoft Windows*. Edmonton, Alberta, CA: Green's Publishing, Inc.

Hiscock, M., & Hiscock, C. K. (1989). Refining the forced-choice method for the detection of malingering. *Journal of Clinical and Experimental Neuropsychology, 11*, 967–974.

Hsieh, S. J., & Tori, C. D. (2007). Normative data on cross-cultural neuropsychological tests obtained from Mandarin-speaking adults across the life span. *Archives of Clinical Neuropsychology, 22*, 283–296.

Jorm, A. F. (2004). The Informant Questionnaire on Cognitive Decline in the Elderly (IQCODE): A review. *International Psychogeriatrics, 16*, 3–19. (This test is downloadable, although your computer would have to have special features for specific languages: http://www.anu.edu.au/iqcode/)

Kiernan, R., Mueller, J., Langston, J., & van Dyke, C. (2009). *2009 Cognistat manual*. Fairfax, CA: Novatek International.

Lai, H. M. (2004). *Becoming Chinese American: A history of communities and institutions*. Walnut Creek, CA: AltaMira Press.

Lee, E. (1996). Asian American families: An overview. In M. McGoldrick, J. Giordano, & J. K. Pearce (Eds.), *Ethnicity and family therapy* (2nd ed., pp. 227–248). New York, NY: Guilford Press.

Lee, T. M., & Chan, C. C. (2000a). Are trail making and color trails tests of equivalent constructs? *Journal of Clinical and Experimental Neuropsychology, 22*, 529–534.

Lee, T. M., & Chan, C. C. (2000b). Stroop interference in Chinese and English. *Journal of Clinical and Experimental Neuropsychology, 22*, 465–471.

Lee, T. M., Cheung, C. C., Chan, J. K., & Chan, C. C. (2000). Trail making across languages. *Journal of Clinical and Experimental Neuropsychology, 22*, 772–778.

Lezak, M. D., Howieson, D. B., & Loring, D. W. (2004). *Neuropsychological assessment* (4th ed.). New York, NY: Oxford.

Lin, C. C., Chen, W. J., Yang, H. J., Hsiao, C. K., & Tien, A. Y. (2000). Performance on the Wisconsin Card Sorting Test among adolescents in Taiwan: Norms, factorial structure, and relation to schizotypy. *Journal of Clinical and Experimental Neuropsychology, 22*, 69–79.

Lu, L., & Bigler, E. D. (2002). Normative data on trailmaking test for neurologically normal, Chinese-speaking adults. *Applied Neuropsychology, 9*, 219–225.

Lynn, R. (1991). Intelligence in China. *Social Behavior and Personality, 19*, 1–4.

Manly, J. J., Miller, W., Heaton, R. K., Byrd, D., Reilly, J., Velasquez, R. J., … Grant, I. (1998). The effect of African-American acculturation on neuropsychological test performance in normal and HIV-positive individuals. *Journal of the International Neuropsychological Society, 4*, 291–302.

Munoz-Sandoval, A. F., Cummins, J., Alvarado, C. G., & Ruef, M. L. (1998). *Bilingual Verbal Abilities Tests*. Itasca, IL: Riverside Publishing.

Nasreddine, Z., Phillips, N., Bedirian, V., Charbonneau, S., Whitehead, V., Collin, S., … Chertkow, H. (2005). The Montreal Cognitive Assessment, MoCA: A brief screening tool for mild cognitive impairment. *Journal of the American Geriatric Society, 53*, 695–699. http://www.mocatest.org/

Qin, B. (2005, December). *Wage earnings of Chinese in the United States: Individual and contextual determinants.* Retrieved October 19, 2007, from http://handle.tamu.edu/1969.1/3213

Shu, B. C., Tien, A. Y., Lung, F. W., & Chang, Y. Y. (2000). Norms for the Wisconsin Card Sorting Test in 6- to 11-year-old children in Taiwan. *Clinical Neuropsychologist, 14*, 275–286.

Tombaugh, T. N. (1996). *Test of memory malingering*. New York, NY: Multi Health Systems.

Tong, B. (2003). *The Chinese Americans* (rev. ed.). Boulder, CO: University Press of Colorado.

Tsai, S. H. (1986). *The Chinese experience in America*. Bloomington, IN: Indiana University Press.

U.S. Bureau of the Census. (2000). *2000 census of population: General population characteristics.* Washington, DC: Author.

U.S. Bureau of the Census. (2001). *Nation's Asian and Pacific Islander population (profile).* Washington, DC: Author.

U.S. Census Bureau. (1991). *Profile of general demographic characteristics.* Washington, DC: Author.

U.S. Census Bureau. (2007). *Selected population profile in the United States, 2006 American community survey, Chinese alone*. Retrieved October 19, 2007, from http://factfinder.census.gov

Wong, M. G. (1980). Changes in socioeconomic status of the Chinese male population in the United States from 1960 to 1970. *International Migration Review, 14*, 511–524.

Wong, T. M. (2000). Neuropsychological assessment and intervention with Asian Americans. In E. Fletcher-Janzen, T. L. Strickland, & C. R. Reynolds (Eds.), *Handbook of cross-cultural neuropsychology* (pp. 43–53). New York, NY: Kluwer Academic/Plenum Publishers.

Wong, T. M., & Fujii, D. E. (2004). Neuropsychological assessment of Asian Americans: Demographic factors, cultural diversity, and practical guidelines. *Applied Neuropsychology, 11*, 23–36.

Wong, T. M., Strickland, T. L., Fletcher-Janzen, E., Ardila, A., & Reynolds, C. R. (2000). Theoretical and practical issues in the neuropsychological assessment and treatment of culturally dissimilar patients. In E. Fletcher-Janzen, T. L. Strickland, and C. R. Reynolds (Eds.), *Handbook of cross-cultural neuropsychology* (pp. 3–18). New York, NY: Kluwer Academic/Plenum Press.

4 Neuropsychological assessments and Filipino Americans
Cultural implications for practice

Kevin L. Nadal and Jennifer Monzones

Introduction

The United States is becoming more multiculturally diverse; by the year 2050, it is predicted that the racial "minority" or people of color will outnumber the "majority," or Whites (Sue & Sue, 2003). However, despite this growing population, the mental health experiences of people of color in the United States have often been invisible, neglected, or disregarded. In fact, several authors have purported that the profession of psychology has been culturally insensitive to the needs of racial/ethnic minorities, and that the services that are provided to people of color are often ineffective and even detrimental to their mental health (Sue, Arredondo, & McDavis, 1992; Sue & Sue, 2003).

Because of this, the American Psychological Association (APA) created its "Ethical Principles of Psychologists and Code of Conduct" (APA, 2002) in order for psychologists to provide appropriate services to culturally diverse populations by attending to the cultural, individual, and role differences related to age, gender, race, ethnicity, and national origin. In 2002, the Council of Representatives of APA endorsed the "Guidelines on Multicultural Education, Training, Research, Practice, and Organizational Change for Psychologists" (APA, 2003), which stated that multicultural competence should not be limited to psychotherapy and practice, but also should embrace facets of psychology including education, training, research, testing, and consulting.

Under these guidelines, psychologists have been summoned to become multiculturally competent through general awareness, skills, and learning about the major minority groups: Asian Americans and Pacific Islanders, Hispanics/Latinos, Black/African Americans, and Native Americans. However, most research and training tends to focus on these groups as homogenous racial categories, failing to appreciate the within-group differences that may occur. For Asian Americans specifically, this may occur through two forms: (1) psychologists homogenize the experiences of 40 distinct Asian ethnic groups, or (2) psychologists assume the experiences of East Asian Americans (Chinese, Japanese, and Korean Americans) to be universal for all

Asian subgroups (David & Okazaki, 2006; Nadal, 2004). This trend is specifically salient in the field of neuropsychology, in which studies that concentrate on Asian Americans fail to decipher between ethnic groups or utilize small sample sizes, which makes it difficult to understand between-group differences.

This chapter will focus on the experiences of Filipino Americans, one group that is often overlooked, invisible, or marginalized by both general society and within the Asian American community. Previous authors have cited that Filipino Americans are different from East Asian Americans in a number of ways, including a unique colonial history, a range of phenotypic appearances, and disparaging socioeconomic and educational experiences that are contrary to the "model minority myth" (Nadal, 2004). Additionally, previous studies have demonstrated that Filipino Americans may have unique cultural values that are significantly different from those of East Asian Americans (Kim, Yang, Atkinson, Wolfe, & Hong, 2001), that they may experience higher frequencies of racial discrimination than East Asian Americans (Alvarez, Juang, & Liang, 2006), and that they may experience similar types of racial discrimination as Black or Latino populations more than East Asian Americans (Nadal, 2008a; Teranishi, 2002). Moreover, within the Asian American community, Filipinos (and other "Brown Asians") are often viewed as the bottom of the social hierarchy (Cordova, 1983; Okamura, 1998), leading many Filipinos to identify with their ethnic origins instead of with a pan-ethnic Asian American identity (Espiritu, 1992; Nadal, 2009). Additionally, Filipino Americans often align themselves with Hispanics/Latinos and African Americans instead of Asian Americans, because they feel more of a connection due to similar colonial histories, sociocultural experiences, or racial oppression. Because of all of these experiences, Filipino Americans are often considered marginalized minorities and advocate against being included in the model minority classification (Halagao & Nadal, 2009).

Filipino Americans are the second largest Asian American/Pacific Islander population in the United States (Barnes & Bennett, 2002), and are projected to become the largest Asian American population by 2010 (Posadas, 1999). According to the most recent census, there were approximately 2.4 million Filipino Americans living in the United States, with about half of the Filipino American population residing in California. (In fact, in many metropolitan areas in California, Filipino Americans outnumber every other racial/ethnic minority group.) The remainder of Filipino Americans reside in Hawaii (about 9% of the total Filipino American population), New York/New Jersey (about 8.5%), and in the Northwest (about 8.3% in Washington and Oregon). The census also reports that there are approximately 1.37 million Filipino-born immigrants living in the United States, making Filipinos the second largest immigrant population behind Mexicans (U.S. Census Bureau, 2000a).

Filipinos have entered the United States at various points of history, and scholars have connoted that there are four major waves of Filipino immigration into the United States (Posadas, 1999). The first wave of Filipinos included its earliest settlers; while the first Filipinos landed in the United States in Morro Bay, California, in 1587 (via Spanish galleon ships), the first documented Filipino settlement was in 1763 on the Louisiana coast. This group consisted mostly of "Manilamen," who escaped the brutality of Spanish galleon ships and created communities along the bayous, focusing on the shrimping industry. When the United States took over the Philippines in 1899, a second wave immigrated to the United States, consisting mostly of *pensionados*—students who were sponsored by the U.S. government to study in American colleges and universities in the early 1900s (locating mainly in the Midwest or East Coast). The third wave of Filipino immigrants included Filipino laborers and nonsponsored students from the 1910s to 1940s. In Hawaii, these laborers were called *sakadas* and worked in the sugarcane plantations; in California they labored as farmworkers, and in Alaska as fish cannery workers. A number of government laws and acts repealed the further immigration of all Asian groups for several years, eventually leading to a quota of 50 per year, until the Immigration Act of 1965 lifted all previous regulations. As a result, a huge wave of Filipinos immigrated to the United States as educated professionals (e.g., nurses, doctors, and engineers) and continued to settle in various parts of the United States. Today, many types of Filipinos migrate to the United States, with the majority being educated professionals, but also including students or undocumented laborers looking for a better life away from frequently impoverished conditions in the Philippines.

In order to understand Filipino Americans, it becomes important to understand the history and culture of the Philippines. The Philippine Islands, which are located southeast of mainland China and west of the Pacific Islands, consist of over 700 islands and 170 languages (Philippine Census of Population and Housing, 2002). The Philippines has a hybrid culture that has been influenced by several different countries and cultures, through Spanish and American colonization, Japanese occupation, and trade from India, the Middle East, China, Malay, the Pacific Islands, Portugal, and Australia. The most pervasive influences to Filipino culture are likely from the Spanish colonization, which lasted for almost 400 years, which is a similar amount of time that many Latin American countries were colonized by Spain. Accordingly, many Tagalog words (mainly nouns) are similar to Spanish words (i.e., *pantalon* means "pants" in Tagalog, while *pantalones* is the equivalent term in Spanish). Additionally, a year after the Philippines gained independence from Spain, in 1898, the United States then colonized the Philippines (along with Puerto Rico and Cuba), for almost 50 years (Strain, 2003). Accordingly, because of Spanish and U.S. colonization, previous scholars have attested that Filipino Americans share a more similar historical and cultural experience with other Latino ethnic groups with the same colonial history than they do with East Asian groups (Agbayani-Siewert, 2004; Mendoza, 1986; Root, 1997).

Colonialism has also resulted in long-lasting effects on Filipino culture. First, because of American colonization, the Philippines is one of the only Asian countries to have English as one of its national languages (Posadas, 1999). Second, because of Spanish colonization, Filipinos are the only Asian ethnic group to be predominantly Roman Catholic (more than 80%), with an additional 10% being Christian (Agbayani-Siewert & Revilla, 1995). As a result, many Filipinos and Filipino Americans may associate religious identity with ethnic identity, making it difficult to decipher between what is considered Catholic, Filipino, or both (Nadal, 2009). This can be demonstrated through the value of *bahala na* (or fatalism) in the Filipino community, in which many individuals believe that God has control of their fate and health (Ponce & Forman, 1980). Many Filipinos, specifically elders or devout Catholics, may believe that it is best to "leave it in God's hands" when they get sick, instead of seeking proper medical attention.

Colonization has also had an impact on the mental health of Filipinos and Filipino Americans, with some authors citing that many Filipinos and Filipino Americans may develop a "colonial mentality." Colonial mentality has been defined as a form of internalized oppression, in which the colonizer's values and beliefs are accepted by the colonized as a belief and truth of their own (David & Okazaki, 2006; Nadal, 2008b). Filipinos with colonial mentality may glorify both Spanish and Americans values (e.g., lighter skin tone, Spanish cultural traditions, or American education) over indigenous values (e.g., darker skin or indigenous Filipino traditions) (Nadal, 2008b, 2009).

Mental health experiences of Filipino Americans

In recent years, there has been a growing body of literature in the fields of psychology and education that outlines the present-day experiences of Filipino Americans. This may be due to the growing population of Filipino Americans, but is more likely due to the influx of Filipino American scholars entering the fields. In psychology, there are several topics that have shed light on the mental health experiences of Filipino Americans (including Filipino immigrants and second-generation Filipino Americans).

Generational issues

As previously suggested, many Filipinos have felt disconnected to the Asian American community because their sociocultural and educational experiences have been contrary to the model minority myth. While this model minority myth may define Asian Americans as being well educated and successful citizens in the United States (Nadal & Sue, 2008), Filipino Americans have experienced many negative social and educational trends that would separate them from this category. Previous research has found that second-generation Filipino Americans (those born and raised in the United States) encounter a disproportionate incidence of teenage and out-of-wedlock pregnancy, with percentages that are more comparable to African American and Latino groups than to other East Asian American populations (National Center for Health Statistics, 2000; Tiongson, 1997). Filipino Americans also have the highest rates of HIV/AIDS infections out of all Asian American/Pacific Islander groups, with AIDS being the leading cause of death for Filipino American males ages 25–34 in the state of California (San Francisco Department of Public Health, 1992). Lastly, studies have shown that Filipino Americans have the highest incidence of suicidal ideations of all Asian Americans (Asian Americans and Pacific Islanders, 2001).

In terms of education, studies have shown that there is a high percentage of both Filipino men and women that possess a bachelor's degree or higher in the United States (Okamura & Agbayani, 1997). At first glance, it may appear that Filipinos are doing very well; however, there are two very important issues that this statistic may disguise: (1) the majority of these individuals received their degrees in the

Philippines before immigrating to the United States (and therefore it does not take into account the number of second-generation Filipino Americans without college degrees), and (2) Filipino Americans do not receive the same levels of income and are often at a lower occupational status than other groups of similar educational qualifications (Okamura & Agbayani, 1997). Additionally, even with college-educated immigrant parents, research has shown that an unexpectedly high number of second-generation Filipino American students are high school dropouts (Alegado, 1987; Okamura & Agbayani, 1997), and that second-generation Filipino Americans have achieved lower rates of college admission and retention than East Asian Americans (Okamura, 1998). The 1990 census revealed that 22% of second-generation Filipino Americans completed a college degree, in comparison to 51% of Chinese Americans (U.S. Census Bureau, 1994). So while Filipino American families may be educated and have above-average household incomes, their experiences are dissimilar to the model minority and more similar to those of oppressed minority groups like Black/African Americans and Latinos (Nadal, 2008a).

Experiences with race and acculturation

Many authors have cited that experiences with race and acculturation perhaps have contributed to negative experiences for Filipino Americans (see Nadal, 2008a, for a review). First, it is important to notice that Filipinos and Filipino Americans are one of the only ethnic groups that have been placed into several racial and ethnic categories at once (Nadal, 2004). According to the U.S. Census 2000, Filipino Americans are currently classified as "Asian American" (Barnes & Bennett, 2002). However, according to the U.S. Department of Education, Filipino Americans are categorized as "Pacific Islanders" (Horn, 1995), while some have classified Filipino Americans as "Hispanic" due to the Spanish colonization of the Philippines (Trevino, 1987). Moreover, California Senate Bill 1813, which was passed in 1988, now requires all California state personnel surveys or statistical tabulations to classify persons of Filipino ancestry as "Filipino" rather than as Asian, Pacific Islander, or Hispanic (Espiritu, 1992). Additionally, several authors have cited that Filipinos have often been mistaken for members of other racial/ethnic groups, including Latino, Pacific Islander, Arab, Asian, or multiracial (Nadal, 2009; Rumbaut, 1995; Uba, 1994). This experience in which Filipinos are placed into several different categories can lead to identity confusion, stress, or any number of negative mental health outcomes (e.g., Nadal, 2008a; Teranishi, 2002).

There have been numerous studies that conclude that racial discrimination (either subtle or blatant) may lead to various levels of stress for Filipino Americans. One quantitative study ($n = 402$) examined how racial microaggressions (or subtle statements or behaviors that send denigrating messages to people of color) may impact Filipino Americans differently than Chinese Americans. Results included that Filipino Americans may experience racial microaggressions related to (1) being treated as an intellectual inferior or (2) being assumed to be a criminal (Nadal, 2008a). Implications for this study support that Filipino Americans may experience race-related stress that may be different than that of East Asian Americans and more similar to that of Latinos or Black/African Americans. One qualitative study examining both Filipino and Chinese American high school students in California yielded similar results. Using interviews, it was reported that Filipino Americans experienced negative encounters with their teachers, in which they felt unsupported in their everyday school experiences and in achieving higher education, while the Chinese American students reported the contrary (Teranishi, 2002). The Filipino American students affirmed that their teachers and counselors often treated them as "gang members" or "academically unqualified," and perceived that their counselors and teachers encouraged them to attend vocational school or community college due to assumptions about their family obligations or financial situations. This study further supports the aforementioned notion that Filipino Americans may be treated differently from their East Asian American counterparts and should be considered "marginalized minorities" instead of model minorities.

There have been a number of studies that support the relationship between acculturation and stress for Asian Americans. However, most of these studies fail to disaggregate between Asian subgroups, and there are no known studies that concentrate specifically on acculturation experiences for Filipino Americans. Concurrently, because of American colonization, acculturation may take a different form than it would for other Asian American groups. For example, because English is one of the two national languages of the Philippines, Philippine school systems teach English to all of their students and Filipino immigrants speak English at more proficient rates than other Asian Americans. Additionally, because of colonial mentality, many Filipino Americans may view being acculturated as a positive aspect, and therefore may prefer to be "more American" than Filipino. These experiences with acculturation and colonial mentality may result in myriad outcomes, including Filipinos trusting in and being receptive to Whites, Filipinos preferring to have tests and assessments conducted in English, and Filipinos wanting to speak to medical and mental health professionals in English (although they may not fully understand American nuances).

Mental health experiences of Filipino Americans

Although most studies on mental health generalize Asian Americans as a group, there have been a few studies that specifically examine depression and stress for Filipino Americans. One study supports that Filipino Americans have higher incidents of depression than the general population (Tompar-Tiu & Sustento-Seneriches, 1995). Another study found that Filipino Americans may possess lower levels of self-esteem and higher depression scores than other ethnic groups in the sample (Rumbaut, 2005). Another study revealed that Filipino Americans were diagnosed with schizophrenia at higher rates than other Asian American groups, but because there have not been any other studies on the subject, it is difficult to generalize (Dela Cruz, McBride, Compas, Calixto, & Derveer, 2002). Other psychological disorders that may be prevalent (and known) in the Filipino American community become hidden, misunderstood, or unknown, due to cultural shame, lack of knowledge, and lack of research on specific mental health issues for Filipino Americans (Nadal, 2004).

Despite this limited knowledge on depression and other psychological disorders for Filipino Americans, there has been a growing body of literature on Filipino Americans and alcohol use. In one quantitative self-report study (n = 3712), it was discovered that while Filipino Americans were the largest abstainers from alcohol, that out of those individuals that did drink, Filipinos drank for pathological reasons significantly more than any other group in the sample (Johnson, Schwitters, Wilson, Nagoshi, & McClearn, 1985). This study matches previous literature (see Nadal, 2000 for a review), which maintains that alcohol is culturally embedded in Filipino family systems and that alcohol often replaces communication or grieving (specifically for Filipino men).

A later analysis of the aforementioned data revealed that alcohol use was lower among international-born Filipinos than those born in the United States; additionally, Filipinos born and raised in Hawaii specifically had higher incidents of drinking than those in the continental United States (Johnson, Nagoshi, Ahern, Wilson, & Yuen, 1987). Implications from these two analyses illustrate three major points: (1) Filipino Americans may turn to alcohol as a coping mechanism, (2) Filipino Americans born and raised in the United States may experience specific stressors that may influence their drinking more than those that are international born, and (3) Filipinos in Hawaii may drink more than both international-born and mainland-born Filipino Americans. Given these findings, it becomes important for psychologists to recognize that Filipino Americans may often rely on alcohol instead of seeking help for their mental health problems.

Help-seeking behaviors and experiences in counseling

Some authors have maintained that there are several factors that may contribute to the underutilization of mental health care services for Filipino Americans, citing that "saving face" or the stigma of mental health may decrease the help-seeking behaviors for the group (Sanchez & Gaw, 2007). These scholars conclude that there may be myriad other factors that influence the perceptions of mental health and illness, specific to Filipinos, including religion, family, support systems, coping styles, and indigenous culture-bound traits. Other researchers have cited that the interaction of "face" and language may influence how Filipino Americans perceive and interact with mental health care systems, citing that Filipino Americans will interact mostly with laypersons instead of other forms of mental health professionals, like specialists, general practitioners, or folk systems (Gong, Gage, & Tacata, 2003). So while individuals may have some form of support, they may be more resistant to traditional forms of mental health services. One study supported that religion may be a factor for help seeking for Filipino Americans, namely, that those who are religious (or subscribe specifically to Catholicism/Christianity) may be more likely to seek help from religious clergy, while those who were highly spiritual (but not necessarily religious) would be more likely to seek help from mental health professionals (Abe-Kim, Gong, & Takeuchi, 2004). This finding may speak to the issue of acculturation; for those who are more traditional, it may be easier for them to turn to religion as a coping mechanism, while those who are less traditional are more open to seeking (and aware of) mental health services.

As a result of these findings, there are several authors who propose different types of treatment methods in order to be most effective with Filipino Americans. Okamura and Agbayani (1991) recommend that counselors be more personable with Filipino American clients, because of the Filipino value of emotional closeness and social acceptance, countering previous research with East Asian Americans that support that individuals may prefer a more directive approach. Enriquez (1982) suggests that therapists be indirect with their counseling, utilizing an "asking around" approach using informal and nonjudgmental inquiries. This supports the value of indirect communication in Filipino families and communities, in which individuals are likely to keep family secrets and refuse to discuss anything shameful or distressing to the family. Finally, Sanchez and Gaw (2007) recommend a structured, culturally sensitive, comprehensive approach utilizing a variety of techniques that address both the individual and the cultural context of the Filipino American client.

Review of neuropsychological research on Filipino Americans

Despite being the second largest Asian American group in the United States, there has been minimal neuropsychological research conducted on Filipinos and Filipino Americans. One author has noted that there have been numerous challenges in practicing clinical neuropsychology in the Philippines, as a result of culturally inappropriate tools in a multilingual country, with limited education and low socioeconomic backgrounds (Ledesma, 2002). Filipino Americans' experiences in clinical neuropsychology have been obscured, as Filipino Americans are often subsumed into the greater Asian American population. With little focus on the differences or distinct needs of the Filipino American community, many authors have described Filipino Americans as the "invisible ethnic group" (Sanchez & Gaw, 2007) or "forgotten Asian Americans" (Cordova, 1983). The limited research conducted specifically with the Filipino community has found significant behavioral trends and specific health issues that may lead to increased vulnerability to neuropsychological impairment or dysfunction. This next section will cite various mental health problems within the Filipino American community and elucidate implications for the field of neuropsychology.

Some authors have noted that drug use has been increasing in the Filipino American community. For instance, there has been a noticeable popularity of methamphetamine use within the Filipino and Filipino American community (LaVilla, 1998) and a greater tendency for Filipinos to engage in high-risk sexual behaviors while using drugs than for other Asian ethnic groups (Nemoto et al., 1999, 2000). One study found that Filipino American methamphetamine users are at high risk for HIV/STD infection (Nemoto, Operario, & Soma, 2002), while another study revealed that Filipino American adolescents have more cases of HIV infection than other Asian-Pacific Islander adolescent groups (Chung et al., 2007). While Asian Americans are typically viewed as model minorities who do not engage in criminal or risky behaviors, these studies indicate that Filipino Americans may be engaging in many life-threatening behaviors, including illicit drug use and unprotected sex. All of these studies suggest a potentially elevated risk for HIV-related neuropsychological impairment or HIV-associated dementia within the Filipino American community.

Additionally, previous research demonstrates that within the Filipino American community there is a high prevalence of coronary heart disease (Gerber, 1980), hypertension (Klatsky & Armstrong, 1991), and subarachnoid hemorrhaging (Klatsky et al., 2005)—all factors associated with stroke and vascular dementia. It has also been suggested that Filipinos underutilize Alzheimer's disease services since they constitute less than 1% (0.8%) of cases seen at the California Alzheimer's Disease Diagnostic and Treatment Centers (Chow, Ross, Fox, Cummings, & Lin, 2000), though they represent approximately 6% of residents in major Californian cities. For example, if 5.2% of San Francisco residents and 6.1% of San Diego residents are Filipino American (U.S. Census Bureau, 2000b), it seems unlikely that only less than 1% of the population would develop Alzheimer's disease. This underrepresentation of Filipino Americans may indicate the community's lack of knowledge of available services, or a lack of awareness of the disease in general. But more importantly, it suggests that a percentage of Filipino Americans are underdiagnosed for Alzheimer's-related dementia.

There has been limited literature on the prevalence of learning disabilities (LDs) in the Filipino American community. Previous authors have cited that Asian Americans are diagnosed with LDs at significantly lower rates than Blacks and Latinos (see McCray & Garcia, 2002, for a review). However, the few studies that focus on Asian Americans and LDs (e.g., Fatimilehin & Nadirshaw, 1994; Poon-McBrayer & Garcia, 2000) fail to account for ethnic group differences within the Asian American group or concentrate on Asian ethnic groups (e.g., Chinese, Koreans, Indians) other than Filipino Americans. Given the differences in experiences due to colonization and other sociocultural factors, it would be important to understand how LDs specifically impact Filipino American clients. However, because one study revealed that Asian Americans had similar experiences of LDs as Mexican Americans (Poon-McBrayer & Garcia, 2000), perhaps culture as a general construct influences LDs for immigrant ethnic groups, more than membership in any particular ethnic group.

Previous authors have maintained that there are very few studies concentrating on autism in the Filipino American community or with Asian Americans in general (Won, Krajicek, & Lee, 2004). However, the lack of documented study should not imply that autism does not occur for Filipino Americans; rather, it should indicate that autism is being underreported for a variety of reasons. For example, there are over 500,000 families affected with autism in the Philippines; however, many cases are undocumented because of poverty (inability to seek help or health care), ignorance (lack of awareness of the disorder), or indifference by family members (Autism Society of the Philippines, 2007). Additionally, many Filipino families may find it shameful or stigmatizing to have a child with a disability (both physical and mental), resulting in the autism of many Filipino children and adults remaining hidden (Autism Society of the Philippines, 2007). Stigma may also lead to underreporting of autism for Filipino Americans in the United States, specifically since Filipinos immigrate to the United States in search of the American Dream; accordingly, when a child has autism in an immigrant family, an extra burden of shame may exist.

Although the literature review on Filipino Americans and neuropsychological issues may be scarce, these studies point to a potentially high risk of cognitive impairment within the Filipino American community (i.e., HIV-associated dementia, vascular dementia, or Alzheimer's-related cognitive dysfunction) that has yet to be addressed or studied. Moreover, it is important to recognize that because of the unique historical and sociocultural experiences of Filipino Americans, further research needs to be conducted on Filipinos as a specific ethnic group, and that generalizations cannot be extrapolated from other Asian American populations or racial/ethnic minorities in general. With the limited number of Filipino American psychologists in the United States and the absence of normative test data for Filipinos and Filipino Americans, the need becomes clear for culturally sensitive assessment practices, testing considerations, and treatment strategies geared toward the specific needs of this fast-growing community.

Testing issues and Filipino Americans

Because of the heterogeneity of the Filipino American population, it is of critical importance to develop an understanding of the Filipino American client's specific cultural and educational background in order to provide an accurate context for test score interpretation. Also of import for adequate assessment of Filipino Americans is an awareness of specific cultural issues that could potentially affect testing, and determining whether or not these issues are relevant to a particular client. The following are issues to carefully consider when assessing Filipino Americans.

Norms and neuropsychology

There has been a dearth of research involving psychological assessments and Filipinos or Filipino Americans. Of these studies, several have focused on the performance of various Filipino samples on intelligence and achievement tests as compared to other (ethnic) groups. For example, Brandon, Newton, and Hammond (1987) conducted a study of Hawaiian grade school students (grades 4, 6, 8, and 10) of Caucasian, Japanese, Hawaiian, and Filipino descent, comparing the students' abilities on math achievement tests. They found that Filipino girls outperformed Filipino boys overall on various mathematics subtests, a pattern found within the other three ethnic Hawaiian groups as well. Other researchers investigating the discrepancies between WISC-R verbal IQ and performance IQ scores within a sample of 4.546 gifted students (from grades 1 to 9) found that Filipino students demonstrated equal verbal IQ and performance IQ scores, whereas the other ethnic groups (African American, Hispanic, and Caucasian) exhibited higher verbal IQ than performance IQ scores (Saccuzzo, Johnson, & Russell, 1992). Another study compared the performance of Filipino (in Manila) and Canadian students (from grades 6 to 8) on a series of cognitive tests, and found a greater disparity in performance for Filipino students than for Canadian students (Flores & Evans, 1972). Similarly, past research has found that as a whole, Filipino American immigrants residing in the United States prior to 1971 were assessed as having lower IQs than White American individuals (Filipino IQ of 85.8 compared to 100 IQ for Whites), though Filipinos exceeded Whites in terms of high-status occupations (e.g., 29.3% of Filipinos held managerial, professional, and technical posts in 1980 compared to 27.0% of Whites; Flynn, 1991). This last finding suggests that intelligence tests utilized at that time may not have adequately captured the true intellectual capabilities of Filipino Americans, or that Filipino Americans utilize other strengths (i.e., strong work ethic, sociability, etc.) to successfully acquire high-level occupations. Taken together, these study findings that included Filipino and Filipino Americans are questionable, given the heterogeneity of the Filipino and Filipino American experience. Further research is necessary to determine the generalizability, validity, and fairness of psychological assessment with various Filipino American populations.

Because many of the tests, screenings, and assessments currently employed in the United States fail to account for cultural differences with Filipinos, some authors have started to develop their own scales with Filipino populations. For example, some psychologists have created culturally appropriate screening tools for Filipino children with learning disabilities (Ledesma, 2002), screening scales for illiterate Filipino adults with dementia (Ledesma, 2002), or even personality assessments using Tagalog words and cultural nuances of personality (Church, Katigbak, & Reyes, 1998). Additionally, while some psychological assessments offer Tagalog versions of their measures (i.e., MMPI), there have not been known studies in which these language-specific tests have been normalized on Filipino or Filipino American populations.

English fluency and education

Unlike other Asian groups, Filipinos generally have adequate to superior command of the English language. In the 2000 census, almost half of U.S. Filipinos age 5 or older reported speaking English "very well," and 29.3% reportedly spoke primarily English at home (U.S. Census Bureau, 2000b); however, this can be misleading, because almost a quarter of Filipino Americans (24.1%) endorsed less than adequate English-speaking abilities (U.S. Census Bureau, 2000b). This varying level of English fluency reflects the diversity in educational experiences within the Filipino American community. For those educated primarily in the United States, English is their first and primary language. For others schooled in the Philippines, English comprehension and speaking ability may have been attained (as English is claimed as the second national language in the Philippines and is an integral part of the country's educational curriculum); however, actual proficiency level varies depending on the type of education received, and therefore is a critical factor to establish for assessment and test interpretation purposes.

For Filipino immigrants in particular, place of education is important to consider during assessment, since regionalism plays a central role in the quality of education provided by Philippine schools. Though primary-school enrollment rates are high overall, completion rates significantly differ between urban and rural areas. For instance, in the capital city of Manila, close to 100% of students completed primary schooling, while completion rates in the provinces of Mindanao or Eastern Visaya were only at 30% (Clark, 2004). This contrast illustrates the significant regional difference in the quality of education that may be present in Philippine schools, which in turn affects the level of English proficiency attained by those educated under the Philippines' system.

Additionally, the amount of education completed is another important factor to consider when working with Filipino and Filipino American clients. For those educated in the Philippines—whose school system is one of the shortest in the world, amounting to a total of just ten years of formal schooling (Clark, 2004)—English fluency will depend on the number of years of schooling finished. For example, during the first few years of school in the Philippines, most classes are taught in the local dialect, rather than in English or Tagalog (the national languages). In contrast, from grade 3 onward, English instruction becomes more prevalent (Clark, 2004). Hence, English exposure and fluency are associated with the level of education obtained. Therefore, when evaluating clients' language proficiency and educational abilities, both the amount and type of schooling should be inquired into and considered. Extra attention should be given to these issues when assessing older Filipino clients (who are most likely educated in the Philippines), and more extensive background information is necessary to acquire a clearer understanding of their educational experiences and English-speaking abilities. Although many Filipino and Filipino Americans may appear to adequately speak English (and might even prefer to speak English to practitioners to prove their abilities), some individuals may misunderstand American nuances, which can result in miscommunication in therapy or less reliability in testing. For those with limited English-speaking abilities, use of a translator may be necessary to communicate, as well as for testing purposes. Detailed guidelines for assessment of the non-English-speaking Asian American client are discussed thoroughly in Wong and Fujii (2004).

Acculturation

Though there is no empirical study of the effects of acculturation on neuropsychological test performance with Filipinos Americans (or Asian Americans in general), one study of African American adults has revealed that acculturation accounted for a significant amount of the variance in neuropsychological test performance (Manly et al., 1998). A recent study of an ethnically diverse nonclinical adult sample (including African American, Hispanic, Asian, and non-Hispanic White individuals) found significant differences in test performance between primary English speakers and English as a Second Language (ESL) speakers, as well as significant associations between cognitive test ability and number of years of U.S. education, age at which conversational English was learned, and number of years residing in the United States (Boone, Victor, Wen, Razani, & Ponton, 2007). Based on these findings and others, it is important to consider Filipino or Filipino American clients' acculturation level during testing and test interpretation, and the potential effects of these (socio)cultural variables on test performance. With Filipino Americans in particular, and perhaps ethnic minority individuals in general, there is still a possibility of a client with low acculturation levels despite having lived many years in the United States. Since there are several Filipino ethnic enclaves in the United States (e.g., San

Francisco, San Diego, Jersey City, NJ, or Queens, NY), it is possible for a Filipino immigrant to reject Western mores, habits and beliefs, and remain a monolingual non-English speaker.

Communication styles and other cultural variables

Filipino culture is a hybrid of various traditions, practices, and beliefs, particularly Malaysian, Spanish, and American cultural influences (Wong & Fujii, 2004). Filipino Americans share certain cultural modes of thinking that may influence their receptivity to or comfort with neuropsychological testing and psychological assessment in general. Among the influences of Spanish tradition are Catholicism, relationship hierarchies, and a strong deference to authority (Ponce & Forman, 1980). These beliefs and practices are important to keep in mind when working with Filipino American clients for their potential effects within the testing environment. For instance, as aforementioned, Filipinos typically have a strong belief in *bahala na*, or fatalism. This mode of thinking, attributed to the strong influence of Catholic tradition, not only contributes to a lack of incentive to help one's self, but may also run counter to proactive thinking and one's drive for advancement (Sanchez & Gaw, 2007). During an assessment, the *bahala na* attitude may negatively affect the Filipino American client's effort or motivation to do well in testing. If a client perceives that his or her situation is hopeless and "out of his or her hands," for example, the client may not fully invest in the assessment and may put forth less than adequate effort on administered tests.

Another common Filipino trait influenced by Spanish culture is *pakikisama*, or avoidance of offending or openly disagreeing with others (Ponce & Forman, 1980). This highly valued ideal, borne out of deference to authority and Catholic tradition, involves Filipino Americans communicating agreement with others, despite contrary feelings, and deferring to those in positions of authority because it is the polite thing to do. Also, either out of respect for authority figures or in order to "save face" and avoid *hiya* (shame or embarrassment), Filipino Americans may avoid questioning authority or asking for clarification despite not being able to fully understand what is being told them (Sanchez & Gaw, 2007). These tendencies are important to keep in mind when assessing a Filipino American client, especially with regard to their understanding of test instructions and verbal communications in general.

Filipinos also exhibit cultural characteristics in common with other Asian ethnic groups. For example, Filipinos are collectivists (Sanchez & Gaw, 2007), often placing the needs of the family or others above one's own personal desires. Decision making is often a family affair, and though Western/European American culture may value individualism, especially when an individual becomes an adult, Filipino Americans at any age may still collectively turn to their families for assistance and guidance. Also similar to other Asian groups, Filipinos and Filipino Americans maintain a strong sense of filial piety. As part of their filial obligations, Filipinos and Filipino Americans are expected to defer to the opinions and decisions of elder family members or parents. As a result, Filipino Americans may especially struggle with decisions that counter their family's beliefs or expectations.

Filipinos also frequently display a fragile sense of self-worth, or *amor propio*. Generally, Filipinos are proud individuals, and are extremely sensitive about criticism or negative comments. Also, Filipinos and Filipino Americans value *utang ng loob* (or debt of reciprocity). This belief—that one must help another as payment for past favors—manifests as Filipinos turning to each other for unconditional support and free-of-charge consultation. Thus, Filipinos tend to seek advice from nonimmediate family members regarding personal concerns, based on the individual's career and personal specialties. For instance, Filipinos and Filipino Americans involved in legal proceedings may seek the opinion of a distant cousin who is employed as a paralegal. Or, a nonimmediate family member who is a nurse or phlebotomist may be consulted on medical issues. These individuals are often appointed as a "spokesperson" for the family, and are involved in disseminating and acquiring information on the family's behalf. The spokesperson role can be designated to someone with the most education, the person who is oldest or has the most seniority, or even to someone who is perceived as the most rational, least emotional, and most capable of managing the situation.

With these cultural considerations in mind, neuropsychologists should take several approaches when working with Filipino and Filipino American clients. Wong and Fujii (2004) recommend that the clinician assume the "expert" role when working with this population, as it complements the Filipino deference to authority. More specifically, taking on the role of "medical expert" and emphasizing the medical benefits of neuropsychological assessment may increase the client's understanding of and motivation toward testing, since Filipino Americans may be more comfortable discussing medical issues but are less familiar with psychological or cognitive disabilities. Psychoeducation about neuropsychology in general may also prove to be beneficial.

When communicating with the Filipino American client, it is helpful to take an active role in clarifying his or her understanding of verbal statements and test instructions. Avoid asking simple yes/no questions to assess his or her understanding since Filipino Americans may automatically agree with the clinician due to *pakikisama*, or out of respect for authority figures. Instead, have the client explain in his or her own words, or choose from a list of options to show that he or she understands what was presented. Additionally, offering the client choices may also help to elicit his or her true opinions and desires (Wong & Fujii, 2004). These communicative strategies are particularly important with this population, who may not spontaneously self-report concerns, emotions, or symptoms, but rather may require active questioning or prompting to disclose. For example, the Filipino client may not ask for breaks during the testing process even though he or she is fatigued, but would welcome the opportunity to take a break if so invited.

When gathering information about the client's personal and cultural background, it is especially useful to invite family members or other trusted individuals (or spokespersons) present at the assessment to participate in the clinical interview. Not only will having a trusted person present in the room be helpful in reducing any anxieties the client may have about the testing situation, but it also allows these individuals access to the client's self-report, which they can later clarify or confirm with the clinician.

Where possible, additional collateral reports concerning the client's premorbid and current cognitive functioning should also be obtained from these individuals.

Finally, when providing feedback to Filipino or Filipino American clients, it is important to keep in mind *amor propio,* or their fragile sense of self-worth. Since Filipinos are especially vulnerable to perceived criticism and negative remarks, test results should be disseminated sensitively in order to avoid offense and maintain rapport. When formulating recommendations for these clients, consider the cultural dynamics of Filipino family systems—which may require a different approach from that utilized with other clients.

Case examples

Case example 1

Ian is a 25-year-old second-generation Filipino American male, who works as an accountant for a large corporation. His parents immigrated to the United States over 30 years ago, and they have lived in a large Filipino community for most of his life. He graduated from college three years ago, and is currently single and living with his parents. Lately, Ian has been noticing some difficulty in being able to concentrate and finds himself making small mistakes in his work projects. Accordingly, he ends up staying up late while working on projects at night and starts to get very frustrated. He has trouble falling asleep at night and eventually starts to feel throbbing headaches every time he goes to work. He starts to take over-the-counter medication to help with the headaches, but the pain persists. He makes an appointment with Dr. Brink, his White American primary care physician (PCP), and after several medical tests, it is determined that he is not exhibiting physical symptoms of any medical ailments. Dr. Brink refers to him to a neuropsychologist for testing.

Ian has an immediate reaction to the testing and the word *psychologist*, telling the doctor, "I'm not crazy. Can't you just give me medication that will stop the pain?" However, after the doctor explains that there might be some psychological issues and gives further details about what a neuropsychologist does, Ian reluctantly agrees to contact the neuropsychologist. That night, Ian speaks with several of his family members (his parents, his siblings, and his cousins) to discuss his trepidations. He even calls some distant relatives in the medical field (whom he hasn't spoken to in years) in an attempt to gather opinions and advice about what else his PCP could be missing. They comfort him, tell him they will pray for him, and encourage him to meet with the neuropsychologist as soon as possible.

Ian was extremely anxious and scared as he met with the neuropsychologist. Four tests were administered: the WAIS-III, the MMPI-2, the Rorschach inkblot test, and the Thematic Apperception Test (TAT), as well as two measures of current depressed and anxious mood—the Beck Depression Inventory–II (BDI-II) and Beck Anxiety Inventory (BAI). Results from the WAIS-III indicate that Ian had an above-average intelligence (full-scale IQ = 115); however, in reviewing his performance subtests, it was noticed that his processing speed negatively impacted his performance IQ score. Results from the MMPI-2 do not indicate any significant scores on any of the clinical subscales (with the exception of a high score on hypochondriasis); however, validity scales suggest that Ian may have a tendency to minimize current emotional problems by portraying himself in a positive light. Scores from the BDI-II and BAI reveal no significant mood disturbances (i.e., both scores were 0). Finally, results from two projective tests (Rorschach inkblot test and Thematic Apperception Test) yield limited answers, in which Ian did not speak or elaborate on his reactions to any of the cards.

Case example 2

Pamela is an eight-year-old Filipina American girl. Her parents are both nurses who were born and raised in the Philippines, met and got married in Cebu, and immigrated to the United States right before Pamela was born. Ms. Jacobson, Pamela's White American third-grade teacher, noticed that Pamela had difficulty reading and learning at the same rates as her classmates; she consulted with the school psychologist, suspecting that Pamela may have some form of learning disability. During a parent-teacher conference, Ms. Jacobson informed Pamela's parents of her concern and they reacted in several ways. First, they didn't initially understand Ms. Jacobson, so they continued to ask her an array of questions to make sure they fully understood the information she presented. Second, they blamed themselves as parents, questioning whether they may have done something wrong in their parenting. Finally, they started to pray to God, believing that prayer would help the situation, but at the same time imagining that God was punishing them and their family for something.

After the meeting, Pamela's parents consulted many family members, including an uncle who is a psychiatrist (and was educated in the Philippines) as well as an American-born cousin with a master's degree in education. They also remained in good contact with the Filipino priest from their local church (who is close to their extended family) and have asked their entire church to pray for their family (without disclosing the situation). Finally, Pamela's parents agree to meet with a neuropsychologist; however, they said they would only feel comfortable if they were able to bring other family members to the appointment.

Pamela was administered a Wechsler Intelligence Scale for Children–IV (WISC-IV), Wechsler Individual Achievement Test (WIAT), and Children's Memory Test (CMT). Results indicated a full-scale IQ of 95, a verbal IQ of 85, and a performance IQ of 105. Her WIAT reading score was at the first-grade level, while her math was at the third-grade level. On memory testing, Pamela scored in the low average range for verbal memory and auditory working memory, and in the high average range for visual memory. Test results were consistent with a reading disorder.

Case example 3

Miguela is an 80-year-old, widowed Filipina immigrant. She was born and raised in the Philippines, living most of her life in Lucena, a rural area in Luzon, until moving to the United States to live with her son 15 years ago. As a child, she was educated in a public school in Lucena, and only completed four years of education. She reported having difficulties in school, and eventually decided to discontinue her studies to work as a cook at a local *turo-turo* (fast-cooked roadside eatery). Since arriving in the United States, she has been employed as a nanny for a Filipino family, and is responsible for the care of two young children, ages 7 and 3. Her English-speaking skills have improved over the years, though her fluency remains below average. However, her lack of English fluency has not been problematic since she rarely communicates or interacts with non-Filipinos.

Over the last three months, relatives have noticed that Lola Miguela (as she is often called) has been quite forgetful and becomes easily confused. Both her immediate and employer families have reported that she has recently been leaving the stove on unattended and has been burning the food she prepares for the children—both attributed to her forgetfulness when cooking. Additionally, she becomes easily confused about whether or not she has eaten, or forgets at what time she is to pick up the older child from the school bus stop. She recently was seen for an annual physical examination, accompanied by her son, who informed her primary care physician about the changes in Lola Miguela's memory abilities. Her physician ordered a full neurological workup and referred Lola Miguela for neuropsychological testing.

Lola Miguela arrived at the office of Dr. Hall, an African American neuropsychologist; she was accompanied by her son, daughter-in-law, and close family friend, Janet, who is a nurse. When asked to enter the testing office, the entire party rose and followed Lola Miguela into the office. After introductions were made, Janet immediately began asking questions about the purpose of and necessity for the day's testing. Having educated herself on Filipino culture, Dr. Hall knew to address the concerns of the family through the spokesperson, and to provide medically focused psychoeducation to address their concerns. Once Dr. Hall explained the nature of neuropsychological assessment and provided a brief explanation of brain–behavior relationships, she offered the client and her family a short break to discuss the new information provided. After a few minutes, the neuropsychologist reunited with the group, who appeared calmer and much more relaxed, and Janet declared that Lola Miguela was ready to begin testing.

During the clinical interview, Lola Miguela had difficulty comprehending questions and would simply stare blankly at the clinician. In order to adequately communicate with Lola Miguela, Dr. Hall asked Janet to act as interpreter, obtaining Lola Miguela's background information (including extensive details about her school, the quality of education provided, and her exposure to and comfort level with English). When Lola Miguela was unsure of how to respond, her son often chimed in and provided additional information about his mother's background and clinical history.

After the clinical interview, Dr. Hall opted to administer the Mini-Mental Status Exam to gain a sense of Lola Miguela's global functioning. She scored 15/30, having difficulties with naming "town," completing serial 7s, recalling three objects, and following commands. After the family left the office, Dr. Hall realized that Lola Miguela would greatly benefit from an assessment with a Tagalog-speaking neuropsychologist who had experience working with Filipino immigrant individuals. She consulted with a Filipino American colleague and shared that perhaps Lola Miguela's difficulty with commands was attributed to fluency issues, but that she was concerned about her other difficulties with orientation, naming, attention, and memory. The colleague asked about her premorbid functioning—specifically her previous math abilities and understanding of the concept of "town." Dr. Hall admitted to failing to ask specifically about her premorbid abilities. Moreover, when asked if she was confident that Lola Miguela understood the test instructions, Dr. Hall said that she assumed her client understood, but she did not probe her further to ensure she really did.

Dr. Hall referred Lola Miguela to Dr. Rocha, a Filipino neuropsychologist. Dr. Rocha learned that Lola Miguela had limited math and spelling abilities due to her low-level education. He screened for depression based upon *Diagnostic and Statistical Manual of Mental Disorders*, fourth edition, text revision (DSM-IV-TR) criteria for major depressive disorder. Lola Miguela did not meet criteria for a depression, with her son only endorsing the items of diminished ability to think or concentrate. The MMSE was readministered in Tagalog while leaving out the attentional items requiring serial subtractions and instead asked her to spell "Luzon" backwards. Lola Miguela earned a score of 17/30, which when corrected for her level of education fell within the range for mild dementia. Lola Miguela was also administered the Clinical Dementia Rating (CDR), a multidimensional dementia staging scale based upon behavioral observation. Based upon her son's rating, Lola Miguela again scored in the mild dementia range.

Discussion of case examples

Through these three cases, we notice that the culture and experiences of being Filipino American may impact the mental health of these three individuals (and their families) in myriad ways. In all three cases, we notice the significance of family. It was important for Ian, an independent 25-year-old adult, to still seek advice from his family members about his situation and to potentially help in his decision-making process. In contrast to the individualist ideals of Western/European culture, Filipino Americans at adult ages may still collectively turn to their families for assistance. In all cases, family members in the medical field were consulted for advice. Because Filipinos and Filipino Americans are the second largest immigrant group who work as medical doctors (American Medical Association, 2007) and first largest immigrant group who work as nurses (Brush, Sochalski, & Berger, 2004) in the United States, and because of the value of *utang ng loob* (or debt of reciprocity), Filipinos turn to each other for unconditional support and free-of-charge consultation based on individuals' career and personal specialties. In the case of Pamela and Lola Miguela, it can be observed that the families wanted to invite family members who they view as experts to meet the neuropsychologist, so that they might obtain the best care available. The two case studies illustrate the importance of enlisting a member of the family to take the lead in decision making, communicating, and information disseminating.

The influence of religion has an impact on how both Ian and Pamela and their families cope with challenging situations. For Western/American cultures, prayer is often viewed as impractical because it is not scientifically based. However, for Filipino Americans who practice Catholicism or Christianity, prayer can be used as a coping mechanism, oftentimes as a way to manage stress, grief, or loss. In Pamela's situation, it appears that religion may play an even greater role, in that the family consulted with a priest and asked for public prayers at the church. While the family may not disclose the exact situation to the community (since doing so may be shameful), asking for support would be a powerful way to influence the situation. Also, the reaction of Pamela's parents reflect one that many Filipinos might experience: To believe that disease or mental disorders are punishments from God might be manifestations of Catholic guilt. As a result, many devout Catholics will attend church regularly and abide by all of the church laws as a way of deflecting any retribution from God. Finally, as aforementioned, many Filipino and Filipino Americans may also believe in *bahala na* (or fatalism). Simply stated, individuals may view disease or mental disorders as "how God intended." When Filipino Americans are diagnosed with various medical or mental disorders, many may stop fighting back or seeking treatment because they assume that their destinies are "in God's hands."

The issue of gender may play a salient role in conceptualizing the case of Ian. Because of Spanish colonization, many Filipino men have learned to value *machismo* or the strict gender role of males acting masculine and emotionally strong. Ian would not want to see any type of psychologist, because doing so might be a sign of weakness or failure—two qualities that would be looked down on in men. Gender might also affect some of his scores on certain tests; for example, it is possible that Ian did not score high on the Depression subscale of the MMPI-2 because he did not self-report depressive symptoms (which would be a sign of vulnerability). His denial of symptoms related to depressed mood (BDI-II score = 0) and tendency to minimize emotional distress (as suggested on the MMPI-2 validity scales) may also be attributed to his adherence to strict gender roles. Concurrently, while the MMPI-2 demonstrates that Ian may score high on the Hypochondriasis subscale, one might take into consideration how physical manifestations might be more culture based and may be coping mechanisms to dealing with psychological and emotional problems.

Generational issues may also be a salient factor in the case of Pamela and Ian. In Pamela's case, the recent immigration of her parents might impact their reaction to the situation. Immigrants with more traditional Filipino and Catholic values might operate in a different manner than acculturated second-generation Filipino Americans. Because previous studies have indicated that acculturation positively impacts help-seeking behavior with both Mexican American (Miville & Constantine, 2006) and Chinese American populations (Tata & Leong, 1994), a similar process may likely occur for Filipino Americans. For example, in the case of Ian (a second-generation Filipino American adult), he agreed to meet with a neuropsychologist; however, if he was an immigrant, one might wonder whether or not he would seek further treatment, especially because of his gender. Additionally, English fluency was a significant factor in the case of Lola Miguela. Because of her less-than-average English-speaking ability and poor comprehension skills, the neuropsychologist opted to refer her to a colleague who was fluent in Tagalog and had experience working with Filipino immigrant individuals. When discussing Lola Miguela's MMSE test results with the colleague, it was evident that additional effort would be necessary for accurate test interpretation, given the client's inability to adequately understand the test instructions. In addition to providing appropriate accommodations for testing, a non-performance-based behavioral scale was also administered to reduce testing bias.

Finally, colonial mentality may take subtle forms in all three scenarios. Filipino Americans are likely to comply with authority figures, especially when authority figures are White and American. For Ian, he may be uncomfortable with the suggestion from his primary care physician to meet a neuropsychologist; however, because he respects his doctor (who is White and American), he complies with the authority figure immediately. Although Ian doesn't make his full decision until he consults with his entire family, he assures the doctor of his appointment prematurely. In the case of Pamela's family, it appears that they do not question her schoolteacher either; they may ask her questions to gather more information, but they leave the meeting not fully understanding all the information they were given. As a result, they then ask "experts" from several members of their family and community to fully explain what a learning disability might be, since all of the information may have been lost in translation.

In the case of Lola Miguela, she and her family did not insist on a Tagalog-speaking neuropsychologist and did not stop the clinician even when it became clear that language was a barrier to the testing. As aforementioned, it is common for Filipinos and Filipino Americans to claim to understand English even when they do not. Not only is this an example of the Filipino deference to authority or avoidance of *hiya* (shame), but it also illustrates colonial mentality because the Filipino may not speak his or her mind because he or she feels inferior to the native English speaker and does not want to be assumed to be uneducated. This is also clear with Pamela's family, who made sure to consult with a family member who was educated in the United States; while this behavior may fall in line with the idea of consulting with family members with various specialties, choosing the spokesperson to be someone who has a U.S. education may also be a form of colonial mentality. They may want the spokesperson to be someone who they trust speaks English fluently and who can fully communicate with everyone involved. So although Pamela's parents fully understand English and speak fluently themselves, they may still feel substandard to Americans and feel unconfident about their abilities.

Conclusion

Filipinos and Filipino Americans present a unique set of challenges and considerations for the neuropsychologist, in large part informed by the particular cultural experiences of this community. The practitioner may expect Filipino clients to be proficient in the English language, but not always acculturated to Western norms; deferential to people in positions of authority, such as psychologists or doctors, but not necessarily comfortable with mental health concepts or even with asking basic questions; and frequently anchored by religious faith, commitments to family, and well-established codes of conduct. By understanding some of the salient influences on Filipino culture and thought, the neuropsychologist can be better positioned to anticipate potential problem areas, and approach Filipino clients in a culturally specific, informed manner. Of course, working effectively with Filipino and Filipino American clients is necessarily more complicated than simply learning phrases or basic concepts. Nonetheless, this introduction to Filipino values, beliefs, and practices can provide a useful context for neuropsychologists working with this community.

References

Abe-Kim, J., Gong, F., & Takeuchi, D. (2004). Religiosity, spirituality, and help-seeking among Filipino Americans: Religious clergy or mental health professionals? *Journal of Community Psychology, 32*, 675–689.

Agbayani-Siewert, P. (2004). Assumptions of Asian American similarity: The case of Filipino and Chinese American students. *Social Work, 49*(1), 39–51.

Agbayani-Siewert, P., & Revilla, L. (1995). Filipino Americans. In P. G. Min (Ed.), *Asian Americans: Contemporary trends and issues* (pp. 134–168). Thousand Oaks, CA: Sage.

Alegado, D. (1987). Profile: U.S. Filipinos in the 1980s. *Katipunan*, p. 11.

Alvarez, A. N., Juang, L., & Liang, C. T. H. (2006). Asian Americans and racism: When bad things happen to "model minorities." *Cultural Diversity and Ethnic Minority Psychology, 12*(3), 477–492.

American Medical Association. (2007). *International medical graduates: Top 20 countries where IMGs received medical training*. AMA Masterfile. Retrieved October 17, 2007, from http://www.ama-assn.org/ama/pub/category/1550.html

American Psychological Association. (2002). Ethical principles of psychologists and code of conduct. *American Psychologist, 57*, 1060–1073.

American Psychological Association. (2003). Guidelines on multicultural education, training, research, practice, and organizational change for psychologists. *American Psychologist, 58*, 377–402.

Asian Americans and Pacific Islanders: A people looking forward. (2001). President's Advisory Committee on Asian Americans and Pacific Islanders. Retrieved December 20, 2001, from http://www.aapi.org

Autism Society of the Philippines. (2007). *Autism in the Philippines*. Retrieved October 18, 2007, from http://autismsocietyph.org/home.htm

Barnes, J. S., & Bennett, C. E. (2002). *The Asian population, 2000*. U.S. Census Brief. http://www.census.gov

Boone, K. B., Victor, T. L., Wen, J., Razani, J., & Ponton, M. (2007). The association between neuropsychological scores and ethnicity, language, and acculturation variables in a large patient population. *Archives of Clinical Neuropsychology, 22*, 355–365.

Brandon, P. R., Newton, B. J., & Hammond, O. W. (1987). Children's mathematics achievement in Hawaii: Sex differences favoring girls. *American Educational Research Journal, 24*(3), 437–461.

Brush, B. L., Sochalski, J., & Berger, A. M. (2004). Imported care: Recruiting foreign nurses to U.S. health care facilities. *Health Affairs, 23*(3), 78–87.

Chow, T. W., Ross, L., Fox, P., Cummings, J. L., & Lin, K. (2000). Utilization of Alzheimer's disease community resources by Asian-Americans in California. *International Journal of Geriatric Psychiatry, 15*, 838–847.

Chung, P. J., Travis, R., Jr., Kilpatrick, S. D., Elliott, M. N., Lui, C., Khandwala, S. B., et al. (2007). Acculturation and parent-adolescent communication about sex in Filipino-American families: A community-based participatory research study. *Journal of Adolescent Health, 40*, 543–550.

Church, A. T., Katigbak, M. S., & Reyes, J. A. S. (1998). Further exploration of Filipino personality structure using the lexical approach: Do the big-five or big-seven dimensions emerge? *European Journal of Personality, 12*, 249–269.

Clark, N. (2004). Education in the Philippines. *World Education News & Reviews, 17*. Retrieved October 1, 2007, from http://www.wes.org/ewenr/04Nov/Practical.htm

Cordova, F. (1983). *Filipinos: Forgotten Asian Americans*. Dubuque, IA: Kendall/Hunt.

David, E. J., & Okazaki, S. (2006). Colonial mentality: A review and recommendation for Filipino American psychology. *Cultural Diversity and Ethnic Minority Psychology, 12*(1), 1–16.

Dela Cruz, F., McBride, M., Compas, L., Calixto, P., & Derveer, C. (2002). White paper on the health status of Filipino Americans and recommendations for research. *Nursing Outlook, 50,* 7–15.

Enriquez, V. G. (1982). *Decolonizing the Filipino psyche: Philippine psychology in the seventies.* Quezon City, Philippines: Philippine Psychology Research House.

Espiritu, Y. L. (1992). *Asian American panethnicity: Bridging institutions and identities.* Philadelphia, PA: Temple University Press.

Fatimilehin, I. A., & Nadirshaw, Z. (1994). A cross-cultural study of parental attitudes and beliefs about learning disability (mental handicap). *Mental Handicap Research, 7*(3), 202–227.

Flores, M. B., & Evans, G.T. (1972). Some differences in cognitive abilities between selected Canadian and Filipino students. *Multivariate Behavioral Research, 7*(2), 175–191.

Flynn, J. R. (1991). *Asian Americans: Achievement beyond IQ.* Hillsdale, NJ: Lawrence Erlbaum Associates, Inc.

Gerber, L. M. (1980). The influence of environmental factors on mortality from coronary heart disease among Filipinos in Hawaii. *Human Biology, 52,* 269–278.

Gong, F., Gage, S. L., & Tacata, L. A. (2003). Helpseeking behavior among Filipino Americans: A cultural analysis of face and language. *Journal of Community Psychology, 31,* 469–488.

Horn, L. (1995). *Minority undergraduate participation in postsecondary education* (National Center for Education Statistics Report 95-166). Washington, DC: U.S. Department of Education.

Johnson, R. C., Nagoshi, C. T., Ahern, F. M., Wilson, J. R., & Yuen, S. H. L. (1987). Cultural factors as explanations for ethnic group differences in alcohol use in Hawaii. *Journal of Psychoactive Drugs, 19*(1), 67–75.

Johnson, R. C., Schwitters, S. Y., Wilson, J. R., Nagoshi, C. T., & McClearn, G. E. (1985). A cross-ethnic comparison of reasons given for using alcohol, not using alcohol, or ceasing to use alcohol. *Journal of Studies on Alcohol, 46,* 283–288.

Kim, B. S. K., Yang, P.H., Atkinson, D. R., Wolfe, M. M., & Hong, S. (2001). Cultural value similarities and differences among Asian American ethnic groups. *Cultural Diversity and Ethnic Minority Psychology, 7,* 343–361.

Klatsky, A. L., & Armstong, M. (1991). Cardiovascular risk factors among Asian Americans living in Northern California. *American Journal of Public Health, 81,* 1423–1428.

Klatsky, A. L., Friedman, G. D., Sidney, S., Kipp, H., Kubo, A., & Armstrong, M. (2005). Risk of hemorrhagic stroke in Asian American ethnic groups. *Neuroepidemiology, 25,* 26–31.

LaVilla S. (1998). Drug craze catches fire: Filipino Americans in Bay Area among biggest users of "shabu." *Asian Week, 20,* 12–13.

Ledesma, L. (2002). The practice of clinical neuropsychology in the Philippines. *INS Net, 10,* 3–4.

Manly, J. J., Miller, S. W., Heaton, R. K., Byrd, D., Reilly, J., Velasquez, R. J., et al. (1998). The effect of African-American acculturation on neuropsychological test performance in normal and HIV-positive individuals. *Journal of the International Neuropsychological Society, 4,* 291–302.

McCray, A. D., & Garcia, S. B. (2002). The stories we must tell: Developing a research agenda for multicultural and bilingual special education. *International Journal of Qualitative Studies in Education, 15*(6), 599–612.

Mendoza, M. T. (1986). *Television, ethnicity, and adolescent values: Socialization of Filipino and other ethnic youths in the United States.* Ann Arbor, MI: University Microfilms International.

Miville, M. L., & Constantine, M. G. (2006). Sociocultural predictors of psychological help-seeking attitudes and behavior among Mexican American college students. *Cultural Diversity & Ethnic Minority Psychology, 12*(3), 420–432.

Nadal, K. L. (2000). Filipino American substance abuse: Sociocultural factors and methods of treatment. *Journal of Alcohol and Drug Education, 46*(2), 26–36.

Nadal, K. L. (2004). Filipino American identity development model. *Journal of Multicultural Counseling and Development, 32*, 44–61.

Nadal, K. L. (2008a). *Ethnic group membership, phenotype, and perceptions of racial discrimination for Filipino Americans: Implications for mental health.* Unpublished doctoral dissertation, Teachers College, Columbia University, New York.

Nadal, K. L. (2008b). Colonialism: Societal and psychological impacts on Asian Americans and Pacific Islanders. In N. Tewari & A. N. Alvarez (Eds.), *Asian American psychology: Current perspectives.* Thousand Oaks: Sage.

Nadal, K. L. (2009). *Filipino American psychology.* Bloomington, IN: Author House.

Nadal, K. L., & Sue, D. W. (2008). Asian/Asian American youth. In C. S. Clauss-Ehlers (Ed.), *Encyclopedia of cross-cultural school psychology.* New York: Springer.

National Center for Health Statistics. (2000). *National vital statistics report 48(16).* Hyattsville, MD: Author.

Nemoto, T., Aoki, B., Huang, K., Morris, A., Le, M. N., Nguyen, H., et al. (2000). HIV risk behaviors among Asian drug users in San Francisco. *AIDS Education Prevention, 12*, 126–140.

Nemoto, T., Aoki, B., Huang, K., Morris, A., Nguyen H., & Wong. W. (1999) Drug use behaviors among Asian drug users in San Francisco. *Addict Behavior, 24*, 823–838.

Nemoto, T., Operario, D., & Soma, T. (2002). Risk behaviors of Filipino methamphetamine users in San Francisco: Implications for prevention and treatment of drug use and HIV. *Public Health Reports, 117*, S30–S38.

Okamura, J. Y. (1998). *Imagining the Filipino American diaspora: Transnational relations, identities, and communities.* New York, NY: Garland Publishing.

Okamura, J., & Agbayani, A. (1991). Filipino Americans. In N. Mokuau (Ed.), *Handbook of social services for Asian and Pacific Islanders* (pp. 97–115). Westport, CT: Greenwood Press.

Okamura, J. Y., & Agbayani, A. (1997). Pamantasan: Filipino American higher education. In M. P. P. Root (Ed.), *Filipino Americans: Transformation and identity* (pp. 183–197). Thousand Oaks, CA: Sage Publications.

Philippine Census of Population and Housing. (2002). *Philippines: Population expected to reach 100 million Filipinos in 14 years.* http://www.census.gov.ph/data/pressrelease/2002/pr02178tx.html

Ponce, D. E., & Forman, S. (1980). The Filipinos. In J. F. McDermott, W. S. Tseng, & T. W. Maretzki (Eds.), *People and cultures of Hawaii: A psychocultural profile* (pp. 155–183). Hawaii: University of Hawaii Press.

Poon-McBrayer, K. F., & Garcia, S. B. (2000). Profiles of Asian American students with LD at initial referral, assessment, and placement in special education. *Journal of Learning Disabilities, 33*(1), 61–71.

Posadas, B. M. (1999). *The Filipino Americans.* Westport, CT: Greenwood Press.

Root, M. P. P. (1997). Contemporary mixed-heritage Filipino Americans: Fighting colonized identities. In M. P. P. Root (Ed.), *Filipino Americans: Transformation and identity* (pp. 80–94). Thousand Oaks, CA: Sage Publications.

Rumbaut, R. G. (1995). The new Californians: Comparative research findings on the educational progress of immigrant children. In R. G. Rumbaut & W. A. Cornelius (Eds.), *California's immigrant children* (pp. 17–70). La Jolla, CA: Center for U.S.-Mexican Studies, University of California, San Diego.

Saccuzzo, D. P., Johnson, N. E., & Russell G. (1992). Verbal versus performance IQs for gifted African-American, Caucasian, Filipino, and Hispanic children. *Psychological Assessment, 4*, 239–244.

San Francisco Department of Public Health. (1992). *AIDS Surveillance report, AIDS cases between 1981–1992*. San Francisco, CA: Author.

Sanchez, F., & Gaw, A. (2007). Mental health care of Filipino Americans. *Psychiatric Services, 58*(6), 810–815.

Strain, T. H. (Director, Producer). (2003). Episode two: The story we tell. In *Race: The power of an illusion* [film]. Available from Independent Television Service at www.itvs.org.

Sue, D. W., Arredondo, P., & McDavis, R. J. (1992). Multicultural counseling competencies and standards: A call to the profession. *Journal of Counseling & Development 70,* 477–486.

Sue, D. W., & Sue, D. (2003). *Counseling the culturally diverse* (4th ed.). New York, NY: John Wiley & Sons, Inc.

Tata, S. P., & Leong, F. T. L. (1994). Individualism-collectivism, social-network orientation, and acculturation as predictors of attitudes toward seeking professional psychological help among Chinese Americans. *Journal of Counseling Psychology, 41*, 280–287.

Teranishi, R. T. (2002). Asian Pacific Americans and critical race theory: An examination of school racial climate. *Equity & Excellence in Education, 35*, 144–154.

Tiongson, A. T. (1997). Throwing the baby out with the bathwater: Situating young Filipino mothers and fathers beyond the dominant discourse on adolescent pregnancy. In M. P. P. Root (Ed.), *Filipino Americans: Transformation and identity* (pp. 257–271). Thousand Oaks, CA: Sage.

Tompar-Tiu, A., & Sustento-Seneriches, J. (1995). *Depression and other mental health issues: The Filipino American experience*. San Francisco, CA: Jossey Bass Publishers.

Trevino, F. M. (1987). Standardized terminology for Hispanic populations. *American Journal of Public Health, 77*, 69–72.

Uba, L. (1994). *Asian Americans: Personality patterns, identity, and mental health.* New York, NY: Guilford Press.

U.S. Census Bureau. (1994). *1990 census of population, general population characteristics, the United States* (CP-1-1). Washington, DC: U.S. Government Printing Office.

U.S. Census Bureau (2000a). *Profile of selected demographic and social characteristics: 2000. Population universe: People born in the Philippines* (Table FBP-1). http://www.census.gov/population/cen2000/stp-159/STP-159-philippines.pdf

U.S. Census Bureau. (2000b). *We the people: Asians in the United States*. Retrieved October 1, 2007, from http://www.census.gov/population/www/cen2000/briefs.html#sr

Won, J. W., Krajicek, M., & Lee, H. (2004). Culturally and linguistically competent care of a Korean-American child with autism. *Illness, Crisis, & Loss, 12*(2), 139-154.

Wong, T. M., & Fujii, D. E. (2004). Neuropsychological assessment of Asian Americans: Demographic factors, cultural diversity, and practical guidelines. *Applied Neuropsychology, 11*, 23–36.

5 Neuropsychology of Hmong Americans

Daryl Fujii and Alyssa Kaying Vang

Brief history

Laos is a Southeast Asian country roughly the size of Utah (91,400 square miles). It is bordered by Thailand, Cambodia, Myanmar, China, and Vietnam. Laos is an ethnically diverse country. The majority Lao live primarily in the lowlands of the country, while the other major ethnic group, the Hmong, inhabit the mountains. The Hmong are slash-and-burn farmers whose primary crops include rice, corn, and opium poppies. They live in small villages and also raise livestock such as cattle and pigs. Other minority ethnic groups are the Mon-Khmer and the Yao.

The Hmong, whose history dates back to 2000 B.C., are originally from the mountainous regions of southern China. For centuries, the Hmong battled with the Chinese government in attempts to maintain their unique ethnic identity. In the 1700s, Chinese generals tricked Sonom, the last Hmong king, to surrender in exchange for peace. Instead, he was executed. Tensions between the societies increased further after China was defeated in the 1842 Opium War and raised taxes to pay their indemnities to the British. The Hmong rebelled by waging a series of wars against the Chinese government between 1850 and 1880. The rebellion was quashed and the Hmong fled south. The majority settled in the mountains of Laos, although many also migrated to Vietnam and Thailand (Bankston, n.d.).

The Hmong faced similar oppression in Laos, which was part of France's Indochinese Empire. French taxation resulted in two major Hmong revolts in 1896 and 1920. The French attempted to pacify the Hmong by allowing them self-government in an autonomous Hmong district. However, instead of empowering the Hmong, division of political power ensued between the rival Fong and Bliayao families. To defuse this volatile situation, the district's first democratic election was held in 1938 with Touby Lyfong declared the winner. Unfortunately, the election did not unite the Hmong and political division continued into the Vietnamese War. Touby Lyfong allied himself with the Americans, who recruited Hmong to fight the "secret war" in Laos, whereby troops were used to block the Ho Chi Minh trail, the main military supply route from North to South Vietnam. His cousin Faydang Lobliayao joined forces with Lao nationalists who supported independence from France. Lobliayao later became a leader of the Pathet Lao Communist forces that overthrew the Laotian government in 1975 (Bankston, n.d.).

When the Pathet Lao took over the government, the Hmong who sided with the Americans were targeted for retribution. About a third of the Hmong were killed, a third fled to refugee camps in Thailand, and the remaining third stayed in Laos. Many of the Hmong refugees immigrated to France, Australia, and the United States (Bankston, n.d.). The first wave of immigrants to the United States were men associated with General Vang Pao's secret army that aligned with American forces during the Vietnamese War. About 30,000 men immigrated from 1976 to 1978. The second wave of Hmong immigrants consisted of families of the secret army that were permitted to enter the United States after the passing of the Refugee Act in 1980. The third wave of Hmong immigrants consisted of persons still living in impoverished Thai refugee camps, which officially closed in 1996. They were resettled in the United States after failed attempts at repatriation of Hmong refugees and a two-decade denial of the secret war by the American government (Wikipedia, 2009b).

Hmong demographics in the United States

According to the 2000 U.S. census, there were 170,049 Hmong living in the United States, which constitutes 1.7% of the total Asian American population (Reeves & Bennett, 2004). About 55.6% of Hmong are foreign born. Of these immigrants, 31.3% of Hmong have become naturalized citizens. The vast majority of Hmong immigrated during the 1980s. The longitudinal pattern of immigration across decades includes 15.2% before 1980, 46.1% from 1980 to 1990, and 38.7% from 1990 to 2000 (Reeves & Bennett, 2004). Given the high percentage of immigrants, it is not surprising that many are not proficient in English. In 95.6% of Hmong households, a non-English language is spoken at home, with many speaking a creole of Hmong and English, or "Hmong-glish." English is "spoken well" in 37% of households, and in only 4.4% of Hmong households is only English spoken at home (Reeves & Bennett, 2004). About 41.3% are considered linguistically isolated (Yang, 2004).

Settlement in the United States has been selective to a few states. Just below 50% of the Hmong population lived in the Midwest. States with the largest number of Hmong include (1) California, 65,095; (2) Minnesota, 41,800; (3) Wisconsin, 33,791; (4) North Carolina, 7,093; (5) Michigan, 5,383, (6) Colorado, 3,000; (7) Oregon, 2,101; (8) Georgia, 1,468; (9) Washington, 1,294; and (10) Massachusetts, 1,127 (Pfeifer, 2001).

The Hmong are more youthful than the Asian and general population. The 2000 U.S. census data reported the median age of Hmong as 16.3, in comparison to all Asians (33.0) and the total population (35.4) (Reeves & Bennett, 2004). In the 2000 census, 55.2% of Hmong were under 18, while 2.6% were over 65.

About 55.2% of Hmong are married (Reeves & Bennett, 2004). As with Asians in general, Hmong (8.3%) are less likely to be separated, widowed, or divorced than the general population (19%). Hmong tend to have more children, with average household sizes estimated to be 6.14 (U.S. average is 2.59). Despite having larger households, the median family income for Hmong ($32,384) is among the lowest for Asians ($59,324), and lower than the general population's ($50,046). There are fewer Hmong (male, 58.5%; female, 46.5%) participating in the workforce than the general population (male, 70.7%; female, 57.5%), and a lower percentage of Hmong (17.1%)

are employed in management, professional, or related occupations than all Asians (44.6%) or the general population (33.6%). Given these figures, it is not surprising that a high percentage of Hmong (37.8) live below the poverty level (total U.S. population, 12.4) (Reeves & Bennett, 2004).

Pertinent cultural variables

Subcultural divisions

The Hmong can be subdivided according to different attributes. One of the primary manners of classifying Hmong is by dialect spoken. The "White Hmong" (Hmong Der) speak Hmoob Dawb, and the "Green" or "Blue Mong" (Mong Leng) speak in the Moob Leeg dialect. Hmong can also be classified by clans. The most common clans are the Chang/Cha, Fang, Hang, Her/Heu/Herr, Khang, Kong, Kue, Lee/Ly, Lor/Lo, Moua/Mua, Phang/Pha, Thao/Thor, Vue, Xiong, Yang, and Vang (Wikipedia, 2009a). Due to intermarriage, blood relatives often have different surnames. However, it is forbidden to marry someone who shares the same clan name, as this would be considered incestuous (Bankston, n.d.). A final manner of identifying different Hmong subgroups is by their traditional clothing. White, Black, Flowery, Red, Striped, and Cowery Shell are some of the subgroups (Bankston, n.d.).

Family structure

The father is the head of the Hmong family and chief decision maker, while the mother has primary responsibility for the household. Families are children centered and small children are viewed as treasures. Elders are highly respected. As with other farming people, the extended family is a basic unit of organization for Hmong in Laos. However, given U.S. government regulations of fire and housing codes and landlord restrictions, it is very difficult for Hmong in America to maintain this tradition. Thus, the nuclear family has become the basic unit for most Hmong families. Still, extended families usually live nearby to provide support (Bankston, n.d.).

Religious values

The most widespread traditional religious belief is a pantheistic form of shamanism. The Hmong believe that spirits reside in all things. Two worlds coexist: the *yeeb ceeb*, or spiritual world, and the *yaj ceeb*, or materialistic world where humans, material objects, and nature exist. Shamans can make contact with the *yeeb ceeb* through spirit allies and do so on behalf of humans wanting to contact their ancestors (Bankston, n.d.).

An example of a typical shamanistic celebration is the three-day incarnation ceremony for newborns. Hmong believe in reincarnation, *Mus Thawj thiab*, which occurs on the third day of life. The role of the shaman in this ceremony is to evoke a soul from the spiritual world to be reincarnated to the newborn. Once accomplished, the shaman will call upon ancestors to join living family members in blessing and protecting the baby (Bankston, n.d.).

Another traditional religion is the *Chao Fa*, which translates to "Lord of the Sky." This religion was founded by the prophet Yang Chong Leu in the 1960s. He announced that a new king would lead the Hmong to salvation against the lowland Laotians and return the people to the ways of their ancestors. Yang Chong Leu was killed in 1971. After his death, followers remained active against the new Laotian government (Bankston, n.d.).

A growing number of Hmong are Christian. Many were exposed to Christianity through missionaries while in Laos. More are being converted after immigrating to the United States. Hmong have been converted to numerous Christian denominations, including Baptist, Catholic, Presbyterian, Latter-Day Saints, Methodist, and Jehovah's Witness (Bankston, n.d.). The Christian and Missionary Alliance (C&MA) is the largest Christian denomination for the Hmong.

Illness beliefs and traditional healing practices

Traditional Hmong healing practices differ considerably from Western medicines and center around herbal medicines, massages, and shamanism. Herbal medicines and massages are common interventions for stomach aches and other minor ailments. Although herbal medicines can be administered by a shaman, most Hmong households have their own herbal gardens. Many women are experts in herbal remedies (Bankston, n.d.).

More serious illnesses are believed to be spiritual in nature, with interventions based upon etiology. For example, one cause of illness is a wandering soul that leaves the body. In this manner the material-world body is alienated from its spiritual essence. This disconnection can result from loneliness, fright, bereavement, and emotional stress from separation. Symptoms of this illness may include loss of weight, loss of appetite, and lethargy. For this type of illness, the shaman would intervene by calling the soul back to the body. For more serious illness, a shaman may engage in animal sacrifice (Bankston, n.d.).

Due to significant differences in Hmong and Western conceptions of illness and treatment, many Hmong often turn to home remedies or traditional healers first for treatment of physical health issues. It is only when these traditional approaches have not been helpful or when the illness has become very serious that Western-trained providers are sought. Even Hmong who are converted Christians generally still practice many of the traditional healing methods and believe it to be linked to the culture, rather than the religion. For instance, when an infant is uncharacteristically inconsolable or simply ill, many Hmong believe this to be a result of fright. Some general approaches to treating this could range from "massaging the fright away" to performing a simple ceremony such as shaking the child's shirt over the stove. These practices are common even for Hmong Christians, even though they may also use prayer as an intervention for serious illness. Moreover, many Hmong (regardless of their religious orientation) are opposed to invasive surgery for fear of the person not fully reincarnating as a whole body. They may also be upset about a physician providing a poor prognosis, believing that such words would "forecast" an unfavorable outcome (Culhane-Pera & Xiong, 2003).

Mental health issues

Many Hmong immigrants have experienced traumas related to war, death of loved ones, maltreatment in refugee camps, and resettlement challenges that have contributed to mental health problems, including major depression, posttraumatic stress disorder, and anxiety (Lie, Yang, Rai, & Vang, 2004). Hmong, however, are very reluctant to seek Western psychiatric services, as mental illness is associated with a significant stigma.

Mental health symptoms such as loss of appetite, sleep problems, anhedonia, and lack of energy have traditionally been attributed to loss of the soul, which is strongly linked to Hmong religious beliefs (Bankston, n.d.). Most Hmong seeking treatment for what is considered by Western thinking to be mental health problems will seek a shaman or others using traditional healing methods such as *tshuaj ntsuab* (herbs), treatment by *kws tshuaj* (medicine doctor) or *kws khawv koob* (ritual healers), and a soul-calling ceremony (*hu plig*) (Culhane-Pera & Xiong, 2003).

If Western treatment is sought, most Hmong will likely seek a medical provider first, as many of them continue to view, describe, and experience their mental health problems through physical symptoms. Even the Hmong words used to describe psychological terminologies reference a body organ. For example, Hmong consider the liver (*siab*) to directly control people's feelings, thoughts, and character, and the word *liver* (*siab*) is used to describe a range of emotions (e.g., feeling worried or depressed is *nyuab siab* or *nyuaj siab*, which in English means "difficult liver"; feeling happy is *zoo siab*, which in English means "good liver"). The Hmong translation for "mental health" is *kev nyuaj siab nyuaj ntsws*, which in English means "ways that cause difficult liver and difficult lungs" (Rader, 2004).

However, with acculturation and through increased exposure to Western treatment, the negative view of Western psychiatric treatment is slowly changing, as more Hmong are beginning to accept treatment for their mental health symptoms. Disorders such as depression are common within the Hmong community, and many currently seek treatment from mental health providers who are often referred to as *thaj maum nyuab siab* ("depression doctors"). A translation of Western health and mental health terminologies into the Hmong language helps facilitate communication (Wisconsin Hmong Mental Health Professional Group, 2003).

Hmong education in Laos

Under French rule, education in Laos was extremely limited. For example, in the 1940s only about 7,000 children attended primary schools in a population of about 1 million people. This situation did not improve significantly when Laos became independent, particularly for the poor. The Royal Lao Government instituted a two-tier system whereby children of the wealthiest classes were overwhelmingly enrolled in schools, while the vast majority of the people were excluded from receiving a public education. A study from 1973 indicated that the wealthiest classes constituted only 1% of the population, but 24% of the students in Laotian schools. In comparison, the poorest classes accounted for 98% of the total population and only 0.4% of the students (Duffy, Harmon, Ranard, Thao, & Yang, 2004).

The situation was much worse for Hmong, as the vast majority of the schools were located in the city and lowlands; thus, public education in the mountainous regions where the Hmong lived was even more limited. Hmong scholar Dr. Yang Dao reported a 99% illiteracy rate in some Hmong-populated provinces during the 1970s (Duffy, Harmon, Ranard, Thao, & Yang, 2004).

Despite the exclusion from the government-sponsored educational system, some fortunate Hmong were able to benefit from other opportunities. Because the Hmong army supported American's secret war in Laos, the U.S. Agency for International Development (USAID) financed the development of schools in remote Hmong villages, building almost 300 elementary schools, 9 middle schools, 2 high schools, and a teacher training school. Thus, Hmong enrollment in school increased from 1,500 students in 20 schools in 1960, to about 10,000 students in 1969. Students learned to read and write in Lao, learned about Lao history, and studied ethics. Students who remained in school were introduced to French (Duffy, Harmon, Ranard, Thao, & Yang, 2004).

Missionaries were also instrumental in educating the Hmong. In the 1940s missionaries created the Romanized Popular Alphabet (RPA), a writing system that was developed for the Hmong language. The RPA was used to translate the Bible and other religious materials to spread Christianity to the Hmong. Some Hmong were taught to read and write RPA in Catholic and Protestant missions near the Sam Neua area (Duffy, Harmon, Ranard, Thao, & Yang, 2004).

Thailand refugee camps were another important teaching institution. Children attended Thai and Hmong schools. Adults received vocational training to assist in managing the refugee camp. Hmong refugees who were accepted for resettlement in the United States received several months of English training as well as Hmong literacy. The RPA achieved more prominence among Hmong refugees in Thailand, as they needed a system to communicate to family who were resettled in Western countries around the world. Thus, thousands of Hmong learned the RPA so that they could correspond with their families. The RPA is still being used in the United States (Duffy, Harmon, Ranard, Thao, & Yang, 2004).

In general, education was reserved for Hmong males, and only a few women were given this opportunity to be educated in Laos. This discrepancy is partly related to the Hmong's patriarchal culture. Upon coming to the United States, many of the women attempted adult school but experienced significant frustration.

Hmong education in the United States

Given the lack of educational opportunities in Laos, it is not surprising that Hmong Americans are poorly educated. About 59.6% have less than a high school education, 16.1% graduated from high school, 16.8% have some college or an associate's degree, and 7.5% have a bachelor's degree or higher (Reeves & Bennett, 2004). It is estimated that 45% of Hmong over age 25 have no formal schooling (Ngo, 2006). Hmong Americans, however, have made great strides in educational attainment, as these numbers are a significant increase from 1990 census data, when only 11% of Hmong graduated from high school, while 3% earned bachelor's degrees. In addition, many interstate differences exist. For example, in California and Alaska more than 50% report no schooling, whereas in states such as Georgia, Oregon, Massachusetts, and Rhode Island less than 25% had no schooling. States with the highest percentages of Hmong with college degrees include Washington, Colorado, Oregon, Georgia, and Rhode Island (Yang & Pfeifer, 2003), although Minnesota and California likely have the most number of college-educated professionals.

The poor academic achievement of the Hmong has been attributed to several factors. First, the lack of formal schooling and English proficiency among many Hmong parents make it difficult for them to assist their children in academics (Lee, 2006; Yang, 2004). Parents are often not familiar with the educational system and thus may be reluctant to involve themselves in school affairs (Ngo, 2006). They may also have different expectations and may assume schools are responsible for discipline as well as moral and academic education, and may become frustrated when schools cannot control their children (Valdes, 1996). Lack of parental guidance continues into college, as many Hmong parents do not understand the process of college admission, and thus students must navigate their own admission processes or rely on friends and older siblings (Ngo, 2000).

Traditional and expanded roles for Hmong children can also negatively affect academic achievement. Hmong girls, who historically have been uninvolved in education, are responsible from a young age for doing chores such as cooking meals, cleaning the house, and babysitting younger siblings, a role that may be more essential to alleviate pressure from parents if both parents work. Another tradition detrimental to obtaining an education is early marriage, as Hmong girls may be encouraged to marry or have marriages arranged while still in their early teens. Boys are often tasked with general maintenance around the house, such as mowing the lawn. In addition, children who are more proficient in English and more acculturated may be utilized as translators, drivers, or intermediaries. At minimum, these multiple responsibilities or the expectations of these responsibilities detract from a child's ability to focus on academics. Hmong children who cannot juggle these multiple roles may forfeit their education altogether (Ngo, 2006).

Another factor is the school systems' inadequate resources to provide Hmong with proper services. Many school districts have a shortage of bilingual teachers. For example, a 1997 California survey found only 28 certified bilingual Hmong teachers for 31,156 students, a ratio of 1 to 1,113 (Yang, 2004). In addition, schools do not tailor curriculums around the special needs of Hmong students. Poor cultural sensitivity also contributes to a lack of communication between teachers and Hmong parents due to different expectations and passive outreach (Yang, 2004).

Recommendations for neuropsychological testing

Currently, there have been no neuropsychological studies based upon an exclusively Hmong sample; thus, the validity of using Western tests with Hmong immigrants is questionable. Without adequate norms, a formal neuropsychological evaluation may not be possible. Still, a conceptual impression from a multimodal assessment based upon social and functional history from client and collateral sources, behavioral observations, limited testing with questionable norms, medical records including neuroimaging if available, and history of progression of cognitive and behavioral changes, in comparison to expectations from neurological disorder, can still be useful for making diagnoses and recommendations for improving functioning.

An assessment based primarily on history, medical data, and presentation may not be sensitive enough to detect subtle cognitive changes from mild brain injuries. However, given Hmong culture in which behavioral or emotional problems are not brought to the attention of professionals until it is very disturbing to family or significantly affecting finances, it is highly likely this type of evaluation can be useful for many Hmong Americans, as their deficits would be noticeable by the time of referral. The following are conceptual issues to consider when providing neuropsychological consultation to Hmong Americans:

Children

1. Western tests are most relevant for Hmong children who are born and educated in the United States and for whom English is their primary language. However, many Hmong American children are bilingual, regardless of whether they were born in the United States. If English is not the child's primary language, then verbal tests could underestimate verbal abilities. Thus, the examiner would have to determine the exposure to and skill level of English. The following are questions to determine English exposure history:
   a. Is Hmong the primary language spoken at home? If so, when did the child learn English? It should be noted that even when Hmong is the primary language spoken at home, many Hmong children are equally fluent in both Hmong and English. Thus, Hmong being the primary language spoken at home should not be relied upon as the only indicator of lack of English fluency.
   b. Is Hmong the primary language spoken with friends? In which language is the child most comfortable conversing? If a child chooses to converse with friends in Hmong, or if he or she is most comfortable speaking in Hmong, there is a greater likelihood that his or her fluency in English is significantly poorer than in Hmong.
   b. Is the child enrolled in English as a Secondary Language (ESL) or English Language Learner (ELL) classes? It should be noted, however, that a disproportionate number of Hmong children are inappropriately placed in ESL/ELL classes simply because they are Hmong. This misplacement results from a lack of culturally specific/sensitive testing, and also a conservative approach to helping Hmong children. At the same time, placement in ESL/ELL classes may be an indicator that the child has a learning disability, is cognitively delayed, or is lower functioning (even by Hmong standards).
   c. What is the child's academic achievement in reading and language? Although poor academic achievement may be due to limited English proficiency, this may not always be the case. Sometimes children do not

excel in reading and language because of a general language disorder. To tease out the cause of poor achievement in reading, it will be helpful to ask parents what the child's language processing skills and speech are in their native language, compared to siblings or peers.

d. Is there a significant discrepancy in English versus math skills? Again, this is not always accurate because to ask this question would be to assume that this is due to limited English proficiency. It is possible that children demonstrate a discrepancy between English and math due to a language disorder or other learning disorders.
e. If Hmong is the preferred language, consider an interpreter. However, since most Hmong American children are bilingual, it is helpful to qualitatively assess their English skills through conversation. This evaluation could be supplemented with school records or talking with the child's teachers. Keep in mind that comprehension (receptive language) is generally better developed than expression (expressive language). Thus it may be that the interpreter would be most useful in eliciting verbal responses from the child or obtaining history information rather than helping the child understand questions asked of him/her.
f. Although there are no specific Hmong norms, clinicians may consider administering the Bilingual Verbal Abilities Test (BVAT) (Munoz-Sandoval, Cummins, Alvarado, & Ruef, 1998). The BVAT evaluates language skills in both English and Hmong and may provide useful information for interpreting neuropsychological test scores on Western tests with a strong language component. The BVAT consists of three subtests from the Woodcock-Johnson Revised Tests of Cognitive Ability and Language Proficiency Battery–Revised: Picture Vocabulary (58 items), Oral Vocabulary Synonyms (20 items) and Antonyms (20 items), and Verbal Analogies (35 items). The test requires a bilingual administrator or interpreter and takes approximately 30 minutes to complete. Items are administered in English, and missed items are then administered in the client's native language. Norms range from 5 to 90.

2. Evaluate for level of acculturation, which is useful for interpretation, particularly to determine if cultural variables could contribute to discrepancies in test performances. It is important to note here that the Hmong community continues to highly value their cultural practices, particularly among those who still practice their traditional religion. Choosing to have exclusively Hmong friends, eating Hmong food, or listening to Hmong music does not necessarily suggest less acculturation or less English proficiency. Many Hmong children are academically accomplished and yet still ascribe to their Hmong values and practices. Nevertheless, assessing for level of acculturation is helpful to gauge whether a person has been exposed to Western concepts. For example, a Hmong child may have Hmong friends, eat Hmong food, practice Hmong traditional religion, and listen to Hmong music, but he or she also may have visited a theme park, gone to the state fair, and engaged in extracurricular activities organized by Westerners.

This child would thus have some understanding of Western culture and could be equally competent in his or her Western environment. On the other hand, a Hmong child who has Hmong friends, eats Hmong food, practices traditional religion, and listens to Hmong music but has never been exposed to any Western culture (besides that through the school), may not do well on Western standardized testing due to limited exposure to Western ways of thinking. Conditions that may limit children's exposure to more Westernized ways of thinking or Western culture include families living in very impoverished conditions, parents who are struggling with their own mental health issues, and parents who do not incorporate any Western values into their lives. Having parents with little or no education or who do not speak English is not necessarily an indicator of a child's low acculturation, as there are many Hmong parents who are uneducated and do not speak English but allow their children to engage in extracurricular activities, and these are the children who do just as well as other children.

3. Obtaining collateral information from primary caretakers or parents (through the use of interpreters if they do not speak English) will be helpful to understand the child's functioning within his or her own culture. Hmong parents are often very keen to their children and know their child's strengths and weaknesses relative to other children. However, to extract this information, it is important to ask specific detailed questions, as Hmong parents may not voluntarily provide this information.
4. If the child suffered a significant illness (or if there is an identifiable precipitant), Hmong parents are more likely to seek treatment. However, if there has not been any significant illness or identifiable precipitant, parents often accept the child's condition as their fate and raise the child as best as they know how—sometimes even to the degree of coddling the child and unintentionally inhibiting that child's adaptive growth.
5. It is most ideal to have a family work with (or child assessed by) a clinician who speaks the Hmong language, for very obvious reasons, such as being able to ask questions directly of the child and parents. Additionally, if a child is confused about a question or not able to provide a response, the clinician can "test limits" by asking the question in Hmong. However, there are few Hmong-speaking psychologists who can directly assess and work with Hmong families, and so having a Hmong-speaking provider is not always possible. In such a case, using an interpreter who is well versed in the mental health field is highly recommended. This is because mental health concepts and terminologies are difficult to interpret in Hmong. Having an interpreter who understands mental health issues can avoid any misunderstandings.

Adults

1. Given that most Hmong who immigrated to America have a poor command of English, it is highly likely that an interpreter will be required. Comprehensive recommendations on how to select and work with

interpreters are beyond the scope of this chapter. Some basic considerations include meeting the interpreter beforehand to familiarize him or her with the purpose and requirements of the evaluation as well as provide guidelines for interaction (for a review see Ponton & Corona-LoMonaco, 2007). Clinicians should avoid using family, particularly children, as interpreters due to potential biases and difficulties that it can cause in Hmong American family dynamics. Perhaps more important, interpreters should be used as cultural guides for both putting behaviors into context and recommendations. Given the small size of the Hmong community, however, clinicians should inform the client and an English-speaking family member beforehand of the identity of the interpreter. It is possible that the interpreter and the client are familiar with one another in some capacity. Thus, the client may prefer a family member over a close acquaintance as the interpreter in order to keep family business within the family. It is helpful to consider that some clients may prefer to not have an acquaintance interpret for them because of confidentiality concerns given the small Hmong community.

2. To obtain a thorough pertinent history and to assist in developing rapport, encourage the client to provide a detailed account of his or her life in Laos, the impact of the war, and the traumas that he or she experienced prior to immigrating to the United States. Hmong often provide information through storytelling rather than responding to a list of questions. If not spontaneously revealed, clients can be prompted for experiences of head injuries, traumatic events, malnutrition, and loss of loved ones.
3. Hmong's concept of time is less driven by calendar days, hours, or minutes. Instead, Hmong recall time in relation to events, seasons of the year, age of children, etc. Therefore, not knowing specific time frames may not always be an indicator that the person is a poor historian. When a patient does not know how long ago things occurred, it may be helpful to ask questions within the context of events, particularly those events or holidays that are important to his or her culture, such as Hmong New Year.
4. Evaluate for acculturation. Of particular importance is age at time of immigration (see children recommendation 2).
5. Evaluate for specific symptoms of posttraumatic stress disorder (PTSD), depression, anxiety, and substance abuse and dependence. If present, inquire about the client's explanation for the symptoms. Many Asian cultural groups somatasize mental health problems (Lin & Cheung, 1999). A denial of mental health symptoms does not necessarily suggest a lack of distress. However, clinicians should not assume that somatization is due to stigma against mental illness, but rather to a lack of awareness that emotional problems can manifest as physical problems. Psychoeducation regarding these phenomena may be very therapeutic for Hmong, whose mental health symptoms are traditionally experienced and explained as spiritual or physical causes.
6. Due to lack of neuropsychological norms for Hmong, for diagnostic referrals, a hypothesis testing approach based upon expectations of presentation

for a specific neurological disorder is recommended (Fujii & Wong, 2005; also see Chapter 1). Hypotheses should be developed from consensus statements or other widely accepted expert-based diagnostic guidelines. Data collected with a multimethod approach utilizes client and collateral interviews describing the onset, quality, severity, and progression of cognitive, behavioral, and emotional symptoms of the presenting problem, as well as any medical and imaging data. This information would be compared to different diagnostic criteria for goodness of fit.

7. For referrals requesting a functionality evaluation after a known neurological disorder, it is recommended that clinicians utilize the literature and consensus statements to guide exploration of associated cognitive, behavioral, or emotional problems. Of particular importance are changes since the onset of a disorder. Inquire about the impact that these symptoms are having on the client and family. Clinicians can also assess for declines in functional behaviors, such as using money, remembering shopping lists, planning meals, or paying bills. For older adults, measures that estimate severity of impairment based on functionality, such as the Clinical Dementia Rating, are also recommended (Hughes, Berg, Danziger, Coben, & Martin, 1982).
8. Although comprehensive neuropsychological testing is not recommended, clinicians may perform limited testing with homemade translated tests to supplement functional assessments. Clinicians should keep in mind that these are gross measurements at best, and would only be significant if performances are highly discrepant from expectations of the most similar normative group.
9. Due to low levels of education, there is a high level of illiteracy among adult Hmong immigrants, particularly women. An implication is that most Hmong adults have also experienced limited exposure to pencil-and-paper tasks. Given the high illiteracy rates, clinicians should be knowledgeable on the literature of how illiteracy affects brain functioning (for reviews see Ardila & Rosselli, 2007; Castro-Caldas, 2007). For example, illiterates were less likely to develop aphasia and more likely to produce semantic versus phonemic paraphasias after left hemisphere lesions than literates (Castro-Caldas, 2007). On testing, illiterates' scores were not significantly different than those of literates of similar socioeconomic status on naming and identification of real versus pictures of objects, verbal fluency of familiar objects such as items in a supermarket, verbal memory recognition, and orientation. Cognitive areas most affected by education and literacy include digit span, verbal abstractions, calculations, and long-term semantic memory (Reis, Guerreiro, & Petersson, 2003). Clinicians should keep in mind that although an adult Hmong is illiterate in English, he or she may be literate in a different language, for instance, Hmong Romanized Popular Alphabet.
10. Given these studies, it would be most prudent to evaluate Hmong adults on tests or evaluations that are least affected by literacy. When testing for verbal memory, although there are no Hmong norms, we recommend using the World Health Organization (WHO) UCLA Auditory Verbal Learning Test

(Maj et al., 1994) as the stimulus, with careful translation into Hmong (word list can be found in Mitrushina, Boone, Razani, & D'Elia, 2005). Words for this list were selected for their commonality across cultures, and the test was validated with samples from several countries, including Thailand.

11. General estimates of premorbid functioning can be based upon several factors: (a) education in Hmong, with quality of education based upon hours in the classroom, subjects learned, availability of school materials, and student-to-teacher ratios; (b) children's academic achievement; and (c) current socioeconomic status. For these indicators, because the expectations would be low for both categories a and c, information would be most significant if education and socioeconomic status is average or higher. It is important to note that many Hmong had to start a new life when they immigrated to the United States.
12. The following are recommendations for writing the report (see Chapter 1): (a) make the implicit explicit by describing the thinking behind your conclusions, (b) don't forget to incorporate the potential contribution of psychological disorders such as PTSD in the formulation and recommendations, (c) indicate your level of certainty given the type of data that you have collected, and (d) describe all nonstandardized test administrations.
13. The following are suggestions for making recommendations and providing feedback: (a) focus on crisis resolution; (b) emphasize community strengths such as reliance on family, ethnic community, and strong individual and group survival skills; (c) describe the rationale for recommendations; (d) avoid interactions that result in a loss of face; (e) be sure that the family is present and the father is involved in decision making; and (f) be respectful of family decisions if nontraditional forms of treatment are selected (Bromley & Chhem Sip, 2003).

Case sample

PY is a 16-year-old Hmong American male who was referred for a neuropsychological evaluation at the recommendation of school personnel because of a significant decline in academic functioning. According to school staff, PY had been doing relatively well in school prior to the 10th grade, but had been gradually failing his classes within the last two years and ceasing to do the work despite attending classes daily. PY had also stopped eating lunch, and was not socializing with anyone, though he had always been described as "shy." Additionally, PY had started to exhibit uncharacteristic behaviors such as growing out his hair (both on his head and on his face). There was concern among school staff that his behavior reflected possible participation in a Hmong gang. Consequently, it took two years for a referral to be initiated. During this time period, PY was only receiving English Language Learners (ELL) services.

When the appointment was scheduled, PY's parents declined an interpreter. At various points of the meeting with PY's parents, they appeared to be unsure about some of the questions answered and offered information that was at times confusing.

The English-speaking psychologist wondered if he could bring in an interpreter to help him understand a few things, to which the parents politely agreed. An interpreter who works exclusively within a mental health setting was asked to participate and was able to clarify symptoms, specific timelines, and concerns. The following information incorporates these data.

PY's parents reported concerns about his social isolation and lack of interest, which they feel have been more concerning and significant within the last two years, even though they acknowledged that PY had always played by himself. They described PY as "lost in his world." His parents reported that when PY started high school, he stopped doing his schoolwork, though he willingly attends school regularly. The parents were also very concerned about PY's declining performance at school. They thought that PY had received special education services in elementary to junior high school, but were not sure as to the specific type.

PY's parents also described a number of behaviors that were concerning them, including compulsive behaviors related to eating, dressing, and hand washing. For instance, PY insists on putting his food in certain places on his plate, without them touching each other. He is also particular about which utensils and silverware he uses. He refuses to drink soda pop unless it has been purchased from a particular convenience store. Additionally, he is very organized and will fold his dirty laundry even though he knows it will be washed. PY is also described as rarely initiating interactions with his family. He does not join the family during meals and prefers to eat alone. He only communicates with the family when he needs something. His parents reported that these behaviors have always been present for PY. His mother also reported that when PY was much younger, he did not seek comfort from her whenever he was upset or hurt.

His parents are not aware of any trauma or stressor preceding this decline in functioning. There is no known medical or neurological history. There is no known head injury or loss of consciousness. There was no known substance use and no known history of physical or sexual abuse.

Hmong is spoken in the home, but PY reportedly prefers to speak English. Early developmental milestones were unremarkable, with the exception of delayed language development and limited social interactions.

At his testing appointment, PY was observed in the waiting area to be away from his parents, standing and staring at a wall. He did not make any eye contact when the neuropsychologist greeted him, though this improved over time as PY became more comfortable. PY spoke minimally throughout the evaluation and did not initiate conversation. There was minimal reciprocal conversation. However, PY was pleasant and compliant with all aspects of the testing.

The following are the test results:

Wechsler abbreviated scale of intelligence (WASI)

Verbal IQ	67
Performance IQ	83
Full-Scale IQ	74

Woodcock-Johnson III tests of achievement

Test	*Grade equivalent*	*Standard score*
Broad Reading	2.7	52
Broad Math	4.4	66

Wechsler memory scale III

Subtest	*Percentile rank or standard score*
Information and Orientation	1%
Mental Control	SS = 1
Digit Span	SS = 8

Oral and written language scales (OWLS)

Subtest	*Standard score*
Oral Expression	41
Listening Comprehension	47
Developmental Test of Visual Motor Integration (VMI)	SS = 86

Grooved pegboard

	Time	*No. drops*	*Standard score*
Preferred (right) hand	123 s	3	0
Nonpreferred hand	114 s	0	20

Trail making test

	Time (in seconds)	*Standard score (z-score)*
Trails A	90 s	–7.3
Trails B	160 s	–7.25

Adaptive behavior assessment system (ABAS)

General Adaptive Composite = 44 (<1st percentile)

Conceptual	SS = 48 (<1st percentile)
Social	SS = 54 (<1st percentile)
Practical	SS = 50 (<1st percentile)

After integrating all the test data and history information, PY's evaluation appeared consistent with a history of autism spectrum disorder (with compulsive features), as well as concerns with speech and language issues (in both Hmong and English). Recommendations were made to the school's educational team to review his eligibility for special education services under the autism spectrum disorder classification.

The case of PY unfortunately illustrates how a child's disorder was missed because of cultural differences. Moreover, any learning or behavioral challenges PY experienced were attributed to his speaking English as a second language and gang involvement. It was later learned that PY never received any special education accommodations throughout his schooling. The only service he received was through the English Language Learner programs.

Conclusion

The case of PY highlights many important cultural issues to consider when evaluating Hmong children:

1. Utilizing interpreters familiar with Hmong culture and mental health issues is important, as PY's interpreter was able to solicit a much more rich and accurate history which ultimately helped to clarify many of PY's specific mental health symptoms. PY's parents were initially vague in describing social and academic problems and were only able to provide pertinent diagnostic information with both culturally and psychiatrically informed questioning.
2. There are no words to capture the mental health disorder of autism Hmong culture. Autistic features are often perceived in isolation of one another. Therefore, with a higher-functioning autistic child, such as PY, early socialization issues, for instance, may be minimized, hoping that the child will "grow out of it." For a lower-functioning autistic child, mental retardation is the general focus, and parents then become more protective of this child, at times coddling them.
3. PY's parents did not understand PY's academic needs or the educational system and therefore could not fully advocate for all of PY's needs. Their limited awareness is not uncommon, as many Hmong parents are not familiar with the American educational system and lack the English skills or educational experience to fully comprehend how the system runs. This can result in the inappropriate or insufficient support of the child's academic growth.
4. Because PY was born and raised in America, having gone through the traditional Western educational system, and because English is his first language, using Western tests and norms to obtain an estimate of PY's current functioning was appropriate.

References

Ardila, A., & Rosselli, M. (2007). Illiterates and cognition: The impact of education. In B. Uzzell, M. Ponton, & A. Ardila (Eds.). *International handbook of cross-cultural neuropsychology* (pp. 181–198). Mahwah, NJ: Lawrence Erlbaum Associates.

Bankston, C. (n.d.). *Hmong Americans.* Retrieved February 9, 2009, from http://www.everyculture.com/multi/Ha-La/Hmong-Americans.html

Bromley, M. A., & Chhem Sip, S. K. (2003). Substance abuse treatment issues with Cambodian Americans. In S. L. Ashenberg Straussner (Ed.), *Ethnocultural factors in substance abuse treatment* (pp. 321–343). New York, NY: Guilford Press.

Castro-Caldas, A. (2007). Relationship between functional brain organization and education. In B. Uzzell, M. Ponton, & A. Ardila (Eds.), *International handbook of cross-cultural neuropsychology* (pp. 199–214). Mahwah, NJ: Lawrence Erlbaum Associates.

Culhane-Pera, K. A., & Xiong, P. (2003). Hmong culture: Tradition and change. In K. A. Culhane-Pera et al. (Eds.), *Healing by heart: Clinical and ethical case stories of Hmong families and Western providers* (pp. 11–68). Nashville, TN: Vanderbilt University Press.

Duffy, J., Harmon, R., Ranard, D. Thao, B, & Yang, K. (2004). The Hmong: An introduction to their history and culture. Washington DC. Retrieved February 16, 2009 from http://www.cal.org/co/hmong/hlit.html.

Fujii, D., & Wong, T. (2005). Neuropsychological assessment with Asian-American immigrants: Recommendations for meeting *Daubert* standards. *Journal of Forensic Neuropsychology, 4*(4), 3–31.

Hughes, C., Berg, L., Danziger, W., Coben, L., & Martin, R. (1982). A new clinical scale for the staging of dementia. *British Journal of Psychiatry, 140*, 566–572.

Lee, S. J. (2006). Additional complexities: Social class, ethnicity, generation, and gender in Asian American student experiences. *Race, Ethnicity and Education, 9*, 17–28.

Lie, G. Y., Yang, P., Rai, K., & Vang, P. V. (2004). Hmong children and families. In R. Fong (Ed.), *Culturally competent practice with immigrant and refugee children and families* (pp. 122–145). New York, NY: The Guilford Press.

Lin, K.M., & Cheung, F. (1999). Mental health issues for Asian Americans. *Psychiatric Services, 50*, 774-780.

Maj, M., Satz, P., Janssen, R., Zaudig, M., et al. (1994). WHO neuropsychiatric AIDS study, cross-sectional phase II: Neuropsychological and neurological findings. *Archives of General Psychiatry, 51*, 51–61.

Mitrushina, M., Boone, K., Razani, J., & D'Elia, L. (2005). *Handbook of normative data for neuropsychological assessment* (2nd ed., pp. 618–622). New York, NY: Oxford University Press.

Munoz-Sandoval, A. F., Cummins, J., Alvarado, C. G., & Ruef, M. L. (1998). *Bilingual Verbal Ability Tests*. Itasca, IL: Riverside Publishing.

Ngo, B. (2000). *Obstacles, miracles, and the pursuit of higher education: The experiences of Hmong American college students*. Unpublished master's thesis, University of Wisconsin–Madison.

Ngo, B. (2006). Learning from the margins: The education of Southeast and South Asian Americans in context. *Race Ethnicity and Education, 9*, 51–65.

Pfeifer, M. (2001). *2000 census shows contrasting growth and settlement patterns of major Southeast Asian origin groups*. Retrieved February 8, 2009, from http://www.hmongstudies.org/4IndochineseGroups.html

Ponton, M., & Corona-LoMonaco, M. E. (2007). Cross-cultural issues in neuropsychology: Assessment of the Hispanic patient. In B. Uzzell, M. Ponton, & A. Ardila (Eds.), *International handbook of cross-cultural neuropsychology* (pp. 265–282). Mahwah, NJ: Lawrence Erlbaum Associates.

Rader, P. (2004). *Lost in translation: The challenge of Hmong mental health counseling*. Retrieved May 29, 2009, from http://cehd.umn.edu/alumni/link/2004Fall/RU-Goh.html

Reeves, T. J., & Bennett, C. E. (2004). *We the people: Asians in the United States*. Washington, DC: U.S. Census Bureau. Retrieved February 9, 2009, from http://www.census.gov/prod/2004pubs/censr-17.pdf

Reis, A., Guerreiro, M., & Petersson, K. M. (2003). A sociodemographic and neuropsychological characterization of an illiterate population. *Applied Neuropsychology, 10*, 191–204.

Valdes, G. (1996). *Con respeto: Bridging the distances between culturally diverse families and schools: An ethnographic portrait.* New York, NY: Teachers College Press.

Wikipedia. (2009a). *Hmong American.* Retrieved February 12, 2009, from http://en.wikipedia.org/wiki/Hmong_American

Wikipedia. (2009b). *Hmong people.* Retrieved February 12, 2009, from http://en.wikipedia.org/wiki/Hmong_people

Wisconsin Hmong Mental Health Professional Group. (2003). *Hmong-English mental health terminology glossary.* Retrieved May 29, 2009, from http://dwd.wisconsin.gov/migrantsandrefugees/pdf_files/hmong_mental_health_terminology_rev_jan_03.pdf

Yang, K. Y. (2004). Southeast Asian American children: Not the "model minority." *The Future of Children, 14*, 127–137.

Yang, K., & Pfeifer, M. (2003). *Profile and Hmong educational attainment.* Washington, DC: Hmong National Development, Inc. Retrieved May 15, 2009, from http://hmongstudies.org/HmongCensusReport.pdf

6 Neuropsychology of Asian Indians

Vaishali S. Phatak, Vidyulata Kamath, and Daryl Fujii

Brief history

India is an ancient and dynamic culture with a continuous civilization since 2500 B.C.E. The people that inhabited the Indus River Valley founded a culture reliant on commerce and dependent on agricultural trade that has continued until the present day (Danielou, 2003). As Aryan-speaking groups of people came into the region from the Northwest, they settled in the middle Ganges River Valley, adapting to the preexisting cultures in the area during the second millennium (Naidis, 1966).

During the fourth and fifth centuries C.E., Northern India was unified under the Gupta Dynasty (Danielou, 2003). What was previously a multitude of kingdoms with changing boundaries was united in a period that would come to be known as the Golden Age of India. In the 700 years that followed, the religion of Islam became common first in North India and eventually expanded across the subcontinent. Between the eleventh and twelfth centuries, invaders from Turkey and Afghanistan established sultanates in the city of Delhi. This was followed by the establishment of the Mughal Empire by the Chaghtai Turkish adventurer Babur at the start of the sixteenth century. The Mughal Dynasty lasted two centuries and had gained influence over large portions of the area (Leonard, 1997). In spite of foreign invasions, many other indigenous kingdoms flourished and managed to remain unaffected by the political upheaval that surrounded them.

Meanwhile, Europeans started to come for trade and took advantage of the divided nature of these kingdoms. Portugal, Netherlands, France, and the United Kingdom all established colonies within India. Britain's first outpost in South Asia was established in 1619 at Surat by the British East India Company. From this presence the British spread their control, ultimately ruling most of present-day India, Bangladesh, Sri Lanka, and Pakistan. In 1857, the British Parliament transferred political power from the East India Company to the British crown after Indian soldiers led an unsuccessful rebellion in North India (Danielou, 2003; Leonard, 1997).

The early twentieth century marked the beginning of the movement for independence. Starting in 1920, Mohandas K. Gandhi changed the Indian National Congress political party into a group protest to vie for independence (Wolpert, 1991). Millions of people united using political and nonviolent resistance to campaign against Britain's rule. As a result of the increasing Indian unity in the quest for sovereignty from Britain, India became a dominion within the Commonwealth on August 15, 1947. Due to Hindu-Muslim conflict and other strategic reasons British India was separated into India and Pakistan. India became a republic within the Commonwealth in 1950 (Kulke & Rothermund, 2004).

Currently, India is the second most populated country and the world's largest liberal democracy. Over 300 languages and dialects are spoken across the Indian subcontinent. The national language is Hindi, but other commonly spoken languages include English, Gujarati, Punjabi, Bengali, Urdu, Marathi, Oriya, Kannada, Tamil, and Malayalam (Benson, 2004). Table 6.1 shows the official recognized languages by each of the Indian states and territories.

Immigration history

The earliest history of Asian Indian migration to the United States can be traced to the turn of the twentieth century. Early immigrants were agricultural workers and unskilled laborers disillusioned with the famine in the British India province of Punjab or university students interested in gaining American support in the movement for a free India (Leonard, 1997; Shukla, 2003). From the beginning, both groups faced the widespread and overt anti-Asian sentiment (Benson, 2004). American laws shifted throughout the early 1900s, at first barring Indians from owning land and later categorizing them as members of the Caucasian race. This privilege of White status allowed early Indian immigrants to own land, become naturalized, and attain increased economic gains. Despite these minor advances, Asian Indians were set back by the Immigration Act of 1917, which largely prevented Asians from entering the U.S. (Benson, 2004). Further setbacks came in 1923 when the U.S. Supreme Court ruled that Indians were not free White persons. As a result of this ruling, established Indians living in the United States lost citizenship and property (Rangaswamy, 2000). Though U.S. laws eventually changed to allow foreign entry, the rates of Asian Indians entering the United States stagnated (Benson, 2004). By the late 1940s, the size of the Indian American community had declined significantly as many immigrants returned to India (Benson, 2004).

The next drastic shift in the immigration came with the passage of new legislation that relaxed immigration laws. The 1965 Immigration and Nationality Act drastically revived Asian Indian immigration (Adler & Gielen, 2003). Professionals and technical workers encompassed over 93% of the incoming population, and their primary goals were to advance economically and educationally. As a result of their professional qualifications, Indian Americans provided a notable contribution to the American labor force (Das, 2002; Rangaswamy, 2000). A major source of heterogeneity among Asian Indians in the United States came with a 1976 statute that removed the number of individuals allowed from each hemisphere. Up until that time, the demographic profile of Indian Americans was largely a highly educated class of medical and technical professionals. With the statute of 1976, relatives of Indian immigrants and other Indians from a variety of educational backgrounds greatly diversified the demographics patterns (Rangaswamy, 2000). There is now substantial variability in educational attainment, English proficiency, and socioeconomic

Table 6.1 Official and Officially Recognized Languages by Indian States and Territories

State/Territory	*Language*
Andaman and Nicobar Islands (terr.)	English, Hindi
Andhra Pradesh	Telgu, Urdu
Arunachal Pradesh	English
Assam	Assamese, Bengali, Bodo
Bihar	Hindi, Urdu
Chandigarh	Punjabi, Hindi
Chhattisgarh	Hindi
Dadra and Nagar Haveli (terr.)	Marathi, Gujarati
Daman and Diu (terr.)	Gujarati, Marathi, English
Delhi (terr.)	Hindi, Urdu, Punjabi
Goa	Kokani, Marathi
Gujarat	Gujarati, Hindi
Harayana	Hindi
Himachal Pradesh	Hindi
Jammu and Kashmir	Urdu
Jharkhand	Hindi
Karnataka	Kannada
Kerala	Malayalam, English
Lakshadweep (terr.)	Malayalam
Madhya Pradesh	Hindi
Maharashtra	Marathi
Manipur	Meitei
Meghalaya	English, Khasi, Garo
Mizoram	Mizo
Nagaland	English
Orissa	Oriya, English
Puducherry (terr.)	Tamil, English, French
Punjab	Punjabi
Rajasthan	Hindi
Sikkim	English
Tamil Nadu	Tamil
Tripura	English, Bengali, Kokborok
Uttarakhand	English, Hindi, Urdu
Uttar Pradesh	Hindi, Urdu
West Bengal	Bengali, Nepali

status (Rangaswamy, 2000). A recent report indicated that 35% of Asian Indians in the central valley area of California have not completed high school, compared to 25% from the general population of individuals living in the central valley (Asian Pacific American Legal Center of Southern California, 2005). This information belies the portrait of Asian Indians as wealthy and educationally advanced professionals. Currently, the Asian Indian community in the United States continues to grow exponentially as evidenced by recent census data.

Population demographics in the United States

Asian Indians represent the third largest Asian American group and the fastest-growing immigrant group in the United States. The exponential growth of the Asian Indians immigrating to the United States continues to increase. Over the past decade, the population doubled to 1.7 million Asian Indian individuals, with over 50% immigrating between 1990 and 2000 (U.S. Census Bureau, 2002). Current census data indicate that Indians in the United States are mostly between the ages of 18 and 64 years, with over 40% classified as foreign-born noncitizens.

Though previously centered primarily in New Jersey and New York, Asian Indians are currently well distributed in urban and metropolitan areas across North America. Currently, New York City; San Jose, California; Chicago, Illinois; Los Angeles, California; and Fremont, California have the largest Asian Indian populations in North America (Benson, 2004). The typical Asian Indian household consists of a married couple with an average of three individuals per household (U.S. Census Bureau, 2004). Asian Indians in the United States vary greatly in acculturation level, socio-economic status, income level, and proficiency of the English language (Ramakrishna & Weiss, 1992). Though a majority of the Asian Indian population has sizable income in comparison to the general population, newly arriving immigrants often live below the poverty level (Benson, 2004). Similarly, employment of Asian Indians ranges from professional degrees and ownership of small businesses and hotels to positions as gas station attendants, taxi cab drivers, and subway newsagents (Benson, 2004; Leonard, 1997). Often Asian Indian business owners recruit incoming Asian Indian immigrants to fill low-paying positions. In many cases, Asian Indian enclaves form as immigrants dwelling in the United States bring family and other associates to the United States and assist in getting them started financially (Benson, 2004).

Generational issues

Migration to the United States is often laden with pressure to minimize differences between the new and native culture (Berry & Annis, 1974; Krishnan & Berry, 1992). Moreover, acculturative stress can occur in varying levels depending on the individual's ability to manage changes in "class, diet, employment, clothing, climate, housing, and family composition" (Roysircar, 2003, p. 259). Within Asian Indian families, interdependence among family members is emphasized. Moreover, the degree of parent assimilation can influence the relationship between first-generation Asian Indian immigrants and their second-generation children. Differences in decision-making style, gender roles, expression of anger, dress, and display of affection between first- and second-generation Asian Indians provide challenges to family relationships (Prathikanti, 1997). Not surprisingly, parents immigrating to the United States struggle with the challenges of raising children in America (Dugsin, 2001). In many cases, parents are operating from a culturally different framework based on values and attitudes oriented to Indian tradition that ignore the challenges of living in a bicultural world (Baptiste, 2005).

Testing issues

Education in India

Education is a highly valued and culturally salient facet of the Asian Indian society. The structure of formal schooling in India is typically divided into primary and secondary school, though it varies from state to state. Lower primary school consists of grades 1 through 5, and upper primary consists of grades 6 through 8. Secondary school consists of grades 9 and 10, and senior secondary school consists of grades 11 and 12. Schools are designated by the language of instruction (e.g., English medium schools, Hindi medium, etc.). UNESCO statistics indicate approximately 89% of children in India are enrolled in a primary school. There is a significant attrition of enrollment by secondary school. Specific data were not available, but estimates are 50 to 60% enrollment rate in secondary school (UNESCO, 2006).

Historically, there has been a reduced societal emphasis of education for girls. Due to this bias, the Indian government has actively pursued programs to facilitate education for girls. Recent educational statistics show improved rates of enrollment for girls. The 2006 data indicated 87% of girls are enrolled in primary school, which is generally comparable to the proportion of boys (90%) enrolled in primary school (UNESCO, 2006). The gap between male and female enrollment slightly widens for tertiary or college-level education. Approximately 10% of female and 14% of male students in India continue on to tertiary-level education (UNESCO, 2006).

The Indian University Grants Commission (UGC) is responsible for determination and maintenance of higher education standards, including teaching, examinations, and research. One hundred twenty-two universities and 2,486 colleges/institutions have been officially accredited by the UGC's National Assessment and Accreditation Council in India. The Times Higher Education Supplement (THES) and Quacquarelli Symonds (QS) World University Rankings, as well as the Shanghai Jiao Tong University Academic Ranking of World Universities, have ranked various Indian Institute of Technology (IIT) campuses and the Indian Institute of Science in its Top 500 world universities (Academic Ranking of World Universities, 2008; Quacquarelli Symonds, 2008).

Cultural factors of Asian Indians in the United States

As stated earlier in the chapter, there has been an increasing demographic diversity among Asian Indian immigrants since the 1980s. It is important for a neuropsychologist to understand the variability of cultural factors, such as educational attainment, occupation, English proficiency, and health practices within the Asian Indian community.

The 2000 U.S. census data show that Asian Indian immigrants as a group continue to be highly educated. The majority of Asian Indians in the United States have a bachelor's degree or higher (63.9%), which is the highest percentage of college-educated individuals compared to other Asians American groups. Further, 12.5% of Indian Americans have some college or an associate's degree, 10.3% are high school graduates, and 13.3% have attained less than high school–level education (U.S. Census Bureau, 2004).

Asian Indians in the United States are more likely to work in professional occupations and have a median earning above the national average. In addition, Asian Indians have the highest proportion of representation (59.9%) in management or professional occupations compared to other Asian Americans. Asian Indians are distributed in several different professions, including sales and office occupations (21.4%); production, transportation, and moving (9.4%); service (7.0%); construction, extraction, and maintenance (2.1%); and farming, and fishing and forestry (0.2%). The median family income of Asian Indians in the United States is $70,708. Asian Indian men have the highest median income of all Asian American males, at $51,904. Asian Indian women have a median salary of $35,173, which is generally comparable to that of Chinese and Japanese American women. Approximately 9.8% of the Asian Indians in the United States are below the poverty level (U.S. Census Bureau, 2004).

Due to the history of British colonialism, English has been a commonly used language in India. Many schools as well as college- and university-level education in India are conducted in English. As a result, many of the Asian Indians immigrants are reasonably proficient in English. The majority of the Asian Indian households (57.6%) in the United States reported speaking in proficient English as well as another language at home, and another 19.3% report speaking exclusively English at home (U.S. Census Bureau, 2004). A total of 23.1% of the Asian Indians reported a non-English language as primarily spoken at home and low proficiency in English. Many of the students and professionals who immigrate to the United States are required to take a standardized exam, the Test of English as a Foreign Language (TOEFL), to demonstrate proficiency in English. Out of a maximum TOEFL score of 300, the Indian examinees' mean score was 246 (Educational Testing Service, 2003). It should be noted that these data do not capture the level of English proficiency of Asian Indians immigrants who came to the United States directly to work or work in nonprofessional settings.

However, it is important to note that nearly a quarter of the Asian Indian households reported a non-English language primarily spoken at home and low proficiency in English.

A survey of health practices of Asian Indian immigrants in the United States over the age of 50 found that 55% of the sample reported aerobic activity in lifestyle, 41% were vegetarians, and 52% were of normal weight. Higher fat intake was associated with higher income, increased bicultural or American ethnic identity, and higher levels of depression. Younger age, longer length of residence in the United States, and increased American ethnic identity were associated with a physically active lifestyle (Jonnalagadda & Diwan, 2005).

Approximately 8% of the middle-aged and older Asian Indian immigrants reported fair or poor health in the health practices survey (Jonnalagadda & Diwan, 2005). Cardiovascular risk factors, particularly hypertension (33%) and diabetes (18%), were the most common chronic diseases in the sample. Epidemiological research has fairly consistently found that Asian Indian adults, both in India and abroad, have a significantly higher risk of coronary artery disease without known behavioral and physiological risk factors (Chadha, Radhakrishnan, Ramachandran, Kaul, & Gopinath, 1990; Enas, Yusuf, & Mehta, 1992; Stoney, Hughes, Kuntz, West, & Thornton, 2002). Asian Indians also have a disproportionately higher rate of mortality associated with coronary heart disease than other ethnicities (Wild, Laws, Fortmann, Varady, & Byrne, 1995). There has been a paucity of research on the prevalence of cerebrovascular disease in Asian Indians. One study comparing Chinese, Malaysians, and Indians in Singapore found similar rates of stroke in the three ethnic groups (Venketasubramanian et al., 2005).

Neuropsychological testing

Familiarity with the formal testing process is a critical consideration for neuropsychological testing. There is a wide spectrum of familiarity with formal testing procedure among Asian Indians. On one end of the spectrum, some of the Asian Indians who came to the United States to pursue higher education have demonstrated their familiarity with formal testing by competitively performing on standardized tests such as Graduate Record Examinations (Educational Testing Service, 2008). On the other end of spectrum, some Asian Indians have been unable to participate in routine or standardized neuropsychological testing due to significant cultural differences. Researchers assessing cognitive functioning in rural areas in India encountered difficulties administering seemingly "culture-free" tests, such as Draw-a-Clock Test or orientation. The investigators realized that clocks were not a relevant part of life in the rural samples, and most of the older subjects did not know how to read a clock. Several researchers also found that older, rural, and less educated individuals often did not know their exact date of birth but were able to give the month and year of birth (Chandra et al., 1998a; Bhatnagar et al., 2002). Although the lack of testing familiarity tends to be most pronounced with less educated individuals, it can also appear with varying levels of educational attainment. A normative study of the Wisconsin Card Sort Test (WCST) using normal adult subjects in India with average education of 13.69 years found that there was a statistically significant difference on the majority of indices of the WCST when compared to a Western sample. The authors qualitatively observed that the Indian subjects had difficulty understanding the inherent task demand and were more likely to randomly sort the cards (Kohli & Kaur, 2006).

As familiarity with formal testing procedures can be a significant concern, the usual cautions that nonverbal tests do not always translate across cultural groups also applies with Asian Indians. Some researchers have used a practice test at the start of the testing session to give the examinee at least brief exposure to testing. Chandra and colleagues recommend the practice test should be "a known neuropsychological test; it should be scorable, simple, not require literacy, have a high probability of success, be arranged in increasing order of difficulty, and such that subject listens and responds" (Chandra et al., 1998b, p. 355).

One of the few standardized neuropsychological measures validated with Asian Indians has been the Mini-Mental Status Exam (MMSE). The MMSE is available in several Indian languages, including Hindi, Gujrathi, Kannada, Malayalam, Marathi, Telugu, and Urdu. There are published UK data for the use of Hindi and Gujarati versions in diagnosing moderate to severe dementia. The translated MMSE was reliable in detecting declined cognitive performance over the course of 26 to 32 months (Shah, Lindesay, & Jagger, 1998). Mild dementia was less effectively detected by the translated versions of the MMSE (Lindesay et al., 1997). It should be noted that the translated MMSE consisted of modifications to make the test more appropriate to the examinee, such as using the translation of the phrase "neither this nor that" instead of "no ifs, ands, or buts," and presenting "close your eyes" orally instead of visually.

The Indo-U.S. Cross-National Dementia Epidemiology Study adapted the Consortium to Establish a Registry for Alzheimer's Disease (CERAD) neuropsychology battery and developed norms with 374 neurologically healthy, predominantly illiterate, older Indian adults from a rural community. This battery consists of the Hindi Mini-Mental Status Exam, Wordlist Learning Test, Semantic Fluency, Object Naming Test, and Constructional Praxis. During battery development, the researchers recognized that performance for the group was at the floor level with standardized administration of the tests. The performance distribution improved on some of the tests by making relatively simple modifications, such as showing actual models of more culturally relevant objects instead of the standard line drawings on the Object Naming Test or having more culturally relevant words on the Wordlist Learning Test. Some tests such as Temporal Orientation Test, Phonemic Fluency, Trailmaking, Draw-a-Clock, and Story Memory were completely eliminated from the battery because performance remained at the floor for the group despite various modification attempts (Ganguli et al., 1996).

The All-India Institute of Medical Sciences (AIIMS) Neuropsychological Battery in Hindi was developed to assess global intellectual and memory abilities of adults. The AIIMS battery consists of 160 items on a Memory scale and Intelligence scale. Each item is scored from 0 to 4 depending on the level of accuracy, frequency, speed, quality, and appropriateness. The Memory scale items include recognition of remote and recent memory items, immediate wordlist recall, digit span (forward and backward), immediate design recall, and wordlist and recall with interference. The Intelligence scale includes items of general knowledge, social comprehension, verbal abstractions of similarities and differences, analogies, numerical logic reasoning, maze learning, and identifying missing visual details. A study with surgical epilepsy patients found significant improvements on Memory and Intelligence scales in patients with good seizure control following right anteromesial temporal lobectomy and a nonsignificant trend of improved Memory and Intelligence scores for patients following left anteromesial temporal lobectomy. The authors draw attention to the AIIMS Memory scale being a global assessment of memory that combines different types of memory, including remote memory, working memory, verbal episodic, and visual episodic memory. Due to the global assessment of memory on the AIIMS, the investigators felt that it was not directly comparable to the epilepsy literature that has routinely found material specific (verbal) episodic memory declines following dominant anterior temporal lobectomy (Sanyal et al., 2005).

There have been several investigations of formal neuropsychological tests with Indian children. A modified version of the Mini-Mental Status Exam (MMSE) was found to be sufficiently sensitive and specific in identifying encephalopathy of varied etiology in a group of Indian children compared to a control group (Jain & Passi, 2005). The Malin adaptations of the Wechsler Intelligence Scale for Children (WISC) and Vineland Social Maturity Scales have been widely investigated with Indian children. These tests have been validated and used with a variety of pediatric populations, including cerebral palsy, learning disability, epilepsy, and so forth. (Agarwal, Sitholey, Kumar, & Prasad, 2001; Kohli, Malhotra, Mohanty, Khehra, & Kaur, 2005; Singhi, Bansal, Singhi, & Persad, 1992). In the United States, Cognistat, a neuropsychological screen, has been translated into Hindi, although there are no specific Indian norms (Kiernan, Mueller, Langston, & van Dyke, 2009).

Neuropsychological norms

Ganguli et al. (1995) developed a version of MMSE in Hindi to be used with a primarily illiterate Indian population. The authors made some alterations in items such as substituting "neither this, nor that" for "no ifs, ands, or buts," a simpler diamond within a square figure for the intersecting pentagons, and to "say a sentence" instead of writing a sentence. The test was administered to 100 subjects living in Ballabgarh, a rural suburb outside of New Delhi. The sample consisted of 100 subjects over the age of 55, with a mean of age 70.7 (sd = 9.7). Seventy-four subjects had no education, while 26 completed some education (10 subjects, 1–5 years; 11 subjects, 6–8 years; 5 subjects, 9–10 years). The mean MMSE score for subjects with no education was 21.8 (sd = 4.6), while the mean score for those with some education was 27.6 (sd = 2.3). By comparison, Crum, Anthony, Bassett, & Folstein (1993) reported the following norms on a comparable U.S. sample in the 70- to 74-year age range: 0–4 years education, M = 22 (sd = 1.7); 5–8 years education, M = 26 (sd = 1.8).

MMSE norms for an urban Indian city are reported by Das et al. (2006). The MMSE was revised similarly to Ganguli et al. (1995). Data were collected from 745 subjects living in Kolkata, a city of primarily Bengali- and Hindi-speaking people with relatively high literacy rates (81%). The mean age of subjects was 66.8 (sd = 10, range = 50–80+), while the mean level of education was 7.7 (sd = 5.5, range = 0–13+). The mean MMSE score for the Indian sample was 28.7 (sd = 2.1). The comparable score for the Crum et al. (1993) sample ages 65–69 and 5–8 years of education was M = 26 (sd = 1.8). Although difficult to compare directly due to inexact demographic matching, such as wider age ranges, the Indian sample with some education appeared comparable or slightly higher than Western norms. The lower education group demonstrated similar scores, although with a higher standard deviation.

Norms for animal naming were reported in two studies. Das et al. (2006) reported a mean of 11.8 (sd = 4.5) for their previously described sample (age, M = 66.8; education, M = 7.7). If using Western norms for a comparable demographic (persons age 60–79 with 0–8 years of education) (Tombaugh, Kozak, & Rees, 1999), the mean of the Indian sample would fall near the 25th percentile. When using the Heaton, Miller, Taylor, and Grant (2004) norms, the sample scored at T = 41 and T = 39 for Caucasian males and females, respectively, and T = 48 and T = 50 for African American males and females, respectively. Lower scores were demonstrated in another study evaluating an urban community sample of 153 elderly ages 55–84 (M = 66.9, sd = 5.6) living in Kerala (Mathuranath et al., 2003). Subjects primarily spoke Malayalam. The mean years of education was 7.2 (sd = 6.1). The literacy rate was reported to be relatively high, at 91%. The overall mean for animal fluency was 7.8 (sd = 3.6), which would translate to a mean score of less than 10% according to Tombaugh et al. (1999) norms. When using age and education norms provided by Heaton et al. (2004), the Mathuranath et al. (2003) sample scored at the T = 28 and T = 26 levels for Caucasian males and females, respectively, and at the T = 36 and T = 38 levels for African American males and females, respectively.

Normative data for a 10-item verbal learning task similar to the Hopkins Verbal Learning Test–Revised (HVLT-R) (Brandt & Benedict, 2001) are reported in two studies. Yepthomi et al. (2006) administered an adapted version of the HVLT-R to a sample of 30 primarily Telegu-speaking subjects with a mean age of 34 (sd = 10.4) who average 9.7 years of education (sd = 4.4). The mean total score of the three immediate recall trials was 21.7 (sd = 5.2), while the delayed score was 8.2 (sd = 2.1). These scores are considerably lower than the HVLT-R normative 30- to 39-year-old sample in the 30- to 39-year-old range (M = 34.5, sd = 2.9), who had a significantly higher education level (M = 13.9, sd = 1.8). The score for the normative Western sample immediate recall was M = 28.0 (sd = 4.4), while the mean score for delayed recall was 9.2 (sd = 2.0). Scores were also lower in the older Das et al. (2006) sample (mean age = 66.8). The immediate total recall score was 16.8 (sd = 3.8), while the delayed recall score was 5.0 (sd = 1.8). In comparison, the scores for the normative sample were 26.7 (sd = 4.5) for immediate total recall and 9.5 (sd = 1.9) for delayed recall. Again, the normative Western sample demonstrated a significantly higher education level (M = 14.32, sd = 3.0) than the Indian sample (M = 7.7, sd = 5.5); however, MMSE scores were comparable (Indian MMSE = 28.7, sd = 2.1; normative sample, MMSE = 28.5, sd = 1.6).

On the Brief Visuospatial Memory Test–Revised (Benedict, 1997), the Yepthomi et al. (2006) sample earned a mean score of 16.1 (sd = 8.0) for total learning and 6.6 (sd = 3.6) for total recall. These scores would fall at the 5th (M = 13.4, sd = 1.8) and 14th (M = 7.8, sd = 13.0) percentiles, respectively, when using norms for the standardization sample. Again, it should be stressed that the Benedict (1997) original sample had a higher level of education (M = 13.4, sd = 1.8), and thus direct comparisons are difficult to make.

Yepthomi et al. (2006) also reported norms for several other commonly used Western neuropsychological tests, including the Grooved Pegboard, Color Trails, and Golden's Stroop Interference trial. In general, the Indian sample demonstrated lower scores when compared to Western norms, although education levels are not always comparable (education, M = 9.7, sd = 4.4). For example, on the Golden Stroop Interference trial, the Indian sample completed a mean of 25.1 cards (sd = 8.9) in 45 seconds, compared to an average of 47.1 cards (sd = 7.9) for the Mitrushina, Boone, Razani, and D'Elia (2005) meta-analysis, where the mean overall education level was 13.5 (sd = 2.33). On the Grooved Pegboard, the Indian dominant-hand mean score was 77.1 (sd = 22.5), while for the nondominant hand the score was 81.9 (sd = 13.8). When using the Heaton et al. (2004) age and education corrected norms, the Indian sample would score at the T = 35 and T = 31 level when using norms for Caucasian males and at the T = 40 and T = 39 level when using norms for African American males, for dominant and nondominant hands, respectively.

Finally, Yepthomi et al. (2006) reported data on Color Trails 1 and 2 with mean scores of 59.8 (sd = 20.5) and 138.5 (sd = 50.1), respectively. Although not entirely comparable in terms of demographics, these scores appear similar to norms collected for a subject with 7–9 years of education in the People's Republic of China (CT 1 M = 55.6, sd = 30.4; CT 2 M = 128.0, sd = 77.2) (Hsieh & Riley, 1997), and a sample of Spanish-speaking males (CT 1M = 49.2, sd = 10.9; CT 2 116.3, sd = 39.4) and females (CT1 M = 49.6, sd = 13.8; CT M = 114.1, sd = 49.8) aged 30–39 with less than 10 years of education who were living in the United States (Ponton et al., 1996).

It should be stressed that these comparative test performances between Asian Indian and Western samples are highly influenced by differences in educational levels and exact age ranges. Thus, clinicians should not automatically assume that Asian Indians will score more poorly on the aforementioned neuropsychological tests. Data comparisons were provided to help guide clinicians in test selection and interpretation and can particularly guard against false positives for determining impairment.

Other Western tests

Other Western neuropsychological tests have been translated into Hindi that may facilitate administration to a primarily Hindi-speaking client. However, these tests do not have norms for a strictly Hindi sample; thus, test scores would have to be interpreted with caution. The Bilingual Verbal Abilities Test (BVAT) (Munoz-Sandoval, Cummins, Alvarado, & Ruef, 1998) evaluates language skills in both English and Hindi, which may provide useful information for interpreting neuropsychological test scores on Western tests with a strong language component. The BVAT consists of three subtests from the Woodcock-Johnson Revised Tests of Cognitive Ability and Language Proficiency Battery–Revised: Picture Vocabulary (58 items), Oral Vocabulary Synonyms (20 items) and Antonyms (20 items), and Verbal Analogies (35 items). The test requires a bilingual administrator or interpreter and takes approximately 30 minutes to complete. Items are administered in English, and missed items are then administered in the client's native language. Norms range from 5 to 90. Cognistat (Kiernan et al., 2009) is a brief 20-minute cognitive screen that evaluates for orientation, language, short-term memory, visual spatial skills, calculations, abstractions, and judgment. Cognistat has been frequently used to evaluate for dementia.

Case sample

Mr. A was a 48-year-old, married, right-handed Asian Indian man with a 14-year history of seizures. He was referred for neuropsychological assessment as part of a larger workup of his intractable epilepsy and consideration of an anterior temporal lobectomy. His other workup revealed complex partial seizures of left temporal origin on EEG and left mesial temporal sclerosis on MRI. Current medications were pregabalin and phenobarbital. Other medical or psychiatric history was unremarkable.

English was Mr. A's third language, with Punjabi and Hindi being first and second languages. He appeared reasonably proficient in English during the clinical interview and indicated much of his formal education was conducted in India in English. The patient reported no learning difficulties in school. He had obtained a bachelor's degree in physics in an English-language curriculum, and had been employed in India as a teacher. He had emigrated from India three years prior to the assessment. He was employed in the United States as a bookkeeper. Mr. A reported having cognitive difficulties in learning new procedures at work as well as slowed processing speed. His wife confirmed greater memory problems and difficulties at work.

For Mr. A's neuropsychological assessment, the following information from background history was considered. The first consideration was English proficiency. Mr. A's English was judged to be adequate for testing based on his English reading skills on formal testing as well as proficiency of English in conversations. However, the battery was structured to limit the English demand on any particular task (e.g., presented Wordlist Memory Test instead of Story Memory Test). A Punjabi interpreter was available during the assessment to ensure comprehension of testing procedures. Second consideration was the patient's level of familiarity with formal testing. Mr. A's history of no learning difficulties in formal schooling and college-level education was felt to demonstrate adequate familiarity with formal testing procedures. The third consideration was previous and current occupational status. It was noted that Mr. A was reporting greater occupational difficulties than at his previous employment in India. The Punjabi Mini-Mental Status Exam was administered to obtain a gross estimate of global cognitive abilities, which was within normal limits. Finally, acculturation level was considered. His recent immigration and socialization primarily within the Asian Indian community suggested a lower level of acculturation. This raised concerns about the cultural relevance of the tests. Effort was made to present more culturally relevant tests. For example, the battery did not include tests that required recognition of items that are more widely prevalent in American society (e.g., "pretzel," "beaver" on Boston Naming Test) or knowledge of American history (Wechsler Adult Intelligence Scale–Information subtest).

The test battery was selected to assess across various cognitive domains, with particular interest in memory and verbal abilities due to the left temporal lobe abnormalities noted in his EEG and MRI studies. Neuropsychological findings estimated premorbid functioning to be in the average range (WRAT-IV Reading SS = 99; Wilkinson & Robertson, 2006) with a low average IQ (FSIQ = 82) on the Wechsler Abbreviated Scale of Intelligence (Psychological Corporation, 1999). His weakest performances were on tests of verbal memory (CVLT-II; Delis, Kramer, Kaplan, & Ober, 2000), psychomotor speed (WAIS-III Processing Speed Index; Wechsler, 1997a), and verbal fluency (DKEFS–Verbal Fluency; Delis, Kaplan, & Kramer, 2001), in the mild to moderately impaired range. He had intact language comprehension. His nonverbal abilities on the Judgment of Line Orientation (Benton, Varney, & Hamsher, 1978), WASI (Block Design, Matrix Reasoning), and Wechsler Memory Scale–III (Faces, Visual Reproduction; Wechsler, 1997b) were low average to average.

Ideally, neuropsychological assessment would be conducted using instruments developed in the patient's primary language and interpreted using normative data with demographic cohorts that match the patient. However, this was not possible with Mr. A. As such, his results should be interpreted cautiously. The primary purpose of the testing was to establish a presurgical baseline of his cognitive abilities. Pattern analysis of Mr. A's test results was consistent with his EEG and MRI findings of left (presumed dominant) temporal lobe dysfunction. It was also felt that his antiepileptic medications were contributing to his reduced processing speed that was noted on testing. While the results may not have been precise, it was felt that a neuropsychological assessment would provide quantitative data of his presurgical cognitive functioning. It was important to establish a presurgical baseline for comparison of potential cognitive morbidity after his temporal lobectomy.

Summary

In summary, Asian Indians in the United States are a diverse cultural group. It is essential that neuropsychologists have an adequate understanding of a range of cultural factors when choosing appropriate neuropsychological assessment tools. The patient's education level, proficiency of English and native languages, gender, socioeconomic status, level of acculturation, and urban or rural background may be important factors that influence testing performance. In the absence of peer-match Asian Indian norms, it may be appropriate to utilize standard American norms with well-educated, English-proficient, and well-acculturated Asian Indian immigrants (Fujii & Wong, 2005). The authors caution that these norm-based data should be interpreted cautiously, particularly taking into account culturally biased items. They recommend the clinician acquire corroborating evidence with school or other testing records for information regarding premorbid functioning. The norm-based approach would not be recommended for Asian Indians with limited knowledge of English, poor acculturation, or lower educational attainment. As evidenced by differences in comparability of Western and Indian norms across tests and for different samples of the Indian population, the diagnostic validity of tests can be threatened by using inappropriate normative information. Fujii and Wong (2005) recommend using a hypothesis testing–based approach with these individuals. The hypothesis testing approach relies on knowledge of brain-behavior relationships and expected consequence of neurological disorder. Cultural considerations and neuroimaging would also need to be integrated to obtain meaningful interpretation of test data. Ideally, using cognitive tests developed in India or normed with the patient's cohort would be desirable.

References

Academic Ranking of World Universities. (2008). *Top 500 world universities.* Retrieved January 3, 2009, from http://www.arwu.org/rank2008/EN2008.htm

Adler, L., & Gielen, U. (2003). *Migration: Immigration and emigration in international perspective.* Westport, CT: Greenwood Publishing Group.

Agarwal, V., Sitholey, P., Kumar, S., & Prasad, M. (2001). Double-blind, placebo controlled trial of clonidine in hyperactive children with mental retardation. *Mental Retardation, 39*, 259–267.

Asian Pacific American Legal Center of Southern California. (2005). *The diverse face of Asians and Pacific Islanders in California.* Retrieved January 4, 2009, from http://apalc.org/demographics/wp-content/uploads/2006/11/caapalc0905.pdf

Baptiste, D. A. (2005). Family therapy with East Indian immigrant parents rearing children in the United States: Parental concerns, therapeutic issues, and recommendations. *Contemporary Family Therapy, 27*, 345–366.

Benedict, R. (1997). *Brief visuospatial memory test-revised.* Odessa, FL: Psychological Assessment Resources.

Benson, S. (Ed.). (2004). *Asian Indian, Korean, and Southeast Asian immigration* (Vol. 2). Detroit, MI: U-X-L.

Benton, A., Varney, N., & Hamsher, K. (1978). Visuospatial judgment: A clinical test. *Archives of Neurology, 35,* 364–367.

Berry, J. W., & Annis, R. C. (1974). Acculturative stress. *Journal of Cross-Cultural Psychology, 5,* 382–406.

Bhatnagar, S., Jain, S., Bihari, M., Bansal, N., Pauranik, A., Jain, D., ... Padma, M. (2002). Aphasia type and aging in Hindi-speaking stroke patients. *Brain and Language, 83*, 353–361.

Brandt, J., & Benedict, R. (2001). *Hopkins Verbal Learning Test–Revised. Professional manual.* Lutz, FL: Psychological Assessment Resources, Inc.

Chadha, S., Radhakrishnan, S., Ramachandran, K., Kaul, U., & Gopinath, N. (1990). Epidemiological study of coronary heart disease in urban population of Delhi. *Indian Journal of Medical Research, 92*, 424–430.

Chandra, V., Ganguli, M., Pandav, R., Johnston, J., Belle, S., & DeKosky, S. (1998). Prevalence of Alzheimer's disease and other dementias in rural India. *Neurology, 51*, 1000–1008.

Chandra, V., Ganguli, M., Ratcliff, G., Pandav, R., Sharma, S., Belle, S., ... Nath, L. (1998). Practical issues in cognitive screening of elderly illiterate populations in developing countries. The Indo-US cross-national dementia epidemiology study. *Aging: Clinical and Experimental Research, 10,* 349–357.

Crum, R., Anthony, J., Bassett, S., & Folstein, M. (1993). Population-based norms for the Mini-Mental State Examination by age and educational level. *Journal of the American Medication Association, 269,* 2386–2391.

Danielou, A. (2003). *A brief history of India.* Rochester, VT: Inner Traditions.

Das, S. (2002). Loss or gain? A saga of Asian Indian immigration and experiences in America's multi-ethnic mosaic. *Race, Gender, & Class, 9*, 131–155.

Das, S., Banerjee, T., Mukherjee, C., Bose, P., Biswas, A., et al. (2006). An urban community-based study of cognitive function among non-demented elderly population in India. *Neurology Asia, 11*, 37–48.

Delis, D., Kaplan, E., & Kramer, J. (2001). *Delis-Kaplan Executive Function System.* San Antonio, TX: The Psychological Corporation.

Delis, D., Kramer, J., Kaplan, E., & Ober, B. (2000). *California Verbal Learning Test* (2nd ed., adult version). San Antonio, TX: The Psychological Corporation.

Davies, K., Bell, B., Bush, A., & Wyler, A. (1998). Prediction of verbal memory loss in individuals after anterior temporal lobectomy. *Epilepsia, 39*, 820–828.

Dugsin, R. (2001). Conflict and healing in family experience of second-generation emigrants from India living in North America. *Family Process, 40,* 233–241.

Educational Testing Service. (2003). *TOEFL test and score data summary.* Retrieved January 3, 2009, from http://ftp.ets.org/pub/toefl/0203test_year_data.pdf

Educational Testing Service. (2008). *Graduate record examination.* Princeton, NJ: Author.

Enas, E., Yusuf, S., & Mehta, J. (1992). Prevalence of coronary artery disease in Asian Indians. *American Journal of Cardiology, 70,* 945–949.

Fujii, D., & Wong, T. (2005). Neuropsychological assessment with Asian-American immigrants: Recommendations for meeting *Daubert* standards. *Journal of Forensic Neuropsychology, 4*(4), 3–31.

Ganguli, M., Chandra, V., Gilby, J., Ratcliff, G., Sharma, S., Pandav, R., et al. (1996). Cognitive test performance in a community-based nondemented elderly sample in rural India: The Indo-U.S. Cross-National Dementia Epidemiology Study. *International Psychogeriatrics, 8,* 507–524.

Ganguli, M., Ratcliff, G., Chandra, V., Sharma, S., et al. (1995). A Hindi version of the MMSE: The development of a cognitive screening instrument for a largely illiterate rural elderly population in India. *International Journal of Geriatric Psychiatry, 10,* 367–377.

Heaton, R., Miller, S., Taylor, M., & Grant, I. (2004). *Revised comprehensive norms for an expanded Halstead-Reitan battery: Demographically adjusted neuropsychological norms for African American and Caucasian adults.* Lutz, FL: Psychological Assessment Resources.

Holmes, R. (2006). The THES university rankings: Are they really world class? *Asian Journal of University of Education, 1*, 1–14.

Hsieh, S., & Riley, N. (1997, November). *Neuropsychological performance in the People's Republic of China: Age and educational norms for four attention tasks.* Paper presented at the National Academy of Neuropsychology, Las Vegas, NV.

Jain, M., & Passi, G. (2005). Assessment of a modified Mini-Mental Scale for cognitive functions in children. *Indian Pediatrics, 42,* 907–912.

Jonnalagadda, S., & Diwan, S. (2005). Health behaviors, chronic disease prevalence and self-rated health of older Asian Indian immigrants in the U.S. *Journal of Immigrant Health, 7*(2), 75–83.

Kiernan, R., Mueller, J., Langston, J., & van Dyke, C. (2009). *2009 Cognistat manual.* Fairfax, CA: Novatek International.

Kohli, A., & Kaur, M. (2006). Wisconsin Card Sorting Test: Normative data and experience. *Indian Journal of Psychiatry, 48,* 181–184.

Kohli, A., Malhotra, S., Mohanty, M., Khehra, N., & Kaur, M. (2005). Specific learning disabilities in children: Deficits and neuropsychological profile. *International Journal of Rehabilitation Research, 28,* 165–169.

Krishnan, A., & Berry, J. W. (1992). Acculturative stress and acculturation attitudes among Indian immigrants to the United States. *Psychology and Developing Societies, 4,* 187–212.

Kulke, H., & Rothermund, D. (2004). *A history of India* (4th ed.). New York, NY: Routledge.

Leonard, K. I. (1997). *The South Asian Americans.* Westport, CT: Greenwood Press.

Lindesay, J., Jagger, C., Mlynik-Szmid, A., Sinorwala, A., Peet, S., & Moledina, F. (1997). The Mini-Mental State Examination (MMSE) in an elderly immigrant Gujarati population in the United Kingdom. *International Journal of Geriatric Psychiatry, 12,* 1155–1167.

Liu, N., Cheng, Y., & Liu, L. (2005). Academic ranking of world universities using scientometrics. *Scientometrics, 64,* 101–109.

Malin, A. (1969). *Manual for Malin's intelligence scale for Indian children (MISIC).* Lucknow, India: Indian Psychological Corporation.

Mathuranath, P., George, A., Cherian, P., Alexander, A., Sarma, S., & Sarma, P. (2003). Effects of age, education and gender on verbal fluency. *Journal of Clinical and Experimental Neuropsychology, 25,* 1057–1064.

Mitrushina, M., Boone, K., Razani, J., & D'Elia, L. (2005). *Handbook of normative data for neuropsychological assessment.* New York, NY: Oxford University Press.

Munoz-Sandoval, A. F., Cummins, J., Alvarado, C. G., & Ruef, M. L. (1998). *Bilingual Verbal Ability Tests.* Itasca, IL: Riverside Publishing.

Naidis, M. (1966). *India: A short introductory history.* New York, NY: The Macmillan Company.

Panicker, A., & Hirisave, U. (2004). WISC-III and MISIC: A comparative study. *Journal of the Indian Academy of Applied Psychology, 30*(1–2), 106–112.

Ponton, M., Satz, P., Herrera, L., Ortiz, F. Urrutia, C., Young, R., et al. (1996). Normative data stratified by age and education for the Neuropsychological Screening Battery for Hispanics (NeSBHIS): Initial report. *Journal of the International Neuropsychological Society, 2,* 96–104.

Prathikanti, S. (1997). East Indian American families. In E. Lee (Ed.), *Working with Asian Americans: A guide for clinicians* (pp. 79–100). New York, NY: Guilford Press.

Psychological Corporation. (1999). *Wechsler abbreviated scale of intelligence.* San Antonio, TX: Author.

Quacquarelli Symonds. (2008). *THE QS World University Rankings 2008.* Retrieved January 4, 2009, from http://www.topuniversities.com/worlduniversityrankings/results/2008/overall_rankings/fullrankings

Ramakrishna, J., & Weiss, M. G. (1992). Health, illness, and immigration. East Indians in the United States. *Western Journal of Medicine, 157,* 265–270.

Rangaswamy, P. (2000). *Namaste America.* University Park, PA: Pennsylvania State University Press.

Roysircar, G. (2003). Religious differences: Psychological and sociopolitical aspects of counseling. *International Journal for the Advancement of Counseling, 25,* 255–267.

Sanyal, S., Chandra, P. S., Gupta, S., Tripathi, M., Singh, V., Jain, S., … Mehta, V. (2005). Memory and intelligence outcome following surgery for intractable temporal lobe epilepsy: Relationship to seizure outcome and evaluation using a customized neuropsychological battery. *Epilepsy & Behavior, 6,* 147–155.

Shah, A., Lindesay, J., & Jagger, C. (1998). Is the diagnosis of dementia stable over time among elderly immigrant Gujaratis in the United Kingdom (Leicester)? *International Journal of Geriatric Psychiatry, 13,* 440–444.

Shaji, S., Promodu, K., Abraham, T., Roy, J., & Verghese, A. (1996). An epidemiological study of dementia in a rural community in Kerala, India. *British Journal of Psychiatry, 168,* 745–749.

Shukla, S. (2003). *India abroad: Diasporic cultures of postwar American and England.* Princeton, NJ: Princeton University Press.

Singhi, P., Bansal, U., Singhi, S., & Pershad, D. (1992). Determinants of IQ profile in children with idiopathic generalized epilepsy. *Epilepsia, 33,* 1106–1114.

Stoney, C., Hughes, J., Kuntz, K., West, S., & Thornton, L. (2002). Cardiovascular stress responses among Asian Indian and European American women and men. *Annals of Behavioral Medicine, 24,* 113–121.

Tombaugh, T., Kozak, J., & Rees, L. (1999). Normative data stratified by age and education for two measures of verbal fluency: FAS and animal naming. *Archives of Clinical Neuropsychology, 14,* 167–177.

UNESCO Institute of Statistics. (2005). *Statistics in brief India.* Retrieved January 4, 2009, from www.uis.unesco.org/profiles/EN/EDU/countryProfile_en.aspx?code=3560

UNESCO. (2006). *UIS statistics in brief (India).* Retrieved January 4, 2009, from http://www.uis.unesco.org

United Nations Educational, Scientific and Cultural Organization. (2003). *Education for all: National plan of action India.* Retrieved January 4, 2009, from http://planipolis.iiep.unesco.org/upload/India/India_EFA_plan.pdf

U.S. Census Bureau. (2002). *Profile of general demographic characteristics: 2000.* Retrieved January 4, 2009, from http://www.census.gov/prod/2002pubs/c2kprof00-us.pdf

U.S. Census Bureau. (2004). *We the people: Asians in the United States.* Retrieved January 4, 2009, from http://www.census.gov/prod/2004pubs/censr-17.pdf

Vas, C., Pinto, C., Panikker, D., Noronha, S., Deshpande, N., Kulkarni, L., et al. (2001). Prevalence of dementia in an urban Indian population. *International Psychogeriatrics, 13,* 439–450.

Venketasubramanian, N., Tan, L., Sahadevan, S., Chin, J., Krishnamoorthy, E., Hong, C., & Saw, S. (2005). Prevalence of stroke among Chinese, Malay, and Indian Singaporeans: A community-based tri-racial cross-sectional survey. *Stroke, 36,* 551–556.

Wechsler, D. (1997a). *Wechsler adult intelligence scale–III.* San Antonio, TX: The Psychological Corporation.

Wechsler, D. (1997b). *Wechsler memory scale–III.* San Antonio, TX: The Psychological Corporation.

Wild, S., Laws, A., Fortmann, S., Varady, A., & Byrne, C. (1995). Mortality from coronary heart disease and stroke for six ethnic groups in California, 1985 to 1990. *Annals of Epidemiology, 5,* 432–439.

Wilkinson, G., & Robertson, G. (2006). *Wide Range achievement test–4.* Wilmington, DE: Wide Range, Inc.

Wolpert, S. (1991). *India.* Berkeley, CA: University of California Press.

Yepthomi, T., Paul, R., Vallabhaneni, S., Kumarasamy, N., Tat, D., Solomon, S., & Flanigan, T. (2006). Neurocognitive consequences of HIV in southern India: A preliminary study of clade C virus. *Journal of the International Neuropsychological Society, 12,* 424–430.

7 Neuropsychology of Japanese Americans

William T. Tsushima, Vincent G. Tsushima, and Daryl Fujii

A review of the neuropsychological literature of the past 25 years suggests that issues of race, ethnicity, and culture have been generally ignored (Puente & Perez Garcia, 2000a). Some neuropsychological reports are available on African Americans and Hispanic Americans, but similar research on Japanese Americans and other Asian Americans is virtually nonexistent. Available data pertinent to the neuropsychological assessment of Japanese Americans appear in publications outside of neuropsychology, such as social psychology, cross-cultural, or educational journals and textbooks. Thus, neuropsychologists, as a whole, are probably uninformed regarding characteristics of Japanese Americans that could be related to their performance on neuropsychological tests.

The aims of the present chapter are to (1) present a brief history of the Japanese in America, (2) describe the status of education in Japan, (3) provide results of psychological testing in Japan, (4) summarize the presence of neuropsychology in Japan, (5) present research that is pertinent to the neuropsychological assessment of Japanese Americans, (6) highlight the psychological and cultural variables that are germane in the neuropsychological assessment of ethnic minority individuals, (7) provide the results of a comparative study of Japanese and Caucasian Americans on varied subtests of the Halstead-Reitan Neuropsychological Battery, and (8) offer some maxims for the examiner of Japanese American patients.

Brief history of the Japanese in America

People from Japan began migrating to the United States following the widespread sociocultural and political changes of the Meiji Restoration (1868–1912), which marked the beginning of the modern era of Japan. In 1869 the first group of people to arrive from Japan was 22 settlers at Gold Hill, California, where they built the Wakamatsu Tea and Silk Farm Colony. The immigrants brought mulberry trees, silk cocoons, tea plants, and bamboo roots. By 1880, 148 Japanese lived in the United States.

Japanese laborers were able to leave their country legally only after 1884, when an agreement was signed between Japan and Hawaiian sugar plantations. Japanese men were recruited for their expertise in agriculture, their work ethic, and their willingness to travel. By 1890, 2,038 Japanese resided in America, providing labor in Hawaii sugarcane and pineapple plantations and California fruit and produce farms. By the turn of the century more than 300,000 men and women left Japan for Hawaii and the U.S. Pacific Coast.

As with the Chinese, the welcoming of Japanese immigrants decreased as their numbers increased. With pressure from the Asiatic Exclusion League and others, President Theodore Roosevelt in 1907 negotiated a "gentlemen's agreement" that called for Japan to issue passports to Japanese coming to the continental United States only if they were joining a parent, husband, or child, or to return to a former home or farm. This agreement greatly diminished Japanese emigration to America, except the many "picture brides"—women who arrived for arranged marriages to Japanese laborers. A movement to exclude Japanese newcomers totally led to the U.S. Immigration Act of 1925, also known as the Oriental Exclusion Act, which banned immigration from Japan until 1952, when 100 immigrants per year were allowed.

The ban on immigration produced well-defined generational groups within the Japanese American community. The generation who migrated to America before 1924 became known as the Issei (first generation), and their U.S.-born children are the Nisei (second generation). The Nisei became a distinct cohort from the Issei generation in terms of age, citizenship, education, and English language ability, as well as the usual generational differences. Many of the Nisei married other Nisei, producing a third distinct generation of Japanese Americans, the Sansei (third generation).

Culturally the Issei spoke Japanese and were strongly identified with Japan, the Nisei acculturated in America but tended to be bicultural, while the Sansei were primarily American in orientation (Kitano, 1993). The generational significances may be fading with advancing generations, such as the Yonsei (fourth generation) and Gosei (fifth generation), who appear to be highly Americanized, particularly with the increasing numbers of interracial marriages among Japanese Americans.

The Japanese immigration that ceased in 1925 resumed after the Immigration Reform Act of 1965, which ended 40 years of bans against immigration from Japan and other countries. In recent years, immigration from Japan has declined and has been similar to Western Europe, on average 5,000 to 10,000 per year, in contrast to the larger numbers migrating from the rest of Asia. The major reasons for the reduced immigration from Japan appeared to be the residual anti-Japanese sentiment following World War II and Japan's robust economy in the latter part of the twentieth century. More recent immigrants have included expatriate professionals and businessmen, former college students who studied in America, and military wives (Gondo, 2009). Additionally, the economic boom in Japan has sent about 100,000 Japanese executives of U.S. subsidiaries of Japanese companies to America, who stay for three to five years while maintaining their Japanese citizenship (Gondo, 2009). Similarly, college students, although technically not immigrants, are a significant group of Japanese nationals living in the United States.

Like other immigrants to the United States, the Japanese encountered discrimination in their new country. In 1905, the Asiatic Exclusion League urged the San Francisco Board of Education to require all Japanese and Korean children to join the Chinese at the segregated Oriental School established in 1884. Beginning in 1909, and continuing until after World War II, anti-Japanese bills were introduced every year into the California legislature. In 1921, California established separate schools for Japanese, Chinese, Indian, and other Asian children, who attended segregated schools until the law was amended in 1947. In 1922, the U.S. Supreme Court ruled in *Takao Ozawa v. United States* that Ozawa, as a Mongolian, did not have the right of naturalization, thus ruling that Japanese were ineligible for U.S. citizenship. The most infamous discriminatory act toward Japanese Americans was Executive Order 9066, signed by President Franklin D. Roosevelt on February 19, 1942, which established 10 relocation centers in California, Idaho, Utah, Arizona, Colorado, New Mexico, and Arkansas during World War II. This wartime decree ordered the incarceration in internment camps of more than 120,000 Japanese Americans, over two-thirds of whom were U.S. citizens. In 1968 the U.S. government acknowledged the injustices and began reparations to Japanese Americans for property they had lost during the war, and in 1988, the U.S. Congress passed legislation that awarded $20,000 to each of the 600,000 surviving internees.

Japanese Americans have historically been among the three largest Asian American communities, but in recent decades they have become the sixth largest Asian group in the United States, behind the Chinese, Asian Indian, Filipino, Vietnamese, and Korean groups. According to the U.S. Bureau of the Census, there are 833,761 Japanese Americans, accounting for 6.7% of all Asians in the United States (U.S. Bureau of the Census, 2005). The largest Japanese American communities reside in California, Hawaii, Washington, New York, and Illinois.

Education in Japan

Japan is known for its well-maintained educational system and outstanding academic achievement. The literacy rate is roughly 95%, compared to 88% in the United States. A Japanese high school diploma is considered to be equal to two years of American college (Ellington, 2001). Japanese children consistently rank at or near the top in international tests of mathematics and science. A comparison of 13-year-olds' average scores in math and science indicated that Japan was ranked fifth, behind Singapore, Taiwan, South Korea, and Hong Kong, while the United States was ranked twelfth (International Association for the Evaluation of Educational Achievement, 2003).

A mathematics test administered to first-grade and fifth-grade children in Japan, Taiwan, and the United States indicated that those from Asia consistently performed at a higher level that their American counterparts (Stigler, Lee, Lucker, & Stevenson, 1982). In a subsequent study, Chinese children surpassed Japanese and American children in scores, while both Chinese and Japanese children obtained higher mathematics scores than American children (Stevenson et al., 1985). However, the children from the three countries performed similarly in a battery of 10 cognitive tasks. The results suggested that the higher academic achievement of Japanese and Chinese children was not attributed to higher intellectual abilities, but to their experiences at home and school.

In a more recent study, first graders in Japan, China, and the United States were given achievement and cognitive tests, and retested 10 years later with achievement tests (Chen, Lee, & Stevenson, 1996). Japanese and Chinese students at both grades had higher mathematics scores than the American students. American and Chinese students received higher reading scores than the Japanese students at both grades. The family's socioeconomic status was the most significant predictive variable pertaining to the academic achievement in all three countries.

In recent decades, the Japanese have accepted English as the current international language, and have included English as a compulsory subject in their schools. Japanese students now have at least six years of English in school, and four more years for those who attend college. It is also common for Japanese parents to have their children from the age of 5 learn English in private, after-school settings. This does not mean that most Japanese can speak English; however, the number of English speakers is increasing.

Psychological test results in Japan

Measures of intellectual functioning in children in Japan have been recorded in a number of investigations. Table 7.1 shows IQs on various American tests of intelligence, largely reported by British psychologist Richard Lynn, who became known for his controversial views on racial and ethnic differences. He asserted that the Japanese have the highest intelligence in the world (Lynn, 1977), and proposed that their abilities should be regarded as genetically programmed (Lynn, 1987), or influenced by early childhood nutrition (Lynn, 2006). Lynn also opined that the Japanese superior perceptual and spatial abilities could be due to advantageous environmental conditions (Lynn & Hampson, 1986b), and their better performance in mathematics was due to superior teaching efficiency in Japanese schools (Lynn, 1987).

While Lynn received recognition and support in some circles (Herrnstein & Murray, 1994; Lykken, 2004), his work has been severely criticized for its lack of scientific objectivity, data misrepresentation, and racism (Kamin, 1995); failure to control for socioeconomic status and location of residence (rural vs. urban) (Stevenson & Azuma, 1983); inappropriate comparisons and data omission (Flynn, 1983); and statistical errors and incorrect assumptions about subtests (Kaufman, McLean, Ishikuma, & Moon, 1989). Other researchers found no overall difference between Japanese, Chinese, and American children on a battery of cognitive tasks and school achievement tests (Stevenson et al., 1985). Suzuki and her associates (1997, 2005) state that the factors associated with intelligence go beyond genetic influences and involve socioeconomic status, home intellectual climate, and educational attainments. They further oppose racial-ethnic generalizations about intelligence, citing numerous studies that demonstrate greater within-group differences than between-group differences. A comprehensive discussion of the issues regarding the intelligence scores of the Japanese is beyond the scope of this chapter.

Neuropsychology in Japan

The field of neuropsychology in Japan has its roots at the end of the nineteenth century, with the first known treatise on aphasia in 1893 by Onishi (Hamanaka, 1994).

Table 7.1 Results of intelligence testing with Japanese children

Subjects	*Tests*	*Results*	*Reference*
Japanese and Ainu 6-year-olds	Goodenough-Harris drawing test	Mean IQ 138	Hilger, Klett, & Watson, 1976
Japanese 13- to 15-year-olds	Differential Aptitude Tests	Mean IQ 104.5 for abstract reasoning Mean IQ 114 for spatial ability	Lynn, Hampson, & Iwawaki, 1987
Japanese standardization sample	WISC Performance (Performance subtests and Digit Span)	IQ 102	Lynn, 1977
Japanese standardization sample	WAIS (Digit Symbol, Block Design, and Digit Span)	IQ 102	Lynn, 1977
Japanese standardization sample	WISC-R	FSIQ 103	Lynn & Hampson, 1986a
Japanese children ages 4–9	Columbia Mental Maturity Scale	IQ 107	Misawa, Motegi, Fujita, & Hattori, 1984
Japanese children ages 2½–8½	McCarthy Scales of Children's Abilities	Average general IQ, low verbal, high perceptual	Lynn & Hampson, 1986b
Japanese children ages 4–5	WPPSI	Average general IQ, low verbal, high perceptual	Lynn & Hampson, 1987
Japanese children grades 1–5	10 cognitive tasks and achievement tests in reading and mathematics	Similar to American and Chinese children	Stevenson et al., 1985

At the beginning of the twentieth century, Japanese neuroscientists examined aphasic patients and their functioning with the dual writing system, kanji and kana. These two distinct systems of letters that have been used in the Japanese language for more than 1200 years continue to be the focus of scientific investigation (Iwata, 2007).

The first neuropsychological monograph in Japan was published in 1935, citing the significance of the apractoagnostic aspects of apraxic disorders (Akimoto, 1976). Ohashi (1960) authored the first comprehensive textbook of neuropsychology in Japan. Contemporary neuropsychology flourished in the 1970s with the establishment of the Japanese Society of Aphasiology in 1975 and the Neuropsychological Association of Japan in 1977 (Murai, Hadano, & Hamanaka, 2002). Several Japanese translations of classic textbooks and authoritative books in European, Russian, and American neuropsychology were published, including the works of Broca, Wernicke, and Luria.

In recent years, neuropsychological research in Japan has been devoted to the dementias, frontal lobe syndromes, and memory disorders. There has been considerable interest in aphasia, alexia, and agraphia, as well as to the disconnection syndrome and specific right-hemisphere syndromes (Hamanaka, 1994; Murai et al., 2002). A number of pioneering efforts by Japanese researchers have appeared in international publications, such as the *Journal of the International Neuropsychological Society* (e.g., Matsui et al., 2007).

Neurolinguistic impairments related to the unique orthographic and grammatical characteristics of the Japanese written language have been the focus of considerable research in Japan. Sasanuma (1986), for example, identified at least four combinations of *kanji* (ideo-phonogram) deficits and *kana* (phonogram) deficits in alexia-agraphia associated with various aphasic syndromes. In a series of case studies, Iwata (2007) reported patients whose kanji reading was severely impaired, while showing no difficulty in reading and writing kana. The kanji alexia and agraphia were attributed to lesions affecting the left posterior inferior temporal area, confirmed by PET scan findings. As a result of these findings, Iwata proposed a new model of neural circuit reading and writing process in the Japanese language. While the Japanese language has unique characteristics, the investigation of linguistic disorders specific to the Japanese language may have implications for neuropsychological assessment in general (Murai et al., 2002).

Various standardized psychological tests developed in the United States and Europe have been translated or adapted for the Japanese, including the Wechsler Intelligence Scales, Stanford-Binet Intelligence Scale, McCarthy Scales of Children's Abilities, Wisconsin Card Sorting Test, Rey Auditory Verbal Learning Test, Mini-Mental State Examination, Raven's Colored Progressive Matrices, Benton Visual Retention Test, Beck Depression Inventory–II, and Minnesota Multiphasic Personality Inventory–2. In addition, to assess the unique orthographic and grammatical impairments in Japanese aphasia, psychologists have constructed and standardized Japanese language tests, such as the Standardized Language for Aphasia (Japanese Society of Aphasiology, 1977) and the Test of Syntactic Processing in Aphasia (Fujita & Miyake, 1984). Other psychological tests developed in Japan are the Hasegawa Dementia Scale–Revised, Kyoto New NX intelligence test, and the Unidimensional Scale for Dementia.

Like the general field of psychology, neuropsychology in Japan is growing but is not as widely developed as in Western countries. An undergraduate major in psychology is available in Japanese universities, although neuropsychology is not yet a formal course in their curricula. The education and training of neuropsychologists have been established and integrated into the medical systems of Japan (Hamanaka, 1994).

Relevant studies of Japanese Americans

Despite the recent interest in understanding cultural variables in neuropsychology (Uzzell, Pontón, & Ardil, 2007), research that can shed light on the neuropsychological assessment of ethnic minorities remains relatively scarce (Puente & Perez-Garcia, 2000b; Wong, 2000).

The educational achievement of Japanese Americans is a relevant factor to address. Kitano (1962) examined the changing school achievement patterns of the Japanese Americans between 1941 and 1959. He noted that the Nisei, or second-generation Japanese Americans who maintained a stereotype of being quiet, studious, and industrious, obtained higher grade point averages than the Sansei, or third-generation Japanese Americans, while their IQs remained essentially the same. Kitano also noted an increasing participation among the Sansei in school social activities, and saw value in the evidence of acceptance and acculturation of Japanese American students.

In a longitudinal study of multiethnic children on the island of Kauai, Hawaii, Werner and Smith (1977) found significant ethnic group differences on school aptitude and achievement tests, with the Japanese obtaining higher scores than Portuguese, Hawaiian, Filipino, and mixed-ethnic students. On aptitude tests, the Japanese scores were at the national average on the verbal scale and above the national norms on the quantitative scale. The achievement tests found the Japanese students with national average reading scores and slightly above-average mathematics and writing scores. Administering the California Psychological Inventory, Werner and Smith also noted that the Japanese American youth on Kauai were from predominantly middle-class homes and appeared to value those personality characteristics that were advantageous in the classroom, for example, responsibility and need for achievement.

In a large-scale study in Hawaii, Caucasian (n = 4,732), Hawaiian (n = 4,292), Filipino (n = 4,039), and Japanese (n = 3,445) children in grades 4, 6, and 8 were administered the Stanford Achievement Test (SAT) (Brandon, Newton, & Hammond, 1987). The Japanese American children were described as high achievers whose mean SAT scores were the highest of the four racial/ethnic groups. Compared with the 1973 SAT norms, the Japanese American scores were from 0.40 to 1.06 standard deviations above the norm group.

The Hawaii Family Study of Cognition evaluated 926 European American and 368 Japanese American families with a battery of tests of verbal ability, spatial ability, perceptual speed, and visual memory (Nagoshi & Johnson, 1987). The Caucasian Americans scored higher than the Japanese Americans on the verbal and visual memory factors, but lower on the spatial and perceptual speed factors. This pattern was also noted by Lynn (1987) in his review of studies that compared Caucasian children with children from Japan. Japanese children appeared superior on visuospatial abilities but relatively weaker on verbal abilities. Nagoshi and Johnson attributed the ethnic differences to genetic factors or pervasive environmental influences independent of education and language background.

The effects of bilingualism were investigated with Japanese American children whose mothers were born and raised in Japan and fathers born and raised in the United States (Tsushima & Hogan, 1975). Aptitude and achievement tests were administered to 142 bilingual Japanese American children in grades 3, 4, and 5, and compared with 265 monolingual American children, whose parents were both born and raised in the United States. The Lorge Thorndike Nonverbal Battery revealed no differences between the bilingual and monolingual children. On the Iowa Test of Basic Skills, the two groups performed similarly at grade 3. By grade 4, monolingual children performed noticeably better than bilingual children on verbal or language type tests, and in grade 5 the differences were even more substantial. The findings revealed a distinct pattern of increasing educational difficulty as the bilingual Japanese American children became older.

A unique effort to study the relation between ethnicity and neuropsychological test performance involved the administration of the Luria-Nebraska Neuropsychological Battery (LNNB) to Americans of Japanese (n = 24), Chinese (n = 24), Filipino (n = 25), and Polynesian (n = 26) ancestry, with no history of neurological or psychiatric disorder (Tsushima, Boyar, Shimizu, & Harada, 1995). No difference was noted between the four ethnic groups across the 11 LNNB clinical scales. The research also found that the LNNB scores of 48 Japanese American neurological patients, mostly with closed head injuries, were substantially worse than the performance of the 24 normal Japanese Americans, although the influence of age and education could not be ruled out. The authors called for similar and larger-scale neuropsychological investigations of other non-White populations.

A study of 201 nondemented Japanese American adults age 70 and older found that education, gender, and language differentially affected the results of the Consortium to Establish a Registry for Alzheimer's Disease (CERAD) neuropsychological assessment battery (McCurry et al., 2001). Those with a high school education or beyond, women, and English-speaking participants scored higher than those with less than high school education, men, and Japanese speakers on various neurocognitive tasks. The investigators observed that older Japanese American adults who spoke Japanese and followed a more traditional Japanese lifestyle had less opportunity to become familiar with certain cognitive activities and problem-solving strategies involved in neuropsychological testing. Thus, in addition to linguistic factors, their relatively lesser acculturation may have also contributed to their lower neuropsychological test results.

The CERAD Neuropsychology Battery was used to compare the baseline performance of demented and nondemented Japanese Americans, age 65 and older (Fillenbaum et al., 2005). The CERAD distinguished nondemented persons from those with dementia, but was less consistent in distinguishing levels of severity of dementia. The battery is considered useful for comparative epidemiological studies of dementia in minority groups. Mention should also be made of the Cognitive Abilities Screening Instrument (CASI), a brief screening instrument for dementia, which was administered to dementia patients and control subjects in two sites in Japan (Osaka and Tokyo) and two sites in the United States (Los Angeles and Seattle). The CASI results did not vary significantly among the four sites despite differences in language, subject characteristics, testing personnel, and settings, demonstrating its cross-cultural applicability (Teng et al., 1994).

The Minnesota Multiphasic Personality Inventory (MMPI), the most frequently used test by clinical psychologists and neuropsychologists (Camara, Nathan, & Puente, 2000), was administered to 67 Japanese American and 97 Caucasian patients diagnosed with somatization disorder or organic brain syndrome (Tsushima & Onorato, 1982). The results revealed no significant differences between the two groups, with diagnostic classifications held constant. Similar results were obtained in two subsequent investigations. The MMPI was administered to 116 Caucasian American, 72 Japanese American, and 50 mixed-ethnic Americans who were chronic pain patients in a biofeedback therapy program (Tsushima & Stoddard, 1990). The three racial/ethnic groups did not differ on any of the MMPI scales, as well as measures of pain, forehead EMG levels, and biofeedback outcome ratings. The Minnesota Multiphasic Personality Inventory–2 (MMPI-2) was completed by 196 White and Japanese American medical patients (Tsushima & Tsushima, 2002). While the two groups of medical patients differed significantly from normal subjects on nearly all of the MMPI-2 scales, multiple regression analyses failed to show significant race differences with the MMPI-2 scales. These findings conflict with other studies of Asian American and White college students, in which Asian Americans had higher MMPI and MMPI-2 scale elevations than White Americans (Sue & Sue, 1974; Sue, Keefe, Enomoto, Durvasula, & Chao, 1996). Sue et al. (1996) submitted that when the MMPI is administered to Japanese Americans, who are the most acculturated among the Asian American groups, ethnic differences may be minimal.

In summary, relevant research on Japanese Americans is scarce but suggests that they are successful in academic achievements and do relatively better on visuospatial tasks than on verbal measures. Bilingualism and acculturation among Japanese Americans remain significant factors that could negatively affect their performance on verbal tasks. Interestingly, the MMPI scores of Japanese Americans have been found to be similar to those of Caucasian Americans, although these data have been obtained primarily in Hawaii. When MMPI studies were conducted on the U.S. mainland, differences between Asian and Caucasian Americans were reported.

Other Western tests translated into Japanese

Other Western neuropsychological tests have been translated into Japanese, which may facilitate administration to a primarily Japanese-speaking client. However, these tests do not have norms for a strictly Japanese sample, and thus test scores would have to be interpreted with caution. The Montreal Cognitive Assessment (MoCA; Nasreddine et al., 2005) is a 30-point dementia screen that incorporates tasks such as draw a clock, verbal fluency, and a mini trailmaking, along with typical orientation, attention, and memory items. The MoCA and Japanese translation is available online at http://www.mocastest.org/. Other instruments used for dementia screening that have been translated into Japanese include Cognistat, which was formerly known as the Neurobehavioral Cognitive Status Examination (Kiernan, Mueller, Langston, & van Dyke, 2009), and the Informant Questionnaire on Cognitive Decline in the Elderly (IQCODE), which is a nonneuropsychological measure of dementia based upon informant report (Jorm, 2004).

The Bilingual Verbal Abilities Test (BVAT) (Munoz-Sandoval, Cummins, Alvarado, & Ruef, 1998) evaluates language skills in both English and Japanese, which may provide useful information for interpreting neuropsychological test scores on Western tests with a strong language component. The BVAT consists of three subtests from the Woodcock-Johnson Revised Tests of Cognitive Ability and Language Proficiency Battery–Revised: Picture Vocabulary (58 items), Oral Vocabulary Synonyms (20 items) and Antonyms (20 items), and Verbal Analogies (35 items). The test requires a bilingual administrator or interpreter and takes approximately 30 minutes to complete. Items are administered in English, and missed items are then administered in the client's native language. Norms range from 5 to 90.

Relevant assessment variables

Various demographic and sociocultural factors can influence the psychological test scores of ethnic minority individuals. As with the majority, the level of educational attainment plays a major role in the performance of neuropsychological tests (Lezak, Howieson, & Loring, 2004; Strauss, Sherman, & Spreen, 2006). Research with diverse populations, such as African Americans (Jencks & Philips, 1998) and Hispanic Americans (Puente & Ardila, 2000), has consistently revealed the detrimental effects of limited education in psychometric and neurocognitive assessments. According to the U.S. Bureau of the Census (2005), 72.5% of Japanese Americans are high school graduates or higher, a rate that supercedes Whites (56.6%) and other Asian Americans—Filipino (59.3%), Asian Indian (54.0%), and Chinese (52.6%). The educational background of Japanese Americans, thus, would seem to favor their performance in standardized psychological testing.

Socioeconomic levels are also positively associated with psychological test results, as greater income, higher educational background, and more cultural opportunities contribute to a person's cognitive development (Mitrushina, Boone, Razani, & D'Elia, 2005). For Japanese Americans, the median annual household income is $51,981, as compared to Whites ($44,687), Asian Indian ($63,669), Filipino ($60,570), and Chinese ($51,444) Americans (U.S. Bureau of the Census, 2005). From a socioeconomic standpoint, Japanese Americans and certain other Asian American groups are not disadvantaged in undertaking psychological tests (Raajpoot, 2000).

Bilingualism has been found to have a detrimental effect on the performance on psychological tests, including both verbal and so-called nonverbal and culture-free tests (Harris, Tulsky, & Schultheis, 2003; Portocarrero, Burright, & Donovick, 2007). Among Whites, only 10.7% speak a language other than English at home, while among Asian Americans 45% of Japanese, 67.4% of Filipinos, 72.8% of Asian Indians, and 79.9% of Chinese speak a second language other than English at home (U.S. Bureau of the Census, 2005). Thus, for Japanese Americans, the bilingual factor may play a role in their psychological examinations, though to a lesser extent than for other Asian Americans.

Acculturation is another significant influence in the neuropsychological assessment of ethnic minorities (Wong, Strickland, Fletcher-Janzen, Ardila, & Reynolds, 2000). Acculturation in the United States is the process whereby individuals learn about and internalize the culture of America. Varied measures of acculturation, such as years educated outside of the United States, the amount of English spoken when growing up, and scores on a formal acculturation scale, have been found to be correlated with neuropsychological test performance (Manly et al., 1998; Razani, Burciaga, Madore, & Wong, 2007). The cultural factors that affect test performance include English verbal skills, familiarity with culture-specific test items, comfort with the testing situation, and test-taking attitude. Although no published acculturation scale specifically constructed for Japanese Americans is available, clinicians can conduct a cultural assessment by administering an Asian acculturation scale (Suinn, Rickard-Figueroa, Lew, & Vigil, 1987; Yamada, Marsella, & Yamada, 1998).

Acculturation is presumably enhanced by duration of residence in America. Presently Japanese have the oldest demographics of any Asian group in the United States. For the Japanese Americans, the proportion that is foreign born (32.4%) is the smallest among all the Asian American groups, compared to the Vietnamese (79.9%), Laotians (79.4%), and Cambodians (79.1%) (U.S. Bureau of the Census, 2005). Furthermore, Caudill (1952) observed that the Japanese Americans have assimilated rapidly into American society because of the compatibility between the values of the Japanese culture, for example, industriousness, and the value system of the American middle class. As the third, fourth, and fifth generations of Japanese Americans increasingly assimilate in the United States, the cultural trend among them is to break away from Japanese traditions and values, and blend into the American cultural fabric. Kitano (1993), observing that fourth- and fifth-generation Japanese Americans readily embrace Western norms and attitudes, anticipates in the near future the possibility of nearly complete acculturation by Japanese Americans.

Acculturation may be affected by geographic location. Uba (1994), in her literature review, noted conflicting findings regarding generational differences in Japanese American ethnic identity, and attributed the disparity to the varying areas where the data were collected, that is, California, Washington, and Hawaii. Japanese Americans comprise different proportions of the population in different states, and experience different social and acculturation influences. These regional factors could affect their ethnic identity and behaviors.

Cultural experiences and practices of diverse populations may also affect test performance. Cultures vary with respect to their familiarity with one-to-one testing and values placed on speed, accuracy, test motivation, and competitiveness (Ardila & Keating, 2007). In Hispanic cultures, for example, taking psychological tests is not a common experience. For many time is valued and speed may not be vital (Puente & Ardila, 2000). These cultural patterns could influence outcomes in a neuropsychological assessment that often includes timed tasks. In view of the traditional Japanese values placed on academic performance and need for achievement, the requirements of psychological testing, with its emphasis on maximum effort in school-like tasks, are compatible with the ingrained lifestyle of the Japanese American.

Neuropsychological test scores of Caucasian and Japanese Americans: A study

The present study was developed to present comparative neuropsychological test results of Caucasian and Japanese Americans that, to date, are not available in the literature. A group of 99 patients (69 Caucasians, 30 Japanese) were administered the Halstead-Reitan Neuropsychological Battery at a medical center in Honolulu, Hawaii, to assess possible deficits in basic adaptive abilities. The patients predominantly suffered closed head injuries (94%) and were involved in motor vehicle accidents (68%) or industrial accidents (19%).

Table 7.2 Age, education, and duration of injury of Japanese and Caucasian patients

	Japanese		*Caucasian*		
	M	*SD*	*M*	*SD*	*F*
Age (years)	44.07	17.21	38.82	12.86	1.04
Education (years)	13.27	1.76	14.12	2.77	3.19
Duration of injury (months)	24.57	19.31	22.84	30.78	0.31

Among the 69 Caucasians were 39 males and 30 females; the 30 Japanese were comprised of 19 males and 11 females.

The mean age of the patients in this study was 40.44 years ($SD = 14.46$). The mean educational level was 13.86 years ($SD = 2.53$). The mean duration of injury was 23.35 months ($SD = 27.80$). The demographic data of the Caucasian and Japanese American patients are presented in Table 7.2. Analyses of variance (ANOVAs) revealed no significant race or gender differences with respect to age, education, and duration of illness.

The Halstead-Reitan subtests under investigation were the Category Test, Tactual Performance Test (TPT), Speech-Sounds Perception Test, Seashore Rhythm Test, Trail Making Test, Finger Tapping Test, and Dynamometer.

Results

The means and standard deviations of the 10 subtests of the Halstead-Reitan Neuropsychological Battery are presented in Table 7.3. ANOVAs were performed to examine race and gender differences on the neuropsychological tests. No race differences were found on any of the 10 subtests, that is, no F score achieved a level of significance at the Bonferroni corrected $p < .005$ level. Significant gender differences were noted on two subtests, the Finger Tapping Test and the dynamometer, in which the males obtained higher scores than the females. This gender pattern

Table 7.3 Neuropsychological subtest scores of Japanese and Caucasian patients

	Japanese		*Caucasian*		
	M	*SD*	*M*	*SD*	*F*
Category	36.39	29.10	37.76	20.87	0.37
TPT time	18.59	9.68	16.56	7.04	0.76
TPT memory	6.96	2.28	7.33	1.66	0.54
TPT location	3.00	2.20	3.70	2.17	0.22
Speech sounds	9.96	7.28	6.96	4.34	3.32
Seashore Rhythm	6.33	5.14	5.00	3.19	2.72
Trail Making A	30.31	10.96	30.90	11.16	0.36
Trail Making B	80.76	37.62	74.46	29.28	0.23
Finger Tapping (both hands)	76.77	18.56	75.21	15.83	0.08
Dynamometer (both hands)	108.84	52.42	119.92	43.17	3.87

has been reported in numerous research on these two measures (Lezak et al., 2004; Mitrushina et al., 2005).

Discussion

The purpose of this study was to examine the neuropsychological test scores of a group of Japanese Americans, primarily mild traumatic brain injury patients, in comparison to a similar group of Caucasian American patients. The data analysis indicated no significant differences between the two groups of patients on a variety of subtests of the Halstead-Reitan Neuropsychological Battery. Similar nonsignificant ethnic differences were found in a study that compared the scores on the Cognitive Abilities Screening Instrument of dementia and control patients tested in the United States and in Japan, although the racial composition of the U.S. patients was not specified (Teng et al., 1994).

The absence of differences between Japanese and Caucasian Americans on neuropsychological measures was not unexpected when considering the major variables that are positively associated with neuropsychological test scores. The relatively high educational attainments and socioeconomic status of Japanese Americans, along with their substantial level of acculturation, were presumed to have a favorable impact on their performance in neuropsychological testing. The present findings suggested that race/ethnicity specific norms, such as those proposed by some for African Americans (Byrd et al., 2006) and Hispanic Americans (Cherner et al., 2007), may not be necessary or appropriate for Japanese Americans.

The present study has notable shortcomings. First, the relatively small number of participants representing the Japanese American group compromised the statistical power of the data analysis and limited any generalizations that can be derived from the data. The number of subjects in both racial groups falls short of the minimum of 100 subjects (or 10 per subtest) needed in each group to assess adequately the 10 subtest scores of the Halstead-Reitan Neuropsychological Battery (Greene, 1987). Without substantial sample sizes, the present findings must be considered highly tentative.

The Japanese American participants were predominantly Sansei or Yonsei, but specific details regarding their generational levels were not obtained. The study also lacked an objective measure of acculturation, for example, the Suinn-Lew Self-Identity Acculturation Scale (Suinn et al., 1987), which would have better identified the sample of Japanese American patients and provided further insight regarding their neuropsychological test performance.

The sample of Japanese Americans in this study was only from Hawaii. It would be desirable to obtain neuropsychological test scores of Japanese Americans in other geographic locations, as different social and environmental factors may produce different neuropsychological test results (Uba, 1994).

Maxims for the neuropsychologist

While Japanese Americans have acculturated in varying degrees to Western society, they continue to retain their own unique identity, social behaviors, and personality characteristics (Vernon, 1982; Marsella, 1993). Their original culture persists in their values, such as deference to authority, as well as in their preference in foods and their ethnic artistry, like the tea ceremony and flower arrangement (Kitano, 1993). To the extent that certain Japanese Americans continue to identify with the cultural patterns of their ancestors, the following maxims are offered for the neuropsychologist evaluating a Japanese American patient:

1. Like other Asians in America, *the Japanese American is generally hesitant to seek psychological assistance* (Rogers & Izutsu, 1980; Fujii, Fukushima, & Yamamoto, 1996). Even among the more acculturated, the possibility of social stigma and the sense of shame may discourage or even prevent one from obtaining mental health consultation. In a psychological examination, the Japanese American patient, out of embarrassment or guilt, may be reluctant to admit to psychological symptoms. Accordingly, the examiner probably needs to encourage the patient to elaborate if a general or open-ended question is asked, or the examiner may have to ask more specific and direct questions.
2. Older Japanese Americans as well as recent immigrants from Japan are expected to maintain the more traditional Japanese characteristics, compared to the younger generation (Wong, 2000). *With the more traditional Japanese, clinicians should address them more formally* ("Mr. or Mrs. Yamamoto" rather than "Hideki" or "Alice"), as they tend to be more formal than Westerners (Hays, 1996). If they are bilingual, the psychologist should speak slowly, listen patiently, and exhibit confidence without being patronizing. It is more important to show care and concern than to be very friendly or humorous. The less acculturated patients may be unfamiliar with neuropsychological testing and contemporary treatments, such as speech, occupational, and psychological therapies. They may need more explanation and encouragement to participate in these important activities.
3. *Japanese Americans hesitate to speak up in the presence of doctors*, in deference to their position of authority (Matsui, 1996). The Japanese patient is known to show respect and deference by quietly listening and not openly disagreeing with a doctor. Thus, he or she may avoid asking for explanations of a diagnosis, or reasons for a test or treatment, even if he or she does not fully understand the nature of his or her condition. It behooves the psychologist to provide a full and detailed explanation of the neuropsychological problem, encourage questions, and inform the client of his or her right to seek a second opinion or refuse treatment.
4. *It is essential to understand the nonassertive and indirect speaking manner of the Japanese American*, who has been socialized to be respectful by being agreeable and avoiding direct expression of opinions (Homma-True, 1997; Wong & Fujii, 2004). Thus, in a neuropsychological examination, he or she may nod or answer yes when he or she does not fully understand the question, or even when he or she is definitely in disagreement (Kitano,

1993). Japanese Americans may respond in a seemingly tangential manner that could be misidentified as a language impairment or a thought disorder. The Japanese indirect speaking style can be puzzling and frustrating to the examiner who wants direct and pertinent answers.

5. The Japanese, like other Asians, emphasize the family unit. Thus, *the practitioner needs to include the patient's family* and involve them in the explanation of the neuropsychological problem and the treatment recommendations (Fujii et al., 1996). While there may be a trend away from the close-knit family system toward Western individualism, the clinician must be aware of this distinct Asian value.
6. In view of the premium attached to school achievement and career advancement among Japanese Americans, *brain injury and its accompanying limitations on career progress may result in turmoil* for the individual because of overwhelming disappointment and shame. The neuropsychologist needs to appreciate these strong cultural values and be prepared to offer acceptable career alternatives that will save face for the impaired person.
7. For many Japanese, *reading and writing skills in English are more developed than speaking English.* Thus, when evaluating verbal skills for some Japanese immigrants, it may be useful to have them read the item and respond by writing.

Case sample

Given that U.S. norms would be appropriate for the vast majority of Japanese Americans, we selected a case of a Japanese national who speaks little English visiting his daughter in America. This case may illustrate how to approach more challenging cases in which the client has a poor command of English and is less acculturated.

Mr. Kono is a 74-year-old Japanese male who has lived his entire life in Osaka, Japan. According to Mr. Kono's wife, Shizuko, her husband began demonstrating forgetfulness about six months ago, which has become progressively more frequent. He often misplaces things and will ask the same questions more than once. Word-finding problems are also apparent. Mr. Kono's activity level has been significantly reduced with poor initiation. Normally a very sociable man, he has become more reclusive and often refuses to leave the home. Shizuko's concerns became more pronounced when she witnessed her husband talking to a bird outside his window.

Despite these behaviors, Mr. Kono continues to be independent in his activities of daily living and will do his routine home chores. His wife has taken care of shopping and bill paying, and thus he does not have these duties.

Mr. Kono is a former president of an accounting firm who has a bachelor's degree in business. He was forced to retire about a year ago due to political maneuverings by his former protégé. Although Mr. Kono never complained, his wife suspects that the manner in which her husband was forced into retirement was highly stressful for him. Shizuko was worried, but did not directly address her concerns with her husband, as he would become very angry when the topic of behavioral changes was brought up. She consulted with their daughter Michiko, who was living in Hawaii after marrying a U.S. citizen 10 years ago. Michiko persuaded her mother to bring her father to Hawaii for a visit with the hope that she could persuade him to get an evaluation. It was Michiko who made the arrangements for a neuropsychological evaluation for possible dementia or depression. Mr. Kono agreed to see "the American doctor" reluctantly, only after Michiko insisted that both he and his wife were to be examined for health status.

Medically, Mr. Kono sustained congestive heart failure about six months ago and was prescribed digoxin for this condition. He was also taking a diuretic for hypertension. Mr. Kono used to drink a small bottle of sake per day (equivalent to about two shots of hard liquor). He smoked a pack a day since he was 20 years old and quit after his heart attack. His eating is fine, but he has gained about 7 pounds due to a reduced level of exercise.

Mr. Kono was interviewed through a professional interpreter. He was neatly groomed and casually attired. His countenance was stoic, which is common for older Japanese males, although it could also be suggestive of depression. Mr. Kono answered questions politely. He reported that his mood was "good" and everything is fine. To increase Mr. Kono's comfort level, his family was allowed to stay during the interview. Later, when Mr. Kono was using the restroom, they commented on how "well behaved" he was during the interview.

Mr. Kono was then administered a short battery consisting of the following instruments, which have either been translated and normed on a Japanese population or in which studies indicate are valid for Japanese: the Cognitive Abilities Screening Instrument (CASI), a multidimensional cognitive screen that has been translated into Japanese and normed on samples in Osaka and Tokyo (Teng et al., 1994); the Wechsler Memory Scale–Revised, which was translated and validated in Japanese (Sugishita, 2001); and an 11-question version of the Centers for Epidemiologic Studies Depression Scale (CES-D) questionnaire that has been used with Japanese Americans (Oba et al., 2009). The Clinical Dementia Rating (CDR), a dementia scale based upon informant observation, was also administered (Hughes, Berg, Danzinger, Coben, & Martin, 1982).

Given Mr. Kono's educational level, particularly for his cohort, and occupation, his premorbid functioning was estimated to be at least in the average range and probably higher. Mr. Kono earned an overall CASI score of 73, which was a borderline level score based upon Osaka norms. Strengths were demonstrated in orientation, attention, and visual constructions, while impairments were demonstrated in concentration/mental manipulation and verbal memory tasks, the latter primarily for encoding with adequate retrieval. Abstractions, animal fluency, and visual memory were below average. On the CDR, Mr. Kono was rated as having questionable impairments in memory, orientation, judgment, and problem solving, and in performing household chores and hobbies, and no impairment in personal care. His score on the CES-D was elevated (7), but not in the depressed range.

Mr. Kono's scores and history were interpreted as a differential between mild cognitive impairment and mild dementia. Potential contributors included dementia of the Alzheimer's type, an adjustment disorder with depressed mood, or medication effects, possibly due to digoxin, that can cause confusion, apathy, depression, as well as visual hallucinations. It was recommended that Mr. Kono be evaluated by a geriatrician and undergo a dementia workup. Family followed up on these recommendations upon returning to Japan. They later reported that a dementia workup was negative with the exception of mild general atrophy on a CT. His digoxin was discontinued and within weeks, Mr. Kono was functioning near baseline. However, his cognition slowly declined over the next three years and he was later diagnosed with dementia of the Alzheimer's type.

Mr. Kono's case is common in traditional Japanese families. He was very reluctant to seek help for a possible mental problem due to shame and stigma. In traditional Japanese culture, the wife does not confront the husband on important issues. Indeed, their Americanized daughter had to make arrangements for testing. In Ms. Kono's case special care was taken to ensure comfort with the procedure by describing the test as a preventative measure that is popular in America. In addition, family was allowed to stay in the office during the evaluation.

Given that Mr. Kono is a Japanese national, test selection was based upon those normed and validated in Japan versus tests validated on Japanese Americans. A problem was that translations of these tests were not available; thus, the interpreter had to translate them. Although not an ideal situation, this was noted in the report, and the possible negative effects on reliability and validity. An estimate of Mr. Kono's premorbid functioning was based upon his education level and high socioeconomic status in a country with a strong education system and economy comparable to the United States. Thus, some confidence could be made that his premorbid functioning was at least average and likely higher. Diagnosis was based upon a multimethod approach as recommended by Fujii et al. (2002, 2005), with cognitive functioning based upon both neuropsychological tests and informant-based questionnaires. In Mr. Kono's case, both evaluation sources were converged. Finally, given that traditional Japanese are reluctant to admit psychological or mental problems, despite denial of depressive feelings and a CES-D score in the normal range, a depressive disorder could not be entirely ruled out and was kept in the differential.

Conclusion

In this chapter, we provided a brief history of the Japanese in America, highlighted the presence of neuropsychology in Japan, summarized the literature regarding relevant variables in the neuropsychological assessment of the Japanese American patient, and presented the comparative results of Japanese and Caucasian American patients who underwent a comprehensive neuropsychological examination. Finally, we offered several maxims regarding the neuropsychological assessment of Japanese Americans, and described a neuropsychological case of testing with an elderly Japanese male who spoke little English. Any chapter dedicated to the description of a particular ethnic group is subject to err on the side of overgeneralization. These characterizations can leave the wrongful impression that there is a homogeneous Japanese American culture that is vastly different from that of other Americans. Cross-cultural experts warn that between-group differences comparing one ethnic group with others are sometimes emphasized, while equally wide or even wider within-group differences are overlooked (Suzuki & Valencia, 1997; Okazaki, 2000). We need to keep in mind the wide spectrum of Japanese Americans who are bilingual and bicultural, along with the fourth- and fifth-generation Japanese Americans who are highly acculturated into the Western world, as well as recent immigrants whose English-speaking abilities are highly variable.

The discussion of Japanese Americans presented here is intended to increase the knowledge and understanding of neuropsychologists who may be otherwise unfamiliar with the psychological and behavioral characteristics of Japanese Americans. Clinicians are cautioned to apply these broad descriptions with sensitivity and judgment in their interactions with individual Japanese Americans.

References

Akimoto, H. (1976). *On apraxias* [in Japanese]. Tokyo, Japan: Tokyo University Press. (Original work published 1935).

Ardila, A., & Keating, K. (2007). Cognitive abilities in different cultural contexts. In B. P. Uzzell, M. Pontón, & A. Ardila (Eds.), *International handbook of cross-cultural neuropsychology* (pp. 109–125). Mahwah, NJ: Lawrence Erlbaum Associates.

Brandon, P. R., Newton, B. J., & Hammond, O. W. (1987). Children's mathematics achievements in Hawaii: Sex differences favoring girls. *American Educational Research Journal, 24,* 437–461.

Byrd, D. A., Miller, S. W., Reilly, J., Weber, S., Wall, T. L., & Heaton, R. K. (2006). Early environmental factors, ethnicity, and adult cognitive test performance. *The Clinical Neuropsychologist, 20,* 243–260.

Camara, W. J., Nathan, J. S., & Puente, A. E. (2000). Psychological test usage: Implications in professional psychological. *Professional Psychology: Research and Practice, 31,* 141–154.

Caudill, W. (1952). Japanese American personality and acculturation. *Genetic Psychology Monographs, 45,* 3–102.

Chen, C., Lee, S., & Stevenson, H. W. (1996). Long-term prediction of academic achievement of American, Chinese, and Japanese adolescents. *Journal of Educational Psychology, 18,* 750–759.

Cherner, M., Suarez, P., Lazzaretto, D., Artiola i Fortuny, L., Rivera Mindt, M., Dawes, S., … Heaton, R. (2007). Demographically corrected norms for the Brief Visuospatial Memory Test–Revised and Hopkins Verbal Learning Test–Revised in monolingual Spanish speakers from the U.S.-Mexico border region. *Archives of Clinical Neuropsychology, 22,* 343–353.

Ellington, J. (2001). *Japanese education in grades K–12* (ERIC Document 458185). Bloomington, IN: ERIC Clearinghouse for the Social Sciences.

Fillenbaum, G. G., McCurry, S. M., Kuchibhatla, M., Masaki, K. H., Borenstein, A. R., Foley, D. J., … White, L. (2005). Performance on the CERAD neuropsychology battery of two samples of Japanese-American elders: Norms for persons with and without dementia. *Journal of the International Neuropsychological Society, 11,* 192–201.

Flynn, J. R. (1983). Japanese intelligence: Now the great augmentation of the American IQ. *Nature, 301,* 655.

Fujii, D., Umetsu, D., Schwartz, T., & Hostetter, G. (2002). Culturally sensitive strategies for practicing neuropsychology in Hawaii. *INSNET, 10*(4), 1–2.

Fujii, D. E., & Wong, T. M. (2005). Neuropsychological assessment with Asian-American immigrants: Recommendations for meeting *Daubert* standards. *Journal of Forensic Neuropsychology, 4*, 3–31.

Fujii, J. S., Fukushima, S. N., & Yamamoto, J. (1996). Psychiatric care of Japanese Americans. In A. Gaw (Ed.), *Culture, ethnicity and mental illness* (pp. 304–345). Washington, DC: American Psychiatric Association.

Fujita, I., & Miyake, T. (1984). *Test of Syntactic Processing in Aphasia (Trial 2A)* [in Japanese]. Tokorozawa, Japan: Japanese Speech-Language-Hearing Association.

Gondo, M. (2009). *Parsing Asian America. Goldsea Asian American demographics*. Retrieved from http://goldsea.com/AAD/Parsing/parsing.html

Greene, R. L. (1987). Ethnicity and MMPI performance: A review. *Journal of Consulting and Clinical Psychology, 55*, 497–512.

Hamanaka, T. (1994). One hundred years of neuropsychology in Japan: Retrospect and prospect. *Neuropsychological Review, 4*, 289–298.

Harris, J. G., Tulsky, D. S., & Schultheis, M. T. (2003). Assessment of the non-native English speaker: Assimilating history and research findings to guide clinical practice. In D. S. Tulsky, D. H. Saklofske, G. J. Chelune, R. K. Heaton, R. J. Ivnik, R. Bornstein, et al. (Eds.), *Clinical interpretation of the WAIS-III and WMS-III* (pp. 343–390). New York, NY: Academic Press.

Hays, P. A. (1996). Culturally responsive assessment with diverse older clients. *Professional Psychology: Research and Practice, 27*, 188–193.

Herrnstein, R. J., & Murray, C. (1994). *The bell curve.* New York, NY: Free Press.

Hilger, S. M. I., Klett, W. G., & Watson, C. G. (1976). Performance of Ainu and Japanese six-year-olds on the Goodenough-Harris drawing test. *Perceptual and Motor Skills, 42*, 435–438.

Homma-True, R. (1997). Japanese American families. In E. Lee (Ed.), *Working with Asian Americans: A guide for clinicians* (pp. 114–124). New York, NY: Guilford Press.

Hughes, C., Berg, L., Danzinger, W., Coben, L., & Martin, R. (1982). A new clinical scale for the staging of dementia. *British Journal of Psychiatry, 140*, 566–572.

International Association for the Evaluation of Educational Achievement. (2003). *Trends in international mathematics and science study.* Amsterdam, The Netherlands: Author.

Iwata, M. (2007). Neural circuit of reading and writing in the Japanese language. In B. Uzzell, M. Pontón, & A. Ardila (Eds.), *International handbook of cross-cultural neuropsychology* (pp. 253–264). Mahwah, NJ: Lawrence Erlbaum.

Japanese Society of Aphasiology. (1977). *Standard Language Test of Aphasia* [in Japanese]. Tokyo, Japan: Hohmeido.

Jencks, C., & Phillips, M. (Eds.). (1998). *The Black-White test score gap.* Washington, DC: Brookings Institution Press.

Jorm, A. F. (2004). The Informant Questionnaire on Cognitive Decline in the Elderly (IQCODE): A review. *International Psychogeriatrics, 16*, 3–19. (Test is downloadable, although your computer would have to have special features for specific languages: http://www.anu.edu.au/iqcode/)

Kamin, L. (1995). Behind the curve. *Scientific American, 272*, 99–103.

Kaufman, A. S., McLean, J. E., Ishikuma, T., & Moon, S. (1989). Integration of the literature on the intelligence of Japanese children and analysis of the data from a sequential simultaneous perspective. *School Psychology International, 10*, 173–183.

Kiernan, R., Mueller, J., Langston, J., & van Dyke, C. (2009). *2009 Cognistat manual.* Fairfax, CA: Novatek International.

Kitano, H. H. L. (1962). Changing achievement patterns of the Japanese in the United States. *Journal of Social Psychology, 58,* 257–264.

Kitano, H. H. L. (1993). *Generations and identity: The Japanese American.* Needham Heights, MA: Ginn Press.

Lezak, M., Howieson, D. B., & Loring, D. W. (2004). *Neuropsychological assessment* (4th ed.). New York, NY: Oxford University Press.

Lykken, D. (2004). The new eugenics. *Contemporary Psychology, 49,* 670–672.

Lynn, R. (1977). The intelligence of the Japanese. *Bulletin of the British Psychological Society, 30,* 69–72.

Lynn, R. (1987). The intelligence of the Mongoloids: A psychometric, evolutionary and neurological theory. *Personality and Individual Differences, 8,* 813–844.

Lynn, R. (2006). *Race differences in intelligence: An evolutionary analysis.* Augusta, GA: Washington Summit Publishers.

Lynn, R., & Hampson, S. (1986a). The rise of national intelligence: Evidence from Britain, Japan and the United States. *Personality and Individual Differences, 7,* 23–32.

Lynn, R., & Hampson, S. (1986b). Intellectual abilities of Japanese children: An assessment of 2½–8½-year-olds derived from the McCarthy Scales of Children's Abilities. *Intelligence, 10,* 41–58.

Lynn, R., & Hampson, S. (1987). Further evidence on the cognitive abilities of the Japanese: Data from the WPPSI. *International Journal of Behavioral Development, 10,* 23–36.

Lynn, R., Hampson, S. L., & Iwawaki, S. (1987). Abstract reasoning and spatial abilities among American, British and Japanese adolescents. *Mankind Quarterly, 27,* 379–384.

Manly, J. J., Miller, S. W., Heaton, R. K., Byrd, D., Reilly, J., Velasquez, R. J., … HIV Neurobehavioral Research Center (HNRC) Group. (1998). The effect of African-American acculturation on neuropsychological test performance in normal and HIV-positive individuals. *Journal of the International Neuropsychological Society, 4,* 291–302.

Marsella, A. J. (1993). Counseling and psychotherapy with Japanese Americans: Cross-cultural considerations. *American Journal of Orthopsychiatry, 63,* 200–208.

Matsui, M., Yuuki, H., Kato, K., Takeuchi, A., Nishiyama, S., Bilker, W.B., & Kurachi, M. (2007). Schizotypal disorder and schizophrenia: A profile analysis of neuropsychological functioning in Japanese patients. *Journal of the International Neuropsychological Society, 13,* 672–682.

Matsui, W. T. (1996). Japanese families. In M. McGoldrick, J. Giordano, & J. K. Pearce (Eds.), *Ethnicity and family therapy* (2nd ed., pp. 268–280). New York, NY: Guilford.

McCurry, S. M., Gibbons, L. E., Uomoto, J. M., Thompson, M. L., Graves, A. B., Edland, S. D., … Larson, E. B. (2001). Neuropsychological test performance in a cognitively intact sample of older Japanese American adults. *Archives of Clinical Neuropsychology, 16,* 447–459.

Misawa, G., Motegi, M., Fujita, K., & Hattori, K. (1984). A comparative study of intellectual abilities of Japanese and American children on the Columbia Mental Maturity Scale. *Personality and Individual Differences, 5,* 173–181.

Mitrushina, M., Boone, K. B., Razani, J., & D'Elia, L. F. (2005). *Handbook of normative data for neuropsychological assessment* (2nd ed.). New York, NY: Oxford University Press.

Munoz-Sandoval, A. F., Cummins, J., Alvarado, C. G., & Ruef, M. L. (1998). *Bilingual Verbal Ability Tests.* Itasca, IL: Riverside Publishing.

Murai, T., Hadano, K., & Hamanaka, T. (2002). Current issues in neuropsychological assessment in Japan. In F. R. Ferraro (Ed.), *Minority and cross-cultural aspects of neuropsychological assessment* (pp. 99–127). Lisse, the Netherlands: Swets & Zeitlinger Publishers.

Nagoshi, C. T., & Johnson, R. C. (1987). Cognitive abilities profiles of Caucasian vs. Japanese subjects in the Hawaii Family Study of Cognition. *Personality and Individual Differences, 8,* 581–583.

Nasreddine, Z., Phillips, N., Bedirian, V., Charbonneau, S. Whitehead, V., Collin, S., … Chertkow, H. (2005). The Montreal Cognitive Assessment, MoCA: A brief screening tool for mild cognitive impairment. *Journal of the American Geriatric Society, 53,* 695–699. http://www.mocastest.org/

Oba, S., Takatsuka, N., Nagata, C., Nagao, Y., Yamamoto, S., Shibuya, C., … Shimizu, H. (2009). Causal attributions to epidemiological risk factors and their associations to later psychological adjustment among Japanese breast cancer patients. *Supportive Care for Cancer, 17,* 3–9.

Ohashi, H. (1960). *Aphasia, apraxia, and agnosia* [in Japanese]. Tokyo, Japan: Igakusho.

Okazaki, S. (2000). Assessing and treating Asian Americans: Recent advances. In I. Cuellar & F. A. Paniagua (Eds.), *Handbook of multicultural mental health: Assessment and treatment of diverse populations* (pp. 171–193). New York, NY: Academic Press.

Portocarrero, J. S., Burright, R. G., & Donovick, P. J. (2007). Vocabulary and verbal fluency of bilingual and monolingual college students. *Archives of Clinical Neuropsychology, 22,* 415–422.

Puente, A. E., & Ardila, A. (2000). Neuropsychological assessment of Hispanics. In E. Fletcher-Janzen, T. L. Strickland, & C. R. Reynolds (Eds.), *Handbook of cross-cultural neuropsychology* (pp. 87–104). New York, NY: Kluwer Academic/Plenum Publishers.

Puente, A. E., & Perez Garcia, M. (2000a). Psychological assessment of ethnic minorities. In G. Goldstein & M. Hersen (Eds.), *Handbook of psychological assessment* (3rd ed., pp. 527–551). New York, NY: Pergamon.

Puente, A. E., & Perez-Garcia, M. (2000b). Neuropsychological assessment of ethnic minorities: Clinical issues. In I. Cuellar & F. A. Paniagua (Eds.), *Handbook of multicultural mental health: Assessment and treatment of diverse populations* (pp. 419–435). New York, NY: Academic Press.

Raajpoot, U. A. (2000). Multicultural demographic developments: Current and future trends. In I. Cuellar & F. A. Paniagua (Eds.), *Handbook of multicultural mental health: Assessment and treatment of diverse populations* (pp. 79–94). New York, NY: Academic Press.

Razani, J., Burciaga, J., Madore, M., & Wong, J. (2007). Effects of acculturation on tests of attention and information processing in an ethnically diverse group. *Archives of Clinical Neuropsychology, 22,* 333–341.

Rogers, T., & Izutsu, S. (1980). The Japanese. In J. F. McDermott, Jr., W. S. Tseng, & T. W. Maretzki (Eds.), *People and cultures of Hawaii: A psychocultural profile* (pp. 73–99). Honolulu, HI: University Press of Hawaii.

Sasanuma, S. (1986). Universal and language-specific symptomatology and treatment of aphasia. *Folia Phoniatrica, 38,* 121–175.

Stevenson, H. W., & Azuma, H. (1983). IQ in Japan and the United States: Methodological problems in Lynn's analysis. *Nature, 306,* 291–292.

Stevenson, H. W., Stigler, J. W., Lee, S., Lucker, G. W., Kitamura, S., & Hsu, C. (1985). Cognitive performance and academic achievement of Japanese, Chinese, and American children. *Child Development, 56,* 718–734.

Stigler, J. W., Lee, S., Lucker, G. W., & Stevenson, H. W. (1982). Curriculum and achievement in mathematics: A study of elementary school children in Japan, Taiwan, and the United States. *Journal of Educational Psychology, 74,* 315–322.

Strauss, E., Sherman, E. M. S., & Spreen, O. (2006). *A compendium of neuropsychological tests: Administration, norms, and commentary* (3rd ed.). New York, NY: Oxford University Press.

Sue, S., Keefe, K., Enomoto, K., Durvasula, R. S., & Chao, R. (1996). Asian American and White college students' performance on the MMPI-2. In J. N. Butcher (Ed.), *International adaptations of the MMPI-2: Research and clinical applications* (pp. 206–220). Minneapolis, MN: University of Minnesota Press.

Sue, S., & Sue, D. W. (1974). MMPI comparisons between Asian-Americans and non-Asian students utilizing a student health psychiatric clinic. *Journal of Counseling Psychology, 21,* 423–427.

Suinn, R. M., Rickard-Figueroa, K., Lew, S., & Vigil, P. (1987). The Suinn-Lew Asian Self-Identity Acculturation Scale: An initial report. *Educational and Psychological Measurement, 47,* 401–407.

Suzuki, L., & Aronson, J. (2005). The cultural malleability of intelligence and its impact on the racial/ethnicity hierarchy. *Psychology, Public Policy, and the Law, 11,* 320–327.

Suzuki, L. A., & Valencia, R. R. (1997). Race-ethnicity and measured intelligence. *American Psychologist, 52,* 1103–1114.

Teng, E. L., Hasegawa, K., Homma, A., Imai, Y., Larson, E., Graves, A., … White, L. R. (1994). The Cognitive Abilities Screening Instrument (CASI): A practical test for cross-cultural epidemiological studies of dementia. *International Psychogeriatrics, 6,* 45–58.

Tsushima, W. T., Boyar, J. I., Shimizu, A. A., & Harada, A. S. M. (1995). Applicability of the Luria-Nebraska Neuropsychological Battery with Asian and Pacific Islander Americans. *Advances in Medical Psychotherapy, 8,* 137–144.

Tsushima, W. T., & Hogan, T. P. (1975). Verbal ability and school achievement of bilingual and monolingual children of different ages. *Journal of Educational Research, 68,* 349–353.

Tsushima, W. T., & Onorato, V. A. (1982). Comparison of MMPI scores of White and Japanese-American medical patients. *Journal of Consulting and Clinical Psychology, 50,* 150–151.

Tsushima, W. T., & Stoddard, V. M. (1990). Ethnic group similarities in the biofeedback treatment of pain. *Medical Psychotherapy, 3*, 69–75.

Tsushima, W. T., & Tsushima, V. G. (2002). Comparison of MMPI-2 scores of White and Japanese American medical patients. *Advances in Medical Psychotherapy and Psychodiagnosis, 11,* 1–8.

Uba, L. (1994). *Asian Americans: Personality patterns, identity and mental health.* New York, NY: The Guilford Press.

U.S. Bureau of the Census. (2005). *Nation's Asian and Pacific Islander population (profile).* Washington, DC: Author.

Uzzell, B. P., Pontón, M., & Ardila, A. (Eds.). (2007). *International handbook of cross-cultural neuropsychology.* Mahwah, NJ: Lawrence Erlbaum Associates.

Vernon, P. E. (1982). *The abilities and achievements of Orientals in North America.* New York, NY: Academic Press.

Werner, E. E., & Smith, R. S. (1977). *Kauai's children come of age.* Honolulu, HI: University Press of Hawaii.

Wong, T. M. (2000). Neuropsychological assessment and intervention with Asian Americans. In E. Fletcher-Janzen, T. L. Strickland, & C. R. Reynolds (Eds.), *Handbook of cross-cultural neuropsychology* (pp. 43–53). New York, NY: Kluwer Academic/Plenum Publishers.

Wong, T. M., & Fujii, D. E. (2004). Neuropsychological assessment of Asian Americans: Demographic factors, cultural diversity, and practical guidelines. *Applied Neuropsychology, 11,* 23–36.

Wong, T. M., Strickland, T. L., Fletcher-Janzen, E., Ardila, A., & Reynolds, C. R. (2000). Theoretical and practical issues in the neuropsychological assessment and treatment of culturally dissimilar patients. In E. Fletcher-Janzen, T. L. Strickland, & C. R. Reynolds (Eds.), *Handbook of cross-cultural neuropsychology* (pp. 3–18). New York, NY: Kluwer Academic/Plenum Publishers.

Yamada, A., Marsella, A. J., & Yamada, S. Y. (1998). The development of Ethnocultural Identity Behavioral Index: Psychometric properties and validation with Asian Americans and Pacific Islanders. *Asian American and Pacific Islander Journal of Health, 6,* 36–45.

8 Neuropsychological assessment of Korean Americans

Mi-Yeoung Jo and Lauren Kwon Dawson

Population demographics

As per the U.S. Census Bureau (2000), there are 1,076,872 Koreans living in the United States. This is an increase of about 35% from 1990, which recorded 798,849 Koreans. Of the approximately 1.1 million Koreans in the United States, 77% were foreign born and speak a language other than English at home. A majority of the Koreans living in the United States are from South Korea, and many live in large urban cities like Los Angeles and New York City. Other states with a significant Korean American presence include New Jersey, Illinois, Texas, Washington, and West Virginia (U.S. Census Bureau, 1990, 2000).

Historical background

Korea is a country with a long history that spans over 5,000 years. The oldest Korean pottery has been dated back to the Neolithic era (Eckert, Lee, Lew, Robinson, & Wagner, 1990). Often referred to as the Land of the Morning Calm, Korea is a peninsula situated on the East Asian continent, with China, Japan, and Russia as its closest neighbors. The Korean spoken language has been traced by some to have its origins in the Altaic language family, which includes the Turkic, Mongolic, and Tungus-Manchu languages (Language Overview, 2007). Koreans had their own spoken language, heavily influenced by the Chinese language, but they did not have a separate writing system prior to the fifteenth century. Korean written language in its modern form, *Hangeul*, was created by King Saejong in the fifteenth century. Hangeul is a phonetic language that consists of 10 vowels and 14 consonants. It is thought to be the first phonetic alphabet in East Asia. The creation of a unique writing system was a major accomplishment of the Korean people, and it allowed the writing down of the Korean spoken language without reliance on Chinese characters. It also set the stage for a rise in literacy rates that cut across class and social lines (Eckert et al., 1990; Nash, 2000). The Korean language has been praised by linguists for its simplicity—each letter has only one sound and there are no silent letters. The high Korean literacy rate is a testament to the simplicity of the language (Kim, 2003;

What Is Hangeul? 2007). According to the World Health Organization (WHO), the Korean literacy rate in 1999 was 97% (WHO, 1999).

Modern Korean history, in the first half of the twentieth century, was characterized by colonial occupation, war, and division of the peninsula into north and south. From 1910 to 1945, Korea was under Japanese occupation and subjected to colonial rule. All things Korean, including its language, names, and culture, were suppressed or forbidden. Following the Japanese surrender on August 15, 1945, during World War II, the Korean peninsula came under divided rule with the Union of Soviet Socialist Republics (USSR) occupying the country north of the 38th parallel and the United States occupying the country south of the 38th parallel. The Korean War broke out on June 25, 1950, when the North Korean Army invaded the southern half of the peninsula. On July 27, 1953, an armistice was signed and the Korean peninsula was divided into North and South, with U.S. forces helping to keep peace at the 38th parallel. North Korea (the Democratic People's Republic of Korea) came under Communist rule while South Korea (the Republic of Korea) followed the model set by Western-style democracy.

More recently, within the past 20 years, Korea's worldwide identity has gone beyond that of wars and the North and South divide. South Korea now has the 13th largest economy in the world (Background Note, 2009). It is the worldwide leader in shipbuilding, electronics, digital displays, and mobile devices. It is also the most wired country in the world and a leader in high-speed Internet access (Onishi, 2006). South Korea has also experienced recognition in other high-profile global arenas. The 1988 Seoul Summer Olympics was one of the first events to bring Korea worldwide recognition as a country other than that embroiled in post–Cold War relations. The South Korean national soccer team's semifinal placement at the 2002 FIFA World Cup was also a source of great national pride. Currently in Asia, and slowly spreading further, South Korean popular culture has been gaining wide recognition and interest. Known as *Hallyu*, or the "Korean wave," many Korean entertainers and celebrities are widely popular outside of Korea, with some quickly gaining mega-star status all over Asia (Lim, 2007). Koreans in leadership positions in high-profile organizations, such as Ban Ki-Moon, secretary general of the United Nations, and local sports figures who have achieved success in overseas baseball and soccer teams, are also bringing attention to South Korea as a country more than the sum of its past political woes.

Immigration history

The history of modern Korean U.S. immigration began on January 13, 1903, when a group of about 100 Korean men, women, and children landed in Hawaii aboard the U.S merchant ship, the S.S. *Gaelic*. Most were farm and field laborers, but the group also included students and political dissidents fleeing from their motherland's political struggles with Japan. In the mid-1950s to 1960s, post–Korean War immigration saw a second surge of Koreans leaving their homeland for better prospects abroad. In the 1970s and 1980s, the third wave of immigrants arrived, with many college-educated professionals and their families (Kim, I. J., 2004). A majority of these immigrants settled in large metropolitan areas such as Los Angeles and New York. Los Angeles has the largest Korean community outside of Korea itself. In 2003, the Korean American community celebrated 100 years of immigration history.

Generational and cultural issues

As it often is with other immigrant groups, Korean American ethnic identity and level of acculturation are heavily influenced by generational factors. First-generation Korean Americans are those who were born in Korea and immigrated to the United States as adults. Many of this generation have minimal or very little English fluency unless they have had some schooling in the United States or have lived and worked in English-speaking communities for many years. Most identify themselves as Korean, rather than as Korean American, and have value systems based on their homeland culture (Chung, 2004). In large metropolitan areas with a thriving Korean community, it is possible for a first-generation Korean to never learn fluent English despite having lived in the United States for many years because of easy access to all things Korean. Members of the "1.5 generation" are those who were born in Korea, but immigrated to the United States as children. They are sometimes referred to as the "knee-high" generation (Gondo, 2003). They have been educated primarily in the United States and are often fluent English speakers. Depending on how young they were when they immigrated and how much exposure and access they had to other Koreans and a larger Korean community while growing up, some may identify with both cultures while others may identify primarily with the dominant U.S. culture. Second-generation Korean Americans are those who were born and raised in the United States. Many in this group identify mostly with the dominant U.S. culture and its value system, especially if they have not had much access to a larger Korean community. They may see themselves mostly as American and may speak very little or no Korean (Chung, 2004). Of course, there is wide intragroup variability within these three major generational groups, and there are always exceptions to the rule, depending on factors such as age at immigration, years of education in the United States, and level of exposure to a larger Korean community, among others.

Koreans have, on average, higher educational levels and higher average household incomes than those of other Asian immigrant groups (Gondo, 2003). Approximately 56% of Korean Americans have high school diplomas and 28% have bachelor's degrees or higher. The median household income for Korean Americans in 1999 was $40,037 (U.S. Census Bureau, 2000). Many Koreans left professional jobs in Korea to move to the United States. However, due to the language barrier, they were often unable to find professional positions commensurate with their educational and occupational backgrounds. Many started small, family businesses that did not require extensive English skills.

Religion, especially Christianity, plays a significant role in many Korean and Korean American families. The largest Presbyterian church in the world is in Seoul (Brozan, 1992). Korean immigrants from the very beginning sought out the church to fulfill their communal and spiritual needs (Kim, H., 2004). It is estimated that approximately 75% of Korean Americans practice Christianity, while the remaining

25% practice Catholicism, Buddhism, or are nonspiritual (Yoo, 2003). Many Korean American churches serve as centers of the Korean community, and it is how much of Korean culture is maintained in the United States (Kim, H., 2004; Nash, 2000).

The 1992 Los Angeles riots had an important role in the Korean American psyche. The riots, which resulted in widespread destruction of Korean-owned businesses in South Central Los Angeles and neighboring Koreatown, brought to light the need for a new, stronger political consciousness for the Korean American community. Many families lost their livelihood in the riots and found they were denied access to mainstream support and rebuilding efforts due to language and other cultural barriers (Chung, 2004). Following the riots, there was a call for more political solidarity in the Korean American community and a call for 1.5- and second-generation leaders, who would have easier access to the mainstream political system by virtue of their English fluency skills. Organizations such as the Korean American Coalition (KAC) and the Korean American Democratic Committee (KADC) came to play a more critical role in the Korean American political arena (Chung, 2004). Many Korean Americans also saw the need for a new social awareness and openness toward the communities that many of their businesses served.

Assessment issues

Education in Korea

South Korea has a highly competitive education system. It was the first nation in the world to provide high-speed Internet access for all its primary, junior, and secondary schools (Onishi, 2006). South Korea follows a 6-3-3-4 educational system, with six years of mandatory elementary education (grades 1–6), three years of junior high school education (grades 7–9), and three years of high school education (grades 10–12). Institutes of higher learning include two- or three-year junior colleges or four-year colleges and universities. Preschool education is carried out in kindergartens (Education System: Overview, 2006). In addition to their regular, full-time school, many students attend private academies (*hak-won*) in order to supplement their education and remain competitive for college entrance exams. Students, even in elementary school, have days that start very early in the morning and end late at night. Where one gets into university has a significant influence on one's career prospects. It is not uncommon for college-bound students to try repeatedly over several years to get into the college or university of their choice rather than settling for a lower-ranked school.

English is taught starting in the third grade in South Korea. English fluency is one of the most desired skills since it often leads to better jobs and better advancement opportunities in the highly competitive professional world in Korea. However, many lament the insufficiency of Korean English education; it has been criticized for emphasizing grammar and rules over practical conversational skills. Most Koreans who have thus been schooled can read and understand written English fairly well, but have significant difficulty speaking and conversing in English. This is referred to by some as "mute English education" (Competitive Power of English, 2000).

Despite the strong Korean education system, many Koreans consider being educated in the United States more desirable than being educated in Korea. Many well-to-do families in Korea send their children abroad to be educated in the United States. Close to 100% of first-generation Korean Americans will cite their children's education as the top reason for immigrating. Strong academic achievement, preferably from elite institutions, continues to be one of the most highly prized goals for Korean American families.

Pertinent cultural variables

Korean culture is traditionally a hierarchical one where respect for elders and those in authority is infused into every aspect of interpersonal relating, from within the family extending to the larger community. This is reflected in the language by the many different titles and ways of address, depending on seniority and rank, even within family members. Elders, or those in high-seniority positions, oftentimes enjoy unchallenged roles, as many of lower rank will avoid confrontations for fear of appearing rude or disrespectful. Children are taught never to talk back to adults; company bosses are often the sole decision makers, and employees are expected to follow along without question. This deference to seniority and authority can often cross over into doctor–patient relationships. Koreans address doctors as "teacher" and see them as authority figures and experts. They will rarely directly challenge suggestions or recommendations made by them (Wong, 2000). Clinicians need to be aware of this dynamic when explaining assessment results and recommendations. Time should be spent explaining and clarifying needs for certain recommendations, as necessary, especially as this may have an impact on compliance and treatment outcome. Need for a second opinion in appropriate cases should be discussed.

Koreans use many different forms of address, depending on one's familiarity with the other person as well as his or her rank compared to the other. In general, Koreans are more formal and reserved in their dealings with professionals than they would be with close friends. Koreans never use first names as a way of address in professional settings, and usually refer to someone by their occupation or title (e.g., president, boss, doctor). When this is not practical, use of last names is preferred over use of first names. Overly familiar or friendly gestures or tone of voice are reserved for family and close friends and can be seen as a lack of respect and intelligence in more formalized settings. Nonverbal communication, such as eye contact, is also modulated by rank and level of familiarity with the other person. It is often perceived as rude to look another directly in the eye. Many children are taught to bow and greet an adult without making eye contact. Employees often do the same with their bosses. When giving or receiving an object, use of two hands is seen to be more respectful and deferential than use of one hand. Additionally, many Koreans do not feel comfortable with overly familiar touches, hugs, or kisses, especially in public.

Koreans traditionally believe in fate and destiny, but also believe that one's fate and destiny can change through luck, chance, or direct effort (Harvey & Chung, 1980; Kim, 1996). When Koreans, especially those of the older and more traditional generation, hear bad news, it is not unusual for their first response to be, "It's my fate." It may lead to passive acceptance of a diagnosis or a condition without realizing the importance or need to be more proactive. Many clinicians faced with this situation should spend more time discussing prognosis, treatment compliance, and treatment effectiveness, especially when outcomes are dependent on these factors.

It would not be unusual for many Korean American families to turn first to traditional Eastern medicine like acupuncture or homeopathic care to deal with everyday medical or mental health issues. In Korea, there are physicians trained in Western medicine (WMD) and those trained in Oriental medicine (OMD), with both requiring the same number of years of medical school and a national licensing examination (Lee, Khang, Lee, & Kang, 2002). Oriental medicine is regulated by the government, and some insurance companies do cover services. Hence, clinicians should understand that from the Korean viewpoint, Eastern, or nontraditional, medicine is not as "alternative" an option as it is often seen to be from a Western viewpoint. Korean American clients, especially those older or less acculturated, should be asked about any use of Eastern medicine and their view on the effectiveness of such treatments. It may provide some insight into the willingness to accept more Western-style practices and recommendations.

Korean culture is very homogenous, and this often spills over into the larger Korean mindset. The Korean American community considers itself one large unit, and the success or failure of one on a national or worldwide level brings a sense of success or failure to the group as a whole. They are quick to praise and elevate those that bring pride and recognition to Korea, and are just as quick to feel ashamed and apologetic for those that set bad examples. Having a family member who is different from expected norms can be a great source of distress and shame for many Korean families, and traditionally, such members have been hidden away from public view. Many Korean families see mental illness as a family problem to deal with privately, and this traditional mindset prevents many from seeking professional services for family members. However, with more public awareness and recent high-profile media cases, such as the recent Virginia Tech shootings, the importance of the need to seek professional mental health services is slowly gaining more acceptance among Korean American families.

Other pertinent cultural variables

Koreans use both a solar calendar and a lunar calendar. It is not unusual for Koreans to have two birthdays, one by the solar calendar and one by the lunar calendar. Those of the older generation will usually consider their lunar calendar birthday to be their primary birthday. Age calculations are also slightly different in the Korean system. A newborn baby is considered to be one year old at the time of birth, so Koreans consider themselves one year older than their Western counterparts born in the same year. Additionally, everyone gets one year older on the same day, January 1, instead of on their birthdays. So a baby who is born in December is considered to be two years old by the New Year, when, according to Western age calculations, he or she is just a month old. This usually means that most Koreans are one to two years younger than their stated age. Awareness of this distinction is particularly important in using age-appropriate norms in neuropsychological testing, as well as understanding age-associated developmental milestones in children. In the United States, many Korean Americans will have adopted "American age" as their official age, but this can also vary according to level of acculturation.

Koreans answer negatively posed questions differently than Americans. They respond yes in agreement with the negative connotation of a question and respond no in disagreement with the negative connotation. For example, when asked "Aren't you tired?" an American would answer, "No, I'm not," but a Korean would answer yes, as in "Yes, I'm not tired." In the clinical context, this difference in asking and answering negative questions may lead to confusion during history gathering, and care must be taken to phrase such questions in the affirmative and as clearly as possible.

Korean neuropsychology and normative data

Psychology as a respected field is still in its infancy in Korea and also among Korean Americans. Neuropsychology is fairly unknown. However, more top Korean universities are incorporating neuropsychology into their psychology departments, and more original research is originating from Korea in this area. KoreaMed (http://www.koreamed.org/) and Korean Medical Database (http://kmbase.medric.or.kr/) are two literature search engines that can provide a view of the current state of neuropsychological research in Korea.

Many of the major Western neuropsychological and psychological test instruments have been translated into Korean with Korean normative data. Some instruments have been developed entirely in Korea. The following is a breakdown of some of the tests available in Korean, along with Korean norms, according to cognitive domains:

- General cognition/intelligence
  - Kaufman Assessment Battery for Children (K-ABC)*
  - Korean Bayley Scale of Infant Development–II (K-BSID-II) (Park, Cho, & Choi, 2003)
  - Korean-Leiter International Performance Scale–Revised (K-Leiter-R)*
  - Korean Wechsler Adult Intelligence Scale (K-WAIS) (Yum, Park, Oh, Kim, & Lee, 1992)
  - Korean Wechsler Intelligence Scale for Children–III (K-WISC-III) (Kwak, 2003)
  - Korean Wechsler Preschool and Primary Scale of Intelligence (K-WPPSI) (Park, Kwak, & Park, 1996)
  - MMSE and modified MMSE (Jeong et al., 2007)
  - Naglieri & Das Cognitive Assessment System (CAS)*
  - Seoul Neuropsychological Screening Battery (Kang & Na, 2003)
- Memory
  - Elderly Memory Disorder Scale (EMS)*
  - Korean California Verbal Learning Test (K-CVLT) (Kim & Kang, 1999)

* Hakjisa catalog; availability: http://www.kops.co.kr.

Korean Memory Test (KMT) for Elderly (Kim et al., 2006)
Korean Rey Auditory Verbal Learning Test (K-RAVLT)
Rey-Kim Memory Test (RKMT) (Kim, 2001a)

Language
Korean version Boston Naming Test (K-BNT) (Kim & Na, 1999)*
Korean version Western Aphasia Battery (K-WAB) (Kim & Na, 2004)

Visual-spatial
Clock Drawing Test (Lee et al., 1997)
Korean Complex Figure Test (Kim et al., 2005)
Korean Developmental Test of Visual Perception (K-DTVP-2)*

Executive function
Children's Color Trails Test (CCTT)*
Kims Frontal Executive Neuropsychological Test (K-FENT) (Kim, 2001b)
Stroop (Color and Word Test, Children's Version)*
Trail Making Test (Seo et al., 2006)

Mood/personality
Adolescent Personality Assessment Inventory (PAI-A)*
Korean Child Adolescent Behavior Checklist (Oh, Hong, Lee, & Ha, 1997)
Korean Depression Scale (KDS)*
Korean version Eysenck Personality Questionnaire (K-EPQ)*
Personality Assessment Inventory (PAI)*
Personality Test for Young Children (PTYC)*

Special populations
Autism Diagnostic Interview–Revised (ADI-R)*
Autism Diagnostic Observation Schedule (ADOS)*
CERAD (CERAD-K) (Lee, Lee, et al., 2002; Lee et al., 2004)
IQCODE–Korean version (IQCODE-K) (Jorm, 2004)
Korean Dementia Rating Scale (K-DRS) (Chey, Na, Park, Park, & Lee, 1999)*
Korean Scales of Independent Behavior–Revised (K-SIB-R)*
Montreal Cognitive Assessment (MoCA) (Nasreddine et al., 2005; Lee et al., 2008; http://www.mocatest.org/)
Seoul-Instrumental Activities of Daily Living (S-ADL/S-IADL)*

There are several studies showing that many East Asian groups, including Koreans, do as well if not better than their Western counterparts on measures of general intelligence and visual-spatial tasks (Kwak, 2003; Lynn & Song, 1994). Factorial structures and mean raw scores between the standardization sample of the original Wechsler Intelligence Scale for Children–III (Wechsler, 1991) and several East Asian translated versions, including Korean, were found to be similar (Chen, Chen, & Zhu, 2003; Kwak, 2003; Ueno & Nakatani, 2003). Hence, one could make a reasonable argument that applying U.S. norms for Korean-speaking patients on tasks such as the nonverbal subtests of the Wechsler scales or other measures of general intelligence, like the Raven's Standard Progressive Matrices (Raven, 1981), could

* Hakjisa catalog; availability: http://www.kops.co.kr.

give a generally reliable estimate of true functioning in those areas. However, one caveat is that nonverbal tests in adults who have less than nine years of education may not be as culturally unbiased as one may assume (Artiola i Fortuny, 2003).

On the other hand, one would have a very difficult time making an argument for using U.S. norms on verbal measures translated into Korean since unavoidable language confounds would likely have a significant impact on test results. Even comparing normative data from the Korean version of a particular verbal test to its parallel English version would be misleading. Several of the Korean norms are available in popular English neuropsychology journals. Clinicians should be aware that most of the tests were modified from their original English version to better reflect the Korean language and culture, so they are not directly equivalent forms. Slight modifications to directions during standardization were also done for several tests. For example, the Korean version of the Boston Naming Test (K-BNT) has 60 items, the same as the original Boston Naming Test (BNT) (Kaplan, Goodglass, & Weintraub, 1983), but many of the items from the original BNT had to be omitted and substituted by other items more appropriate for a Korean-speaking population. K-BNT normative data were also based on administration of all 60 items to subjects without regard to basal or ceiling rules. However, as in many studies of the original BNT, significant age and education effects (but no gender effects) emerged on the K-BNT as well, with the best performance from the 15–44 age group with 13+ years of education ($M = 53.93$, $SD = 3.06$) and the worst from the 75+ age group with no years of education ($M = 27.42$, $SD = 8.22$) (Kim & Na, 1999).

Comparisons of normative data for parallel versions of another commonly used neuropsychological instrument, the California Verbal Learning Test (CVLT) (Delis, Kramer, Kaplan, & Ober, 1987), also highlight another potential problem. The Korean version of the CVLT (K-CVLT) was modeled after the CVLT but modified to be more appropriate for a Korean-speaking population. Comparing K-CVLT norms to the original CVLT norms, Kim and Kang (1999) reported that "CVLT norms were generally inflated compared to the K-CVLT norms." Differences in normative sampling were cited as possible reasons for the discrepancy, with the CVLT normative group having a mean educational level of 14 years, which was not seen to be representative of the U.S. population, while the K-CVLT included subjects in each educational group (0, 0–6, 6–9, 9–12, 12+) as representative of the national distribution in Korea. However, there are a few other parallel tests that seem to lend more favorably to direct comparison of normative data. When the CERAD (Welsh et al., 1994) was translated into Korean (CERAD-K (N)), the authors found the CERAD-K (N) to be very similar to the CERAD and indicated that their normative data "might be useful for the clinical interpretation of the CERAD neuropsychological tests in the Korean elderly or the elderly who have emigrated from Korea" (Lee et al., 2004).

A good understanding of a patient's acculturation level is important in determining the appropriateness of any normative data set, whether it be Korean or Western based. There have been several measures of acculturation developed for Asian Americans that may be helpful in determining a Korean American patient's level of acculturation (Lee, Yoon, & Liu-Tom, 2006). To determine level of English skills, a measure such as the Bilingual Verbal Ability Test (Munoz-Sandoval, Cummins,

Alvarado, & Ruef, 1998) could be utilized. This instrument, which takes approximately 30 minutes to administer through use of an interpreter, assesses one's English skills compared to his or her native language skills. It is available in several languages, including Korean. English fluency and level of acculturation are often highly correlated (Wong, Strickland, Fletcher-Janzen, Ardila, & Reynolds, 2000). However, conversational fluency does not necessarily translate into higher-level verbal skills, such as those often tested by the Wechsler verbal scales. Understanding the patient's level of formal, school-based training in English may provide useful information in determining the appropriateness of using Western-based normative data for more fluent and seemingly more acculturated Korean American patients. However, studies have also shown that fluent English speakers who learned English as a second language can have a differential pattern of test scores compared to those who learned English as their primary language (Boone, Victor, Wen, Razani, & Pontón, 2007; Razani, Burciaga, Madore, & Wong, 2007). Hence, even for Korean American patients who appear to be more acculturated, clinicians should be aware of potential bias when using a Western-based normative data set.

The use of translators in neuropsychological evaluations has been known to present several problems, and the clinician should always consider multiple factors before deciding if use of a translator is the best possible option (Sandoval & Duran, 1998; Wong, 2000). This issue has been discussed in depth in other works, but briefly, some of the major factors to consider include availability of native-speaking clinicians, availability of properly trained translators, and the reliability of translated test results given the referral question. Translators may be best utilized in situations where gathering collateral information from family members who are not fluent English speakers would provide the best information about disease course and duration and the presence or absence of cognitive deficits (Fujii, Umetsu, Schwartz, & Hostetter, 2002).

Estimating premorbid IQ

Estimating premorbid IQ can pose a challenge. Korean language has no silent letters or irregularly spelled words, and thus it is not possible to develop a reading test analogous to the Wechsler Test of Adult Reading or the National Adult Reading Test to assess premorbid cognitive levels. Studies have been done using K-WAIS norms to predict premorbid intelligence, but the effectiveness of such methods is still under debate (Kim, 2001c). Best-practice methods for nonfluent, less acculturated patients would be through getting a detailed history of school performance, educational attainment, and occupational history prior to immigration. Because of the competitive nature of the Korean educational and occupational system, the clinician can be fairly secure in deriving baseline cognitive estimates from such demographic information. However, cohort effects, such as disrupted schooling and work history due to the Korean War, for example, may provide more of a challenge in determining premorbid cognitive levels for older Korean patients. In these cases, the question of whether there have been changes in cognitive status may best be gleaned from information such as ability to manage household finances, ability to access community resources, and engagement in regular cognitive activities as well as data from more easily available tests, such as the Korean versions of the MMSE (Jeong et al., 2007) and IQCODE (Jorm, 2004).

Interpretation of results: Best practices

Evaluation of culturally diverse patients brings with it unavoidable confounds and inherent limitations in interpretation of test results, and thus determining the presence or absence of brain damage can be quite challenging. Fujii et al. (2002) proposed a multimethod approach to interpreting neuropsychological test results with multicultural patients. Briefly, consistency of clinical presentation given what is known about onset, course, and progression of a particular disease or disorder is important to note. Use of multiple collateral sources may also be a key source of information in these types of cases. Ultimately, the limitations of neuropsychological data must be stressed, and the clinician must be particularly mindful of cultural factors in integrating multiple sources of information, both standardized and nonstandardized, into the final case formulation.

Other recommendations

Likely, the fastest way to develop rapport and patient confidence is to understand and respect him or her as an individual and not as one fitting squarely into any given cultural category. The clinician should always be aware of preconceived stereotypes based on popular media or personal experiences. Many immigrants, including Korean Americans, have had negative experiences with assumptions, stereotyping, and "racial microaggressions," and clinicians who seem insensitive to this can quickly lose their patient's respect, confidence, and cooperation (Sue et al., 2007). Seemingly harmless examples include assuming that a Korean patient is from another East Asian culture, assuming that a patient does not speak any English, and assuming foreign birth. Genuine respect and curiosity regarding one's experiences, even if the clinician is not familiar with most things Korean, can go a long way in building rapport and trust.

Case sample

The following case is that of a Korean-speaking male who sustained a traumatic brain injury after a fall. The patient was first evaluated by a non-Korean-speaking neuropsychologist and then subsequently by a Korean-speaking neuropsychologist. The case highlights the advantages of having a same-culture clinician, while it also outlines some difficulties that remain when evaluating a nonacculturated Korean patient, even if patient and clinician are from the same cultural background and speak the same language. In either case, best-practice guidelines discussed earlier would be the best procedure to follow.

Mr. S.K. is a 42-year-old, married, right-handed, Korean male with 12 years of education who was referred for a neuropsychological evaluation following a moderate to severe traumatic brain injury (TBI). He was a recent immigrant from South Korea, where he grew up in a city 20 miles south of Seoul. Mr. S.K. graduated high school in Korea. He described himself as an average student who had no problems learning to read, write, or spell. He was never held back in school or diagnosed with a learning disability. Mr. S.K. was a car mechanic in Korea. He immigrated with his wife of 11 years and two young children to a predominantly Korean community in one of the boroughs of New York City. Family dynamics could be described as "traditionally Korean," where Mr. S.K. was head of the household and primary breadwinner.

Mr. S.K.'s English fluency was basically limited to what he had learned while a student in Korea. On the WRAT-3, English reading skills were at the seventh-grade level, but in Mr. S.K.'s case, as with most Koreans who have learned English in Korea, this did not translate to an equivalent conversational fluency. Mr. S.K. lived in a large Korean community, and thus he did not have the opportunity, necessity, or drive to further his English language skills.

Mr. S.K. suffered his TBI approximately one year following his move to the United States. He was working on a rooftop refrigeration unit when he fell approximately 20 feet through a ceiling onto the ground. Initial Glasgow Coma Scale (GCS) reported by paramedics was 15, but he rapidly decompensated, became minimally responsive, obtunded, and lethargic. Subsequent GCS was 8. His left pupil was noted to be fixed and dilated. Mr. S.K. was taken immediately to neurosurgery when a CT scan revealed a right subarachnoid hemorrhage, a large left frontotemporal parietal epidural hematoma with midline shift left to right, a small right convexity epidural hematoma, a small left parietal convexity epidural hematoma, and multiple skull fractures. He underwent a left frontotemporal parietal craniotomy and ICP monitor. Mr. S.K. also had multiple severe peripheral/orthopedic injuries. The length of post-traumatic amnesia was a few hours. Mr. S.K.'s last memory was of working on the refrigeration unit prior to the accident, and his next memory was that of waking up in the hospital.

Significant changes in personality were noted by Mr. S.K.'s wife following his accident. According to her, Mr. S.K. was "an entirely different person," who lost his sense of humor and initiative or "drive." Premorbidly, he was a real "go-getter," but postinjury, he was listless, lethargic, and depressed. Mr. S.K. also reportedly felt a strong sense of shame about (1) having to talk about his problems, (2) admitting that there were any problems at all, and (3) being unable to do what he could do premorbidly. Although his personality changes post-TBI were not seen to be significantly mediated by cultural factors, and were consistent with TBI-related changes, Mr. S.K.'s reaction to his TBI was certainly seen to have been mediated by cultural factors, particularly his shame in being put in a position to have to deal with them. Mr. S.K.'s treatment course included months of rehabilitation, including speech, occupational, physical, and recreational therapies. He reportedly made good progress and was eventually discharged home to his family.

Mr. S.K. did not return to work after his injury. Social support was limited to his immediate family. Mr. S.K. had a sister living in the United States, in another state, but all other relatives were back in Korea, which is not unusual for many Korean American families. Mr. S.K. reported that he had some friends in town, but had no contact with them since his accident. This again was likely mediated, in part, by cultural factors, as it is often the case that many Koreans will choose to keep it "in the family" and not involve or seek out nonfamily members for support, advice, or information following an adverse psychological or neuropsychological event.

Mr. S.K. underwent neuropsychological testing as part of a clinical follow-up two years following his TBI. He was evaluated by a non-Korean-speaking neuropsychologist who required the use of an interpreter. The examiner noted significant cognitive deficits related to processing speed, visuomotor function, visual memory processing, auditory memory processing, attention and "verbal regulation of the motor act," and "persistent neuroemotional factors related to traumatic brain injury involving stimulus reduction, constriction of life, and irritability." He also noted "positive effort in terms of memory processing" as an indicator of adequate effort necessary for test validity. No formal validity measures were administered. Verbal memory was tested via the interpreter but not incorporated into final impressions. Extensive testing of language functions was not done. Results of the evaluation were noted to be consistent with Mr. S.K.'s TBI. However, no mention was made of possible cultural factors that may be mediating his adjustment post-TBI, and no special recommendations were made that referred to possible barriers due to culture or language when accessing treatment.

Mr. S.K. underwent a repeat neuropsychological evaluation in the context of an independent medical exam one year later by one of the authors, a neuropsychologist fluent in Korean. Behaviorally, Mr. S.K. presented as being in a great deal of distress, both emotionally and physically. His wife was also in a lot of distress, but she was able to connect easily with the examiner and provide a much more comprehensive history of the presenting complaints and premorbid history because the barrier of having to speak through another person was removed. For example, she shared that her husband had not been intimate with her in a long time and avoided physical contact, information that was not shared with the prior neuropsychologist. It is acknowledged that, in this instance, it also likely helped that the examiner was female. Mr. S.K.'s wife was able to directly verbalize to the examiner her positive feelings about having an examiner who was familiar with their culture.

Tests (U.S. standardized and normed) were selected to measure all the major domains of cognitive functioning, and all test instructions and test items were translated directly into Korean by the neuropsychologist whenever possible/appropriate. Certain tests, like Vocabulary and Information from the Wechsler Adult Intelligence Scale–III, that required knowledge that was uniquely American in nature were not administered. Ideally, it would have been best to use normative data for Korean-speaking U.S. residents in assessing Mr. S.K.'s test performance. However, as there were no such norms available, the standard norms used for English-speaking persons of Mr. S.K.'s age and education were utilized to reference his performance to a group of neurologically healthy controls. Given knowledge of the strong educational system in Korea, 12 years of education in Korea was seen to be generally equivalent to 12 years of education in the United States. Qualitative and descriptive data were presented whenever possible to elaborate on Mr. S.K.'s performance from a clinical perspective. Moreover, consideration of his entire pattern of results, including strengths and weaknesses in specific areas, was emphasized to determine his level of cognitive functioning overall. Pattern of performance was evaluated in the context of what is typically known about TBI-related neuropsychological sequelae.

Mr. S.K. passed two formal measures of effort as well as embedded measures of validity. Test results revealed that Mr. S.K. was demonstrating moderate cognitive deficits in the areas of fine motor dexterity, information processing speed, new learning and memory, and executive systems functioning. Results were consistent with cerebral dysfunction secondary to his traumatic brain injury. Recommendations were made for neurorehabilitation with access to a Korean-speaking interpreter in order to be able to fully participate in therapy if there were no Korean-speaking therapists available. Korean-speaking therapists may have been an option in a large city like New York, but would be most certainly difficult to get in many other areas of the United States. Mr. S.K.'s ability to engage in treatment and benefit from it was seen to be severely limited by language barriers, and culturally, there were also concerns that he may not participate fully in therapies that involved personal disclosure (e.g., group therapy) or demonstration of weakness, particularly in front of others. Hence, recommendations were carefully made with these factors in mind to maximize recovery.

References

Artiola i Fortuny, L. (2003, February). *Clinical neuropsychology, low education, and illiteracy*. Presented at the International Neuropsychological Society 31st Annual Meeting, Honolulu, HI.

Background Note: South Korea (2009, October 30). U.S. Department of State. Retrieved May 7, 2010 from http://www.state.gov/r/pa/ei/bgn/2800.htm

Boone, K. B., Victor, T. L., Wen, J., Razani, J., & Pontón, M. (2007). The association between neuropsychological scores and ethnicity, language, and acculturation variables in a large patient population. *Archives of Clinical Neuropsychology, 22*, 355–365.

Brozan, N. (1992, March 12). Chronicle. *New York Times*. Retrieved October 21, 2007, from http://query.nytimes.com/gst/fullpage.html?res=9E0CE3D9173CF931A25750C0A964958260

Chen, H. Y., Chen, Y. H., & Zhu, J. (2003). Taiwan. In J. Georgas, L. Weiss, F. J. R. van de Vijver, & D. H. Saklofske (Eds.), *Culture and children's intelligence: Cross-cultural analysis of the WISC-III* (pp. 241–252). San Diego, CA: Academic Press.

Chey, J. Y., Na, D. R., Park, S. H., Park, E. H., & Lee, S. A. (1999). Effects of education in dementia assessment: Evidence from standardizing the Korean-Dementia Rating Scale. *Clinical Neuropsychologist, 13*, 293–302.

Chung, A. Y. (2004). The dawn of a new generation: The historical evolution of inter-generational conflict and cooperation in Korean-American organizational politics. In I. J. Kim (Ed.), *Korean-Americans: Past, present, and future* (pp. 101–120). Elizabeth, NJ: Hollym International Corp.

The competitive power of English. (2000, June 9). *The Chosun Ilbo*. Retrieved October 8, 2007, from http://www.chosun.com/w21data/html/news/200006/200006090279.html

Delis, D. C., Kramer, J. H., Kaplan, E., & Ober, B. A. (1987). *The California Verbal Learning Test* (research ed.). San Antonio, TX: Psychological Corporation.

Eckert, C. J., Lee, K., Lew, Y. I., Robinson, M., & Wagner, E. W. (1990). *Korea old and new: A history*. Seoul, Korea: Korea Institute, Harvard University.

Education System: Overview. (2006). Retrieved October 22, 2007, from the Korean Ministry of Education and Human Resources Development Web site: http://english.moe.go.kr/main.jsp?idx=020101

Fujii, D., Umetsu, D., Schwartz, T., & Hostetter, G. (2002). Culturally sensitive strategies for practicing neuropsychology in Hawaii. *INSNET, 10*(4), 1–2.

Gondo, M. (2003). *Parsing Asian America. Goldsea Asian American demographics.* Retrieved October 3, 2007, from http://goldsea.com/AAD/Parsing/parsing.html

Harvey, Y. S. K., & Chung, S. H. (1980). The Koreans. In J. F. McDermott, W. S. Tseng, & T. W. Maretzki (Eds.), *People and cultures of Hawaii: A psychocultural profile* (pp. 135–154). Honolulu, HI: University of Hawaii Press.

Jeong, S. K., Lim, E. S., Nam, H. S., Kweon, S. S., Park, K. S., Shin, M. H., & Choi, J. S. (2007). Population-based norms for the Korean Mini-Mental State Examination and Korean version of modified Mini-Mental State Examination [in Korean]. *Journal of the Korean Neurological Association, 25,* 1–9.

Jorm, A. F. (2004). The Informant Questionnaire on Cognitive Decline in the Elderly (IQCODE): A review. *International Psychogeriatrics, 16,* 3–19. (http://www.anu.edu.au/iqcode/)

Kang, Y., & Na, D. L. (2003). *Seoul Neuropsychological Screening Battery.* Incheon, South Korea: Human Brain Research & Consulting Co.

Kaplan, E., Goodglass, H., & Weintraub, S. (1983). *The Boston Naming Test.* Philadelphia, PA: Lea & Febiger.

Kim, A. (2003). *South Korea and Korean-Americans in the United States.* Retrieved October 3, 2007, from http://www2.bc.edu/~brisk/korea.htm

Kim, H. (2001a). Assessment of memory disorders using Rey-Kim Memory Test [in Korean]. *Journal of Rehabilitation Psychology, 8,* 29–48.

Kim, H. (2001b). Clinical evaluation of the frontal lobe syndrome using Kims Frontal Executive Neuropsychological Test [in Korean]. *Journal of Rehabilitation Psychology, 8,* 173–190.

Kim, H. (2001c). Use and misuse of premorbid intelligence estimation [in Korean]. *Korean Journal of Clinical Psychology, 20,* 145–154.

Kim, H. (2004). The Korean independence movement in the United States: Syngman Rhee, Ahn Ch'ang-Ho, and Pak Yong-Man. In I. J. Kim (Ed.), *Korean-Americans: Past, present, and future* (pp. 63–98). Elizabeth, NJ: Hollym International Corp.

Kim, H., & Na, D. L. (1999). Normative data on the Korean version of the Boston Naming Test. *Journal of Clinical and Experimental Neuropsychology, 21,* 127–133.

Kim, H. H., & Na, D. L. (2004). Normative data on the Korean version of the Western Aphasia Battery. *Journal of Clinical and Experimental Neuropsychology, 26,* 1011–1020.

Kim, I. J. (2004). A century of Korean immigration to the United States: 1903–2003. In I. J. Kim (Ed.), *Korean-Americans: Past, present, and future* (pp. 13–37). Elizabeth, NJ: Hollym International Corp.

Kim, J. K., & Kang, Y. (1999). Normative study of the Korean-California Verbal Learning Test (K-CVLT). *Clinical Neuropsychologist, 13,* 365–369.

Kim, L. I. C. (1996). Psychiatric care of Korean Americans. In A. Gaw (Ed.), *Culture, ethnicity, and mental illness* (pp. 347–375). Washington, DC: American Psychiatric Press.

Kim, T. Y., Kim, S. Y., Kim, J. W., Yoo, B. G., Lim, B. H., Ihn, Y. K., … Kim, S. H. (2006). The Korean Memory Test (KMT) for elderly: Estimating validity and reliability [in Korean]. *Journal of the Korean Geriatrics Society, 10,* 77–85.

Kim, T. Y., Kim, S. Y., Sohn, J. E., Lee, E. A., Lim, B. H., & Ihn, Y. K. (2005). Study of validity and reliability of the Korean Complex Figure Test [in Korean]. *Journal of the Korean Geriatrics Society, 9,* 30–38.

Kwak, K. (2003). South Korea. In J. Georgas, L. Weiss, F. J. R. van de Vijver, & D. H. Saklofske (Eds.), *Culture and children's intelligence: Cross-cultural analysis of the WISC-III* (pp. 227-240). San Diego, CA: Academic Press.

Language Overview. (2007). Retrieved October 3, 2007, from the Korean Overseas Information Service Web site: http://www.korea.net/korea/kor_loca.asp?code=A020301

Lee, D. Y., Lee, K. U., Lee, J. H., Kim, K. W., Jhoo, J. H., Kim, S. Y., ... Woo, J. J. (2004). A normative study of the CERAD neuropsychological assessment battery in the Korean elderly. *Journal of the International Neuropsychological Society, 10,* 72–81.

Lee, J. H., Lee, K. U., Lee, D. Y., Kim, K. W., Jhoo, J. H., Kim J. H., et al. (2002). Development of the Korean version of the Consortium to Establish a Registry for Alzheimer's Disease Assessment Packet (CERAD-K): Clinical and neuropsychological assessment batteries. *Journals of Gerontology Series B: Psychological Sciences and Social Sciences, 57,* 47–53.

Lee, J. Y., Lee, D. W., Cho, S. J., Na, D. L., Hong, J. J., et al. (2008). Brief screening for mild cognitive impairment in elderly outpatient clinic: Validation of the Korean version of the Montreal cognitive assessment. *Journal of Geriatric Psychiatry and Neurology, 21*(2), 104–110.

Lee, R. M., Yoon, E., & Liu-Tom, H. T. (2006, April 1). Structure and measurement of acculturation/enculturation for Asian Americans using the ARSMA-II (Acculturation Rating Scale for Mexican Americans). *Measurement and Evaluation in Counseling and Development.* Retrieved October 15, 2007, from http://www.accessmylibrary.com/coms2/summary_0286-32939350_ITM

Lee, S., Khang, Y., Lee, M., & Kang, W. (2002). Knowledge of, attitudes toward, and experience of complementary and alternative medicine in Western medicine- and Oriental medicine-trained physicians in Korea. *American Journal of Public Health, 92,* 1994–2000.

Lee, S. H., Park, W. M., Kim, S. H., Kang, Y. S., Ha, J. Y., & Lee, H. L. (1997). The usefulness of Clock Drawing Test as screening for dementia on the basis of the correlation between clock drawing and MMSE-K [in Korean]. *Journal of the Korean Academy of Family Medicine, 18,* 785–792.

Lim, L. (2007). South Korean culture wave spreads across Asia. Retrieved October 21, 2007, from NPR Web site: http://www.npr.org/templates/story/story.php?storyId=5300970

Lynn, R., & Song, M. (1994). General intelligence, visuospatial and verbal abilities in Korean children. *Personality and Individual Differences, 16,* 363–364.

Munoz-Sandoval, A. F., Cummins, J., Alvarado, C. G., & Ruef, M. L. (1998). *Bilingual Verbal Ability Tests*. Itasca, IL: Riverside Publishing.

Nash, A. (2000). Korean Americans. In J. Lehman (Ed.), *Gale encyclopedia of multicultural America* (2nd ed., Vol. 2, pp. 1071–1090). Detroit, MI: Gale Group.

Nasreddine, Z., Phillips, N., Bedirian, V., Charbonneau, S., Whitehead, V., Collin, S., ... Chertkow, H. (2005). The Montreal Cognitive Assessment, MoCA: A brief screening tool for mild cognitive impairment. *Journal of the American Geriatric Society, 53,* 695–699.

Oh, K. J., Hong, K. E., Lee, H. R., & Ha, E. H. (1997). *Korean Child and Adolescent Behavior Checklist*. Seoul, Korea, Chung-Ang Publisher.

Onishi, N. (2006, April 2). In a wired South Korea, robots will feel right at home. *New York Times*. Retrieved September 8, 2007, from http://www.nytimes.com/2006/04/02/world/asia/02robot.html

Park, H., Cho, B., & Choi, H. (2003). *Korean Bayley Scale of Infant Development–II*. Institute for Bayley Scale of Infant Development II. www.bayley.co.kr

Park, H., Kwak, K., & Park, K. (1996). *Manual for Korean Wechsler Primary & Preschool Scale of Intelligence (K-WPPSI)*. Seoul, Korea: Special Education Publishers.

Raven, J. (1981). *Manual for Raven's Progressive Matrices and Mill Hill Vocabulary Scales* (Research Supplement 1). London, UK: H. K. Lewis.

Razani, J., Burciaga, J., Madore, M., & Wong, J. (2007). Effects of acculturation on tests of attention and information processing in an ethnically diverse group. *Archives of Clinical Neuropsychology, 22*, 333–341.

Sandoval, J., & Duran, R. P. (1998). Language. In J. Sandoval, C. L. Frisby, K. F. Geisinger, J. D. Scheuneman, & J. R. Grenier (Eds.), *Test interpretation and diversity: Achieving equity in assessment* (pp. 181–212). Washington, DC: American Psychological Association Press.

Seo, E. H., Lee, D. Y., Kim, K. W., Lee, J. H., Jhoo, J. H., Youn, J. C., … Woo, J. I. (2006). A normative study of the Trail Making Test in Korean elders. *International Journal of Geriatric Psychology, 21*, 844–852.

Sue, D. W., Capodilupo, C. M., Torino, G. C., Bucceri, J. M., Holder, A. M. B., Nadal, K. L., et al. (2007). Racial microaggressions in everyday life: Implications for clinical practice. *American Psychologist, 62*, 271–286.

Ueno, K., & Nakatani, I. (2003). Japan. In J. Georgas, L. Weiss, F. J. R. van de Vijver, & H. Saklofske (Eds.), *Culture and children's intelligence: Cross-cultural analysis of the WISC-III* (pp. 215–225). San Diego, CA: Academic Press.

U.S. Census Bureau. (1990). *Profile of general demographic characteristics.* Washington, DC: Author.

U.S. Census Bureau. (2000). *2000 Census of population: General population characteristics.* Washington, DC: Author.

Wechsler, D. (1991). *Wechsler Intelligence Scale for Children* (3rd ed.). San Antonio, TX: The Psychological Corporation.

Welsh, K., Butters, N., Mohs, R. C., Beekly, B. S., Edland, S., Fillenbaum, G., et al. (1994). The Consortium to Establish a Registry for Alzheimer's Disease (CERAD) Part V: A normative study of the neuropsychological battery. *Neurology, 44*, 609–614.

What is Hangeul? (2007). Retrieved October 22, 2007, from the Korean Overseas Information Service Web site: http://www.korea.net/korea/kor_loca.asp?code= A020302

Wong, T. (2000). Neuropsychological assessment and intervention with Asian Americans. In E. Fletcher-Janzen, T. L. Strickland, & C. R. Reynolds (Eds.), *Handbook of cross-cultural neuropsychology* (pp. 43–53). New York, NY: Kluwer Academic/Plenum Publishers.

Wong, T. M., Strickland, T. L., Fletcher-Janzen, E., Ardila, A., & Reynolds, C. R. (2000). Theoretical and practical issues in the neuropsychological assessment and treatment of culturally dissimilar patients. In E. Fletcher-Janzen, T. L. Strickland, and C. R. Reynolds (Eds.), *Handbook of cross-cultural neuropsychology* (pp. 3–18). New York, NY: Kluwer Academic/Plenum Publishers.

World Health Organization. (1999). *World Health Report 1999* (pp. 84–87). Geneva, Switzerland: Author.

Yoo, D. (2003, July 26). Cultural tug of war: The Korean immigrant family and church in transition—Korean Americans and their religions: Pilgrims and missionaries from a different shore [Book review]. *Christian Century*. Retrieved October 8, 2007, from http://findarticles.com/p/articles/mi_m1058/is_15_120/ai_106098107

Yum, T. H., Park, Y. S., Oh, K. J., Kim, J. K., & Lee, Y. H. (1992). *Korean Wechsler Adult Intelligence Scale (K-WAIS) manual.* Seoul, Korea: Korea Guidance.

9 Neuropsychology of Laotian Americans

Daryl Fujii

Brief history

Laos is a Southeast Asian country that is slightly larger than the state of Utah. It is bordered by Thailand, Cambodia, Myanmar, China, and Vietnam. The northern part of the country is mountainous, while much of the southern part is lowlands, except for the southeast border with Vietnam, which is also mountainous. Historically, Laotians have been farmers, although there are some natural resources, such as copper, gold, and wood. Many, particularly in the less fertile mountain areas, have been sustenance farmers engaging in slash-and-burn farming.

Laotians are diverse in ethnic identity. The culturally dominant group is the Lao or Lao Loum, who live in the lowlands. The highlands are inhabited by the Hmong or Lao Sung, and the Mien or Hmong-Yao. The Lao Theung, comprised of the Mon-Khmer and Viet-Muong tribes, live in the mid-slope region. This chapter will focus on the Lao.

Laotians are descendants of the T'ai people of southern China, who migrated to Laos in the sixth century. Laos was originally part of Cambodia. It became an independent country in 1353 under Prince Fa Ngum, who established Lan Xang, or "The Kingdom of a Million Elephants." Under Prince Fa Ngum, Laos enjoyed great power and prosperity and extended into most of modern Thailand. Luang Prabang was the nation's capital until 1563, when King Setthalhiralh moved the capital to its current location at Vientiane (Bankston, 2000). Laos subdivided into three separate kingdoms after the death of King Souligna Vongsa in 1694. By the mid-1800s, most of the weakened country, with the exception of Luang Prabang, was taken over by Vietnam and Thailand. A few decades later, the French colonized Southeast Asia, controlling Vietnam, Thailand, and Laos at the end of the nineteenth century (Bankston, 2000). French occupancy was briefly interrupted during World War II, when Japan conquered much of Indochina. When the Japanese surrendered in 1945, Laos claimed independence under the *Lao Issara* (Free Laos) banner. However, this movement was short lived as the French reoccupied the country by early 1946.

Laos regained independence in the 1954 Geneva peace conference after France was defeated by the Vietnamese Communists (Wikipedia, 2009a). The first years of Laotian independence were characterized by high instability, with rivalries between the neutralists, right wing, left wing, and future prime minister Kaysone Phomvihane's group. Elections were held in 1955, and the first coalition government was headed by neutralist Prince Souvanna Phouma in 1957. This government collapsed the next year and in 1960, when Captain Kong Lac staged a coup to reform the neutralist government. Prince Souvanna briefly regained control only to be driven out by rightist forces led by General Phoumi Nosavan later that year (Wikipedia, 2009b).

A second Geneva conference held in 1961–1962 reestablished Laos' independence and also its neutrality in the Indochina war being fought in Vietnam. The agreement was not binding and civil war ensued from 1962 to 1975 between the Royal Lao Government, supported by the United States, and the rebellious Pathet Lao, supported by the Communist North Vietnamese.

The main battlefield was along the Ho Chi Minh trail, which was a supply lifeline for the North Vietnamese while infiltrating South Vietnam. The Pathet Lao supported the North Vietnamese to protect this strategic trail, while the Royal Lao Government Army, lead by Hmong leader General Vang Pao, attempted to capture this area (Wikipedia, 2009b).

The United States eventually withdrew from Vietnam in 1973, and South Vietnam fell to the North in April 1975. With the backing of North Vietnam, the Pathet Lao, led by Kaysone Phomvihane, gained control of the coalition government and formed the Lao People's Democratic Republic (LPDR). The LDPR immediately imprisoned many members of the previous government and Royal Lao Army in "reeducation camps." These policies prompted about 10% of the population to leave the country, and many initially settled in Thai refugee camps before moving on to other countries. Early Laotian immigrants to the United States consisted of former government administrators, soldiers from the royal army, and shopkeepers. Later immigrants were less educated and included farmers and villagers (Bankston, 2000).

Laotian population demographics in the United States

According to the 2000 U.S. census, there were 167,792 Laotians living in the United States, which constituted 1.6% of the total Asian American population (Reeves & Bennett, 2004). About 68.1% of Laotians are foreign born, of which 45.6% have become naturalized citizens. The vast majority of Laotians immigrated during the 1980s: 16.9% immigrated before 1980, 65.7% from 1980 to 1990, and 17.4% from 1990 to 2000 (Reeves & Bennett, 2004). Given the high percentage of immigrants, it is not surprising that many are not proficient in English. In Laotian households, 92.9% speak a non-English language, while 40.1% report speaking English "very well." It is estimated that 26.3% of Laotian households meet criteria for being linguistically isolated (Yang, 2004). Laotian households only speaking English are reported to be 7.2% (Reeves & Bennett, 2004).

Settlement in the United States has been selective to a few states, with almost half living in California and the west. States with the largest number of Laotians are as follows: (1) California, 55,456; (2) Texas, 10,114; (3) Minnesota, 9,940; (4) Washington, 7,974; (5) North Carolina, 5,313; (6) Illinois, 5,235; (7) Georgia, 4,531; (8) Wisconsin, 4,469; (9) Oregon, 4,349; and (10) Tennessee, 4,214 (Pfeifer, 2001).

Similar to other Asian American ethnic groups, Laotians are located in urban areas (96%) (Bankston, 2000).

The Laotian American population is more youthful than the Asian and general population. The 2000 U.S. census data reported the median age of Laotians as 26.1, in comparison to all Asians (33.0) and the total population (35.4) (Reeves & Bennett, 2004). In the 2000 census, 34.3% of Laotians were under 18 years of age, while 3.4% were older than 65.

About 53.1% of Laotians over age 15 were married (Reeves & Bennett, 2004). As with Asians in general, Laotians (10.5%) are less likely to be separated, widowed, or divorced than the general population (19%), and have more children, with average household sizes estimated at 4.23 (U.S. average is 2.59). Despite having larger households, the median family income for Laotians ($43,542) is among the lowest for Asians ($59,324), and lower than the general population's ($50,046). There are fewer Laotians (male, 65.5%; female, 56.3%) participating in the workforce than the general population (male, 70.7%; female, 57.5%), and a lower percentage of Laotians (13.4%) are employed in management, professional, or related occupations than all Asians (44.6%) or the general population (33.6%). Given these figures, it is not surprising that a high percentage of Laotians (18.5) live below the poverty level (total U.S. population, 12.4) (Reeves & Bennett, 2004).

History of education in Laos

Education in Laos was traditionally provided by monks at Buddhist wats until the mid–twentieth century. Most villages had a wat, and only males were allowed in these schools. Curriculums included reading Lao and Pali scripts, arithmetic, religion, and other social subjects. When the French colonized Laos, they established a secular education system primarily for the elite in urban centers. Members of the royal family and households, and children of Vietnamese immigrants who were sent to Laos to oversee the country, constituted the majority of these students. The education was patterned after the French system, which was divided into primary and secondary educational systems. Courses were taught in French from the second or third grade. Postsecondary education was unavailable in Laos, and advanced students had to travel to Vietnam and Cambodia for specialized training, or to France for university-level studies (Wikipedia, 2008).

Laos developed its own educational system when it gained independence in the 1950s. The Pathet Lao provided instruction in Lao, and the Royal Lao Government (RLG) implemented a Laotian curriculum in the 1960s. The educational system grew steadily, and by 1970 about a third of the civilian employees of the government were primary school teachers, although most were poorly paid and trained. At this time, about 36% of primary school–age children, or approximately 200,000 students, were enrolled in the RLG schools (Wikipedia, 2008).

When the Lao People's Democratic Republic (LPDR) was established in 1975, one of the goals was to institute a universal primary educational system by 1985. To implement the plan, the government built and staffed schools within each village. However, due to limited resources, most schools only had one or two grades, teaching materials were sparse, and classes were held irregularly, overcrowded, and conducted for only a few hours per day by one or two teachers in thatched huts. Due to the paucity of resources, most students took about 11–12 years to complete a primary school curriculum. Repetition rates ranged from 40% for the first grade to 14% for the fifth grade. Dropout rates were also high, with 22% of first-graders leaving before the second grade and a 55% dropout rate for all students (Wikipedia, 2008).

Quality of education and enrollment varied across urban–rural areas, gender, and ethnicity. Enrollment and education quality were higher in urban areas, where there were more resources and an education was more valued than in rural areas, where farming was the major industry. Boys were more likely to attend schools than girls, with an initial 37% female enrollment that increased to 44% by 1989. In addition to urban–rural factors, due to language barriers, Lao from the lowlands had higher rates of enrollment than their Hmong counterparts, who spoke a different language and did not have a literacy tradition. Enrollment of Hmong girls was even lower, at about 26% (Wikipedia, 2008).

Secondary educational schools also expanded under the LPDR, but are much less prevalent than primary schools. By 1992–1993, only about 130,000 students were enrolled in postprimary educational programs, including secondary schools, vocational programs, and teacher training schools. Secondary education institutions are concentrated in urban centers, with most located in provincial capitals and to a lesser extent district centers. The vast majority of secondary education students come from the cities, as students from rural areas must board in makeshift facilities (Wikipedia, 2008).

Postsecondary educational institutions are even scarcer, with the majority of schools located in the capital of Vientiane. Institutions of higher learning include the National Teacher's Training School at Dong Dok, the Irrigation College at Tad Thong, the Agriculture College at Na Phok, the National Polytechnic Institute, and the University of Medical Sciences. The academic rigor of these universities lags behind other Asian countries, as none of the Laotian institutions are ranked in the top 100 Asian universities (Webometrics, n.d.). To supplement the limited availability of local institutes of higher learning, between 1975 and 1990, the LPDR granted over 14,000 scholarships for study in Socialist countries, with over 7,000 educated in the Soviet Union, 2,500 in Vietnam, and 1,800 to East Germany (Wikipedia, 2008).

Another educational goal of the RLG was to increase literacy in adults. A national adult literacy campaign was initiated in 1983–1984 that recruited educated citizens to teach basic reading skills to over 750,000 adults. National literacy increased to about 44%. Rates were much higher for adults between the ages of 15 and 45, with 92% of men and 76% of women reported to be literate in 1985. Unfortunately, due to the lack of reading materials, particularly in rural areas, many newly literate adults lost their proficiency after a few years (Wikipedia, 2008).

Although still a work in progress, the LDPR's attempts to expand the educational system in Laos have been successful, as evidenced by a steady increase in enrollment and literacy rates. Primary school enrollment increased from 100,000 students in 1959, to 317,000 in 1976, to 603,000 in 1992 (Wikipedia, 2008). The youth literacy rate (literacy defined as "with understanding, both read and write a short simple statement on everyday life") has increased from 62.6% in 1980 to 78.5% in 2004. Literacy for Laotian adults increased from 33.2% in 1980 to 60.2% in 2003, while for males it increased from 74.4% in 1980 to 81.1% in 2003 (Globalis, n.d.).

Education history in the United States

In comparison to the general population and other Asians, Laotian Americans are poorly educated. About 49.6% have less than high school, 24.4% are high school graduates, 18.3% completed some college, while only 7.7% earned a bachelor's degree or higher (Reeves & Bennett, 2004). Low academic achievement for Laotian adults is not surprising given that 68.1% of Laotians are foreign born and the lack of educational opportunities in Laos. Unfortunately, the limited available data also indicate that Laotian children experience significant difficulties in American schools (Yang & Niedzwiecki, 2003).

There is a paucity of studies with a specific non-Hmong Laotian American population, and thus little hard evidence of reasons for the poor academic achievement of Laotian Americans. Yang and Niedzwiecki (2003) propose several potential causes. First, a significant number of Laotian students have limited English proficiency, which makes it difficult to learn in schools where English is the medium of communication. Second, systematic miscommunication between students, parents, and teachers can affect a Laotian student's ability to learn. Parents who are poorly educated and lack adequate English skills are ill-equipped to serve as educational mentors to their children or communicate concerns with teachers. In addition, differences in expectations and values between foreign-born parents who emphasize cultural traditions and American-born children who focus on assimilation exacerbate the generation gap between parents and children. Third, Laotian students experience discrimination from policy makers and teachers. Policy makers who are removed from the classroom tend to overlook the special needs of Southeast Asians due to the model minority image of Asians. Thus, much-needed programs for Southeast Asians are not adequately funded or supported. Simultaneously, teachers who are closer to the Laotian students may feel they are not college material and indirectly communicate this assessment of their ability to them. This powerful combination can result in Laotian children giving up due to an internalization of their learning problems. Finally, Laotian students may experience widespread feelings of alienation from mainstream schools. Very few schools have sufficient numbers of Southeast Asians on staff, or curriculum to assist the students in understanding themselves and their culture.

Pertinent cultural variables

Family structure

In a traditional Laotian family, the family is headed by the husband or oldest male, who is the primary decision maker, although elders of both genders are highly respected (Keovilay & Kemp, n.d.). The man represents the household in community affairs, while the woman runs the household and oversees the finances. In America, these roles are less well defined, as it is common for Laotian women to work, and thus many Laotian men assist with household tasks, while women can also be active in the community (Bankston, 2000). Children are expected to remain quiet and respectful in their interactions with elders and visitors (Keovilay & Kemp, n.d.).

The most common family arrangement in the United States is the nuclear family living in close proximity to extended family. Extended family is important for both social and financial support (Bankston, 2000).

Religious values

Religious beliefs of most Laotians appear to be a combination of Theravada Buddhism and animism (Keovilay & Kemp, n.d.). All Buddhists equate life to suffering caused by one's desires, and that suffering in one's current life results from misdeeds in previous lives. Two core Buddhist values are harmony and balance, and conflicts are to be avoided at all costs. Theravada Buddhism is a more individualistic denomination that stresses personal development and individual good behavior to attain enlightenment before helping others. Thus, males are strongly encouraged to become Buddhist monks for a brief period (World Culture Encyclopedia, 2008).

Many Laotians also believe in spirits, or *phi*. Nature is filled with spirits that inhabit places such as rivers, rice fields, or groves of trees. Laotians worship *phi* by offering them food in outdoor shrines (Keovilay & Kemp, n.d.). A small number of Laotians have converted to Protestant Christianity, particularly in areas where the Laotian community is small (Keohavong, 1996).

Illness beliefs and traditional healing practices

Laotian beliefs about illnesses are directly related to their religious and spiritual beliefs. For example, illnesses can be caused by malevolent spirits or result from an offensive deed done to a deceased ancestor (World Culture Encyclopedia, 2008; Keohavang, 1996). Another common belief is that each person has 32 spirits, or *kwhan*, associated with different parts of the body. Illnesses occur when a spirit abandons the person, resulting in an imbalance in spirits (De Voe, 2009). Spirit loss is often associated with travel, as spirits can be left behind. Similar to other Southeast Asians who are influenced by Chinese medicine models, balances among the four human elements, wind, water, earth, and fire, are important for health. Of these elements, wind is the most salient for medical illnesses (Graham & Chitnarong, 1997).

Traditional Laotian healing practices include different forms of massages and herbal treatments, of which the latter can be taken orally, inhaled through the mouth or nose, or applied directly to wounds (Keohavong, 1996). If illness is believed to result from spirit loss, a family member, elder, or *acharn* (teacher/healer) will pray to the spirits of the different body parts to return to the body. When health is returned, the *acharn* may reward the returning spirit with rice and chicken, which is given to the patient (Keovilay & Kemp, n.d.).

Laotian Americans primarily look to family and community for support, and traditional treatments are tried first. If these interventions are not successful, the family will take the person to a Western clinic or hospital. In many cases, traditional practices continue even if the ill person is being treated with Western medicines. In general, Laotians focus on treating acute illnesses. Prevention or health promotion is not valued (Keovilay & Kemp, n.d.).

Mental health issues

Many Laotians experienced significant trauma during the Vietnamese war and political aftermath. Sources of trauma included leaving the country, living in refugee camps, and immigrating to a foreign country. In a study evaluating mixed Indochinese Americans living in California, Gong-Guy (1987) reported that 50% of the Laotian population demonstrated a need for psychiatric services, while 10% of the entire sample met criteria for posttraumatic stress disorder (PTSD). Kinzie and Leung (1996) reported that Laotians may experience depressive symptoms due to loss of country, social position in their home country, and difficulties due to language barriers.

Despite a need for treatment, Laotians are generally reluctant to seek psychiatric services due to shame and fear of stigmatization to the family. In Laos, psychiatrists only treat the insane (Keohavong, 1996). Thus, Laotians will only seek treatment for mental illness if behaviors of a family member are impossible to ignore, the person is too difficult to manage, or families experience significant levels of distress (Kinzie & Leung, 1996). For example, typical symptoms of PTSD, such as nightmares, startle reactions, irritability, and reexperiencing traumas, are not worth mentioning to physicians, and many do not seek treatment for this disorder (Bromley & Chhem Sip, 2003). Emotional problems are generally manifested in vague and multiple somatic complaints, such as poor sleep, pain, gastrointestinal problems, or physical weakness; thus, Laotians who do seek treatment by Western practitioners are often seen by medical doctors (Kinzie & Leung, 1996).

Similar to medical illnesses, Laotians believe that there are numerous causes of mental illness, including spirit loss (Keovilay & Kemp, n.d.), supernatural causes, physical causes, social problems, and psychological causes (Westermeyer, 1988). Factors are generally outside the control of the individual (Westermeyer, 1988).

Health issues

Refugees from Southeast Asia are at high risk for numerous illnesses, including nutritional deficits, hepatitis B, tuberculosis, parasites, malaria, HIV, Hansen's disease, and PTSD (Keovilay & Kemp, n.d.). In a California study, Laotian men were found to have high rates of lung and liver cancer, while the most common cancer found in Laotian women was cervical cancer. Compared to other ethnic minorities, Laotians had the highest teen pregnancy rate, as 19% of pregnant Laotian women were teenagers (Asian and Pacific Islander American Health Forum, n.d.).

Neuropsychological literature

The neuropsychological literature on Laotians is sparse and focuses on test scores with children. Boivin et al. (1996) administered the Kaufman Assessment Battery for Children (K-ABC) and Tactual Performance Test (TPT) with two samples of Laotian children ages 5–12. The first sample was comprised of urban children of medical staff and administrative professionals in Vientiane (n = 24) whose mothers and fathers had mean education levels of 13.4 (sd = 3.56) and 14.7 (sd = 2.3) years, respectively. The other sample consisted of children living in Nai Sai Tong, a rural village (n = 22). Their mothers' mean level of education was 7.6 (sd = 5.3), while their fathers' education level was M = 8.8 (sd = 5.0).

Results indicate that the urban sample scored significant on all global scales and subtest scores (see Table 9.1 for mean scores). Subtest scores for the urban sample were generally within the average range, with the exception of performances on Number Recall, a test similar to Digit Span, that fell within the very superior

Table 9.1 K-ABC and TPT scores for urban and rural Laotian children

	Urban (n = 24)		*Village (n = 22)*	
Measures	*M*	*SD*	*M*	*SD*
Kaufman Assessment Battery for Children (K-ABC)				
Global scales				
Sequential	123	8.4	107	11.1
Simultaneous	108	13.9	87	13.0
Nonverbal	111	13.2	90	11.7
Mental Processing	116	12.4	94	12.7
Sequential subtests				
Hand Movements	11	1.6	8	2.3
Number Recall	17	1.8	16	2.1
Word Order	13	2.3	9	2.4
Simultaneous subtests				
Gestalt Closure	9	2.7	5	2.6
Triangles	13	2.8	9	3.8
Matrix Analogies	11	2.6	8	2.4
Spatial Memory	11	2.4	10	2.6
Photo Series	11	3.1	7	6.6
Tactual Performance Test (TPT)				
Dominant hand[a]	101.2	125.1	107.0	92.2
Nondominant hand	60.3	61.2	71.8	64.9
Both hands	26.8	19.4	39.2	36.1
Memory	4.3	1.7	3.4	1.6
Location	3.4	1.8	2.1	1.6

Source: Boivin, M., et al., *Neuropsychology, 10*, 588–599, 1996.

[a] Values represent time per block.

range, and high average level scores on Word Order and Triangles. The rural sample also generally performed within the average range, although within the lower levels. Exceptions include a superior level score on Number Recall, a low average performance on Photo Series, and a borderline level score on Gestalt Closure.

The finding of stronger sequential versus simultaneous processing was also demonstrated in a Laotian American immigrant sample in Texas ($n = 70$) (Utairatanakit, 1987). The score for the Lao immigrant children on the K-ABC Sequential Composite was $M = 100.8$ ($sd = 13.6$), while that for the Simultaneous Composite was $M = 101.6$ ($sd = 11.4$). Although there were no differences between these scores, the researcher indicated that 39/70 children had limited English proficiency, and thus projected that the Sequential Composite would have been higher if the test had been administered in Lao.

Conant et al. (2003) compared K-ABC Sequential processing subtests scores of the aforementioned Laotian sample with a sample of children from rural southeast Michigan. Using an ANCOVA to control for age and education, differences were found in the Hand Movements subtest $F(3, 96) = -4.55$, $p = .005$, with the American sample performing significantly stronger than the Laotian sample, and Number Recall, which indicated significantly stronger Laotian performances, $F(3, 96) = 30.87$, $p < .001$. Group differences on the Word Order subtest approached significance, with stronger performances for the American sample, $F(3, 96) = 2.68$, $p = .051$.

On the TPT, the urban and village samples performed similarly on trials for dominant, nondominant, both hands, and memory. A significant difference was found for location ($p = .02$), with the urban sample scoring higher than the village sample. It is difficult to compare the performances of the Laotian children with American norms, as the ages of the Laotian sample ranged from 5 to 12, whereas American norms are based upon a specific age. With this caveat, the memory and location scores for the urban sample ($M = 8.3$ years, $sd = 1.9$) were very similar to norms for eight-year-old American children (memory, $M = 4.44$, $sd = 1.2$; location, $M = 3.22$, $sd = 1.7$) (Nussbaum & Bunner, 2009).

Recommendations

Due to the paucity of neuropsychological norms on an exclusively Laotian sample, Western tests would most likely not be valid to estimate actual cognitive functioning. An exception would be use of the K-ABC and possibly TPT with children under 12. The lack of norms would indicate that for a majority of adult cases, a formal neuropsychological evaluation may not be possible. Still, a conceptual impression from a multimodal assessment based upon social and functional history from client and collateral sources, behavioral observations, medical records, including neuroimaging if available, and history of progression of cognitive and behavioral changes, in comparison with expectations from neurological disorder, can still be useful for making diagnoses and recommendations for improving functioning.

This type of assessment based on history and presentation would be insufficient to determine subtle cognitive changes from mild brain injuries. However, given Laotian culture, in which behavioral or emotional problems are not brought to the attention of professionals until it is very disturbing to family or significantly affecting finances, it is highly likely this type of evaluation can be useful, as for many Laotian Americans, their deficits would be noticeable by the time of referral. Although ideally a Laotian American neuropsychologist would perform the evaluation, due to the paucity of these professionals in combination with the pressing need for such an evaluation when a referral is finally made, it is likely a non–Laotian American would be asked to perform a neuropsychological evaluation on a Laotian American. The following are conceptual issues to consider when providing neuropsychological consultation to Laotian Americans:

Child

1. Western tests are most relevant for Laotians born and educated in the United States and for whom English is their primary language. However, many Laotian American children are bilingual, as Lao is spoken in over 92% of households (Reeves & Bennett, 2004). If English is not the child's primary language, then verbal tests would underestimate verbal abilities. Thus, the examiner would have to determine the exposure to and skill level of English. The following are questions to determine English exposure history:
   a. Is Lao the primary language spoken at home? If so, when did the child learn English? Is Lao the primary language spoken with friends? In which language is the child most comfortable conversing?
   b. Is the child enrolled in English as a Secondary Language (ESL) classes? What is the child's academic achievement in reading and language? Is there a significant discrepancy in English versus math skills?
   c. If Lao is preferred, consider an interpreter. However, since most Laotian American children are bilingual, you should qualitatively assess their English skills through conversation. This evaluation could be supplemented with school records or talking with the child's teachers. Keep in mind that comprehension is generally more advanced than expression, and thus it may be that an interpreter would be most useful for facilitating maximal verbal responses or obtaining history versus basic understanding.
2. Evaluate for level of acculturation, which is useful for interpretation, particularly to determine if cultural variables could contribute to discrepancies in test performances (Ponton & Corona-LoMonaco, 2007). Aside from language spoken (see 1a), other indicators of culture include (a) ethnicity of friends, (b) foods eaten or preferred, (c) preferred music, (d) religion, (e) reading preferences, (f) cultural values, and (g) age when immigrated to the United States.
3. School records are a good resource to assist in determining premorbid functioning. However, when evaluating grades it would be important to review attendance, enrollment in mainstream classes, and enrollment in remedial English. Be sure to explore reasons for poor attendance.

4. Given that most parents have low levels of education and work at menial jobs due to poor English skills, parents' education and occupations may not be helpful to estimate premorbid abilities, particularly if both are low. More significant would be parents who have a relatively high level of education in Lao; for example, those who attended secondary schools. Parents who were educated in the city, speak French, or who held relatively high positions in Laos would suggest higher abilities. Similarly, low socioeconomic class would not be as significant as if the family were middle class.
5. In understanding the behavior or emotional state of Laotian American children, it would be important to evaluate the emotional state of the parents. Clinicians should evaluate for the presence of PTSD or depression in the parents, which could significantly affect the home environment or ability to carry out recommendations.
6. The K-ABC and TPT are recommended tests, as there are some norms for Laotian Americans and Laotians so that scores can be interpreted within a cultural context. Although the sample sizes are small, there are norms for children of highly educated parents and more rural areas. It should be mentioned that the Sequential Processing score for both Laotian populations is skewed by an extremely high Number Recall score, which is comparable to Digit Span. When interpreting data, it is recommended that more emphasis be placed on individual subtest scores versus composite indices.

Adults

1. Given that most Laotians who immigrated to America have a poor command of English, it is highly likely that an interpreter will be required. Interpreters would also be important as a cultural guide for placing behaviors in context and to make recommendations. Given the small Laotian community, it may be prudent to inform the family of the identity of the interpreter prior to the interview, as it is possible the family may know the interpreter in another capacity and may feel uncomfortable with this person serving this function. Thus, the family may prefer a family member providing interpretive functions to keep the family business within the family. Comprehensive recommendations on how to select and work with interpreters are beyond the scope of this chapter. Some basic considerations include meeting the interpreter beforehand to familiarize him or her with the purpose and requirements of the evaluations as well as providing guidelines for interaction (for a review see Ponton & Corona-LoMonaco, 2007). Clinicians should avoid using family, particularly children, as interpreters due to potential biases and difficulties that it can cause in Laotian American family dynamics.
2. Females are more comfortable with female interpreters and clinicians, and likewise for males (Keohavong, 1996).
3. Traditionally, Laotians who receive Western medical treatment would see a generalist due to lack of resources, with only the most severe cases referred

to a specialist (Kinzie & Leung, 1996). Thus, to ease possible worries, the clinician may have to thoroughly explain the reason for referral and purpose of evaluation.

4. Laotians tend to be reserved in interactions, particularly when revealing medical history; thus, history may need to evolve over time as the relationship evolves. To obtain a thorough pertinent history and to assist in developing rapport, encourage the client to provide a detailed account of his or her life in Laos, the impact of the war, and the traumas that he or she experienced prior to immigrating to the United States. Explaining the link between questions pertaining to symptoms and medical problems may also assist in eliciting information. If personal, communicating that the information is confidential and not for public discussion may help to alleviate anxieties (Keovilay & Kemp, n.d.).
5. Evaluate for acculturation. Of particular importance is age at time of immigration (see children recommendation 2).
6. Evaluate for specific symptoms of PTSD, depression, anxiety, and substance abuse and dependence. If present, inquire about the client's explanation for the symptoms.
7. Due to lack of neuropsychological norms for Laotian adults, for diagnostic referrals, we recommend a hypothesis testing approach based upon expectations of presentation for a specific neurological disorder (Fujii & Wong, 2005). Hypotheses should be developed from consensus statements or other widely accepted expert-based diagnostic guidelines. Data collected with the multimethod approach utilize client and collateral interviews describing the onset, quality, severity, and progression of cognitive, behavioral, and emotional symptoms of the presenting problem, as well as any medical and imaging data. This information would be compared to different diagnostic criteria for goodness of fit.
8. For referrals requesting a functionality evaluation after a known neurological disorder, it is recommended that clinicians utilize the literature and consensus statements to guide exploration of associated cognitive, behavioral, or emotional problems. Of particular importance are changes since the onset of a disorder. Inquire about the impact that these symptoms are having on the client and family.
9. As mentioned previously, because there are no known norms with Laotian adults, comprehensive neuropsychological testing is not recommended. However, clinicians may perform limited testing with homemade translated tests, keeping in mind that these are gross measurements at best, and would only be significant if performances are highly discrepant from expectations of the most similar normative group.
10. Due to low levels of education, there is a high level of illiteracy among adult Laotian immigrants. Thus, clinicians should be knowledgeable on the literature of how illiteracy affects brain functioning (for reviews see Ardila & Rosselli, 2007; Castro-Caldas, 2007). For example, illiterates were less likely to develop aphasia and more likely to produce semantic versus phonemic paraphasias

after left hemisphere lesions than literates (Castro-Caldas, 2007). On testing, illiterates' scores were not significantly different than those of literates of similar socioeconomic status on naming and identification of real versus pictures of objects, verbal fluency of familiar objects such as items in a supermarket, verbal memory recognition, and orientation. Cognitive areas most affected by education and literacy include digit span, verbal abstractions, calculations, and long-term semantic memory (Reis, Guerreiro, & Petersson, 2003).

11. Given this study, it would be most prudent to evaluate Laotian adults on tests or evaluations that are least affected by literacy. When testing for verbal memory, although there are no Laotian norms, we recommend using the World Health Organization (WHO) UCLA Auditory Verbal Learning Test (Maj et al., 1994) as the stimulus, with careful translation into Laotian (word list can be found in Mitrushina, Boone, Razani, & D'Elia, 2005). Words for this list were selected for their commonality across cultures, and the test was validated with samples from several countries, including Thailand.
12. We also recommend measures that estimate severity of impairment based on functionality, such as the Clinical Dementia Rating (Hughes, Berg, Danziger, Coben, & Martin, 1982).
13. General estimates of premorbid functioning can be based upon several factors: (a) education in Laos, with quality of education based upon hours in the classroom, subjects learned, availability of school materials, and student-to-teacher ratios; (b) children's academic achievement; and (c) current socioeconomic status. For these indicators, because the expectations would be low for both categories a and c, information would be most significant if education and socioeconomic status are average or higher.
14. The following are recommendations for writing the report: (a) make the implicit explicit by describing the thinking behind your conclusions, (b) don't forget to incorporate the potential contribution of psychological disorders such as PTSD in the formulation and recommendations, (c) indicate your level of certainty given the type of data that you have collected, and (d) describe all nonstandardized test administrations.
15. The following are suggestions for making recommendations and providing feedback: (a) focus on crisis resolution; (b) emphasize community strengths, such as reliance on family, ethnic community, and strong individual and group survival skills; (c) describe the rationale for recommendations; (d) avoid interactions that result in a loss of face; (e) be sure that the family is present and the father involved in decision making; and (f) be respectful of family decisions if nontraditional forms of treatment are selected (Bromley & Chhem Sip, 2003).
16. Be cognizant of traditional Southeast Asian values of harmony and balance and the avoidance of conflict. It is possible that a Laotian American client may become angry or upset if he or she perceives the clinician to be too confrontational. In this case, the client may politely tell the clinician that he or she will not return due to lack of transportation or work responsibilities, or just not show up at all for a follow-up appointment (McKenzie-Pollock, 1993).

Illustrative case sample

SP is a 51-year-old Laotian female who was the chief cook in the family restaurant specializing in Thai cuisine. SP's husband and four children, ages 23 to 30, also work in the restaurant. The restaurant is successful to the point where the family live in a middle-class, predominantly White neighborhood. About eight years ago, SP began to experience intermittent episodes of motor weakness in her right arm and mild slurring of speech. Episodes have progressively been getting more frequent, with symptoms becoming worse. SP has also been getting slower in preparing meals and experiencing difficulties keeping up with the orders when the restaurant is busy. SP has also become more fatigued, and once appeared to fall asleep while cutting vegetables. She has also made more mistakes while cooking, sometimes forgetting ingredients.

The family believed SP's symptoms were due to spirit loss, as the family had just moved from the Laotian neighborhood to their new home when her symptoms began. The family initially sought treatment from an *acharn*, who prayed to the spirits to return to SP's body. This intervention appeared to work; however, as SP's symptoms began to progress, the family decided to seek treatment from a community clinic serving the Laotian population. The general practitioner suspected SP had multiple sclerosis (MS) and referred her to a neurologist. The neurologist confirmed the diagnosis through MRI, which revealed scattered white matter lesions with focal lesions in the left frontal and temporal areas.

Since SP was the chief cook, the family was concerned about her ability to work or teach cooking skills to her family. To address this concern, the neurologist referred SP to a neuropsychologist, Dr. F, for assessment and to make recommendations for vocational rehabilitation. Dr. F employed an interpreter from the clinic where SP was initially seen. They met before the evaluation so that Dr. F could explain the purpose of the evaluation to the interpreter, inquire about important cultural factors, and develop a game plan for the evaluation. It was decided that the evaluation would take two days, with another day to provide feedback. The first day of the evaluation would focus on establishing rapport, answering family questions, and data gathering. Testing would be administered on the second day.

SP was accompanied by her husband and oldest son. The purpose of the evaluation was explained to the family as information to assist SP in improving work skills. Both family members stayed during the history-taking session. SP spoke in broken English, which the interpreter described as above average for many first-generation Laotians. To establish rapport, Dr. F asked SP about the family business, her memories of Laos, differences between Laos and the United States, and how difficult it must have been to immigrate. Dr. F got the following background information. SP was born and raised in Vientiane. Her father worked as a teacher, while her mother was a housewife. She has an eighth-grade education and married the son of a government official in Laos. After the Pathet Lao took over the government in 1975, SP escaped to a Thai refugee camp and immigrated to the United States in 1978, shortly after the birth of her first son. SP and family settled in California. They worked in menial jobs in housekeeping and restaurant help before opening their own restaurant about 15 years after immigrating. SP is literate in Laotian and reads Laotian newspaper and books. Initially she did the accounting for the business, until they were able to hire a bookkeeper. SP's oldest son graduated from a four-year college in business, and her youngest son is enrolled part-time.

Given SP's father's occupation, her educational background, middle-class socioeconomic status, children's educational attainment, and relatively good English abilities, Dr. F and the interpreter estimated that her premorbid functioning to be high for Laotian standards. Dr. F decided to use tests from the World Health Organization battery, which, although not validated on a Laotian sample, were validated in several countries in an international HIV study (Maj et al., 1994). Tests included RAVLT (translated to Laotian), Color Trails 1 and 2, Digit Symbol, Digit Span, Animal Fluency, Grooved Pegboard Dominant and Nondominant Hands, and Block Design. To supplement, these tests, WMS-III Visual Reproduction I and II, and WAIS-III Similarities were also administered. Given the lack of validation, results would be interpreted cautiously with broad strokes. Norms for below high school were used for interpretation.

Tests results indicate borderline level functioning on tests of verbal memory, processing speed (Color Trails, Digit Symbol, and Animal Fluency), and fine motor functioning for her dominant right hand. Working memory was in the average range (Digit Span), while abstractions (Similarities), nonverbal reasoning (Block Design), and visual memory (VR I and II) fell within the low average to average range. Test results were interpreted to be consistent with MS and SP's MRI.

In the feedback session, Dr. F explained symptoms of MS and test results. He described the different types of progression in MS and recommended the family consider applying for Social Security disability if SP's condition worsened to the point where she could not work. To facilitate her ability to work, Dr. F recommended that SP reduce her role to assistant cook, limit her working hours, and train family members to cook. Family should allow SP to rest when tired and avoid cooking, carrying items, cutting with knives, or working near the stove.

References

Ardila, A., & Rosselli, M. (2007). Illiterates and cognition: The impact of education. In B. Uzzell, M. Ponton, & A. Ardila (Eds.), *International handbook of cross-cultural neuropsychology* (pp. 181–198). Mahwah, NJ: Lawrence Erlbaum Associates.

Asian and Pacific Islander American Health Forum. (n.d.). *Asian Americans and Pacific Islanders in California*. Retrieved June 6, 2009, http://www.cpehn.org/pdfs/APIAHF%20-%20Fact%20Sheet.pdf

Bankston, C. (2000). Laotian Americans. In J. Lehman (Ed.), *Gale encyclopedia of multicultural America* (Vol. 2, pp. 1091–1100). Detroit, MI: Gale.

Boivin, M., Chounramany, C., Giordani, B., Xaisida, S., Choulamountry, L., Pholsena, P., et al. (1996). Validating a cognitive ability testing protocol with Lao children for community development applications. *Neuropsychology, 10*, 588–599.

Bromley, M. A., & Chhem Sip, S. K. (2003). Substance abuse treatment issues with Cambodian Americans. In S. L. Ashenberg Straussner (Ed.), *Ethnocultural factors in substance abuse treatment* (pp. 321–344). New York, NY: Guilford Press.

Castro-Caldas, A. (2007). Relationship between functional brain organization and education. In B. Uzzell, M. Ponton, & A. Ardila (Eds.), *International handbook of cross-cultural neuropsychology* (pp. 199–214). Mahwah, NJ: Lawrence Erlbaum Associates.

Chu, N. V. (1997, Winter). Re-examining the model minority myth: A look at Southeast Asian youth. *McNair Journal, 5*. http://www-mcnair.berkeley.edu/97Journal/Chu.html.

Conant, L., Fastenau, P., Giordani, B., Boivin, M., Chounramany, C., Xaisida, S., et al. (2003). Environmental influences on primary memory development: A cross-cultural study of memory span in Lao and American children. *Journal of Clinical and Experimental Neuropsychology, 25*, 1102–1116.

De Voe, P. A. (2009). The role of ethnic leaders in the refugee community: A case study of the lowland Lao in the American Midwest. In H. Ling (Ed.), *Emerging voices: Experiences of underrepresented Asian Americans* (pp. 52–70). New Brunswick, NJ: Rutgers University Press.

Fujii, D., & Wong, T. (2005). Neuropsychological assessment with Asian-American immigrants: Recommendations for meeting *Daubert* standards. *Journal of Forensic Neuropsychology, 4*(4), 3–31.

Globalis. (n.d.). *Laos*. Retrieved March 3, 2008, from http://globalis.gvu.unu.edu/indicator_detail.cfm?Country=LA&IndicatorID=124

Gong-Guy, E. (1987). *The California Southeast Asian mental health needs assessment*. California State Department Mental Health Contract 85-7682-2A-2.

Graham, E. A., & Chitnarong, J. (1997). *Ethnographic study among Seattle Cambodians: Wind illness*. Online. Retrieved January 7, 2008, from http://ethnomed.org/ethnomed/clin_topics/cambodian/ethno_wind.html

Hughes, C., Berg, L., Danziger, W., Coben, L., & Martin, R. (1982). A new clinical scale for the staging of dementia. *British Journal of Psychiatry, 140*, 566–572.

Keohavong, S. (1996). *Voices of the Lao community*. Retrieved June 6, 2009, from http://www.comm.ohio-state.edu/pdavid/preparedness/docs/crosscultural/lao.pdf

Keovilay, L., & Kemp, C. (n.d.). *Laotians: Culture, health, refugees, immigrants*. Retrieved June 6, 2009, from http://bearspace.baylor.edu/Charles_Kemp/www/laotian_health.html

Kinzie, J. D., & Leung, P. K. (1996). Psychiatric care of Indochinese Americans. In A. Gaw (Ed.), *Culture, ethnicity, and mental illness* (pp. 281–304). Washington, DC: American Psychiatric Press.

Maj, M., Satz, P., Janssen, R., Zaudig, M., et al. (1994). WHO neuropsychiatric AIDS study, cross-sectional phase II: Neuropsychological and neurological findings. *Archives of General Psychiatry, 51*, 51–61.

McKenzie-Pollock, L. (1993). Cambodian families. In M. McGoldrick, J. Giordano, & J. K. Pearce (Eds.), *Ethnicity and family therapy* (pp. 307–315). New York, NY: Guilford Press.

Mitrushina, M., Boone, K., Razani, J., & D'Elia, L (2005). *Handbook of normative data for neuropsychological assessment* (2nd ed., pp. 618–622). New York, NY: Oxford University Press.

Ngo, B. (2006). Learning from the margins: The education of Southeast and South Asian Americans in context. *Race Ethnicity and Education, 9*, 51–65.

Nussbaum, N., & Bunner, M. (2009). Halstead-Reitan neuropsychological test batteries for children. In C. Reynolds & E. Fletcher-Janzen (Eds.), *Handbook of Child Clinical Neuropsychology* (2nd ed., pp. 247–266). New York, NY: Springer.

Pfeifer, M. (2001). *2000 census shows contrasting growth and settlement patterns of major Southeast Asian origin groups*. Retrieved February 9, 2009, from http://www.hmong-studies.org/4IndochineseGroups.html

Ponton, M., & Corona-LoMonaco, M. E. (2007). Cross-cultural issues in neuropsychology: Assessment of the Hispanic patient. In B. Uzzell, M. Ponton, & A. Ardila (Eds.), *International handbook of cross-cultural neuropsychology* (pp. 265–282). Mahwah, NJ: Lawrence Erlbaum Associates.

Reeves, T. J., & Bennett, C. E. (2004). *We the people: Asians in the United States*. Washington, DC: U.S. Census Bureau. Retrieved February 9, 2009, from http://www.census.gov/prod/2004pubs/censr-17.pdf

Reis, A., Guerreiro, M., & Petersson, K. M. (2003). A sociodemographic and neuropsychological characterization of an illiterate population. *Applied Neuropsychology, 10*, 191–204.

Utairatanakit, D. (1987). Construct and concurrent validity of the Kaufman Assessment Battery for Children (K-ABC) with a Laotian sample (Doctoral dissertation, Texas Women's University, 1986). *Dissertation Abstracts International, 48*, 884.

Webometrics. (n.d.). *World universities' ranking on the web: Top Asia*. Retrieved March 4, 2008, from http://webometrics.info/top100_continent.asp?cont=asia

Westermeyer, J. (1988). Folk medicine in Laos: A comparison between two ethnic groups. *Social Science Medicine, 27*, 769–778.

Wikipedia. (2008). *Education in Laos*. Retrieved August 9, 2008, from http://en.wikipedia.org/wiki/Education_in_Laos

Wikipedia. (2009a). *History of Laos*. Retrieved February 8, 2009, from http://en.wikipedia.org/wiki/History_of_Laos

Wikipedia. (2009b). *Laotian civil war*. Retrieved March 1, 2009, from http://en.wikipedia.org/wiki/Laotian_Civil–War

World Culture Encyclopedia. (2008). *Lao: Religion and expressive culture*. Retrieved June 6, 2009, from http://www.everyculture.com/East-Southest-Asia/Lao-Religion-and-Expressive-Culture.html

Yang, K. Y. (2004). Southeast Asian American children: Not the "model minority." *The Future of Children, 14*, 127–137.

Yang, K. Y., & Niedzwiecki, W. R. (2003). *Southeast Asian Americans and higher education*. Retrieved June 8, 2009, from http://www.serac.org/sea-he-tst6-17-03.pdf

10 Neuropsychology of Thai Americans

Daryl Fujii, Tony Wu, and Kattiya Ratanadilok

Population demographics

Thailand is a Southeast Asian country with an area of 198,456 square miles, which is approximately twice the area of the state of Wyoming (Mulder, 2000). The population of Thailand is 65,068,149, with an ethnic composition of 75% Thai, 14% Chinese, and 11% other, the latter including Malaysian, Laotian, Cambodian, Indian, and Vietnamese. Thai is the official language. Other languages spoken include English, Chinese, and Malay (Ratner, 2000). Roughly 94.6% of the population is Buddhist, 4.6% Muslim, and 0.7% Christian.

Brief political history

Thailand has a rich history. The country, originally known as Siam, was unified during the fourteenth century (Ratner, 2000). Although never known to be a strong military state, Thailand is the only Southeast Asian country that has never been colonized by Western nations (Central Intelligence Agency, 2007). Osborne (2000) attributed Thailand's ability to maintain independence to several factors. First, Thailand was seen as a buffer zone among conflicting European nations. Second, Thai kings were excellent diplomats with an astute understanding of European culture. Finally, Thai rulers had a history of acquiring Western technology through oversea educational training and foreign consultants. Interestingly, Siam formally changed its name to Prathet Thai, or Thailand in English, in 1949, which translates to "Land of the Free."

Economy and education

Up until the latter part of the twentieth century, Thailand was considered a third-world country (Jones, 2003). Its primary exports were agricultural products such as rice and timbers along with handicrafts and gems. Correspondingly, Thailand imported most of the manufactured goods from other countries. However, during the past few decades, manufacturing has dominated the Thai economy, and Thailand is now considered a newly industrialized country (NIC). The economy demonstrated solid growth during the 1980s, and by 1988 its GNP rate achieved 13% per annum

(Cummings & Martin, 2001). It was one of the world's fastest-growing economies during the 1990s, with a surge of foreign investment, and was projected to join Asia's elite "Four Tigers" of Hong Kong, Singapore, South Korea, and Taiwan (Cummings & Martin, 2001). However, in 1997 Thailand's economic surge plummeted when businesses and banks overborrowed and the Thai baht drastically declined in value. Thailand's economy is currently in recovery.

Immigration to the United States

Similar to other Asian countries, immigration to the United States generally did not occur until after the 1965 Immigration Act. The first wave of about 5,000 Thai immigrants arrived during the 1970s. Early immigration was greatly impacted by American presence in Thailand as one of the largest sectors of immigrants was Thai women who married U.S. Air Force personnel. Thus, the gender ratio of the earliest immigrants was three women to one man (Ratner, 2000). Many of the other early immigrants were professionals, such as medical doctors and entrepreneurs who were motivated by educational and economic opportunities (Ratner, 2000; Ramisetty-Mikler, 1993). Immigration increased during the 1980s with an average of 6,500 Thais arriving per year.

According to the 2000 U.S. census, 150,283 Thais were living in the United States (U.S. Census Bureau, 2000). Most Thais reside in or near U.S. urban centers, with the greatest concentration (66%) living in California, primarily in the Los Angeles and San Francisco areas. In fact, the only Thai town in the United States is located in Los Angeles. Other states with large Thai populations include Texas (7,384), New York (6,658), Florida (6,233), and Illinois (5,833) (U.S. Census Bureau, 2000).

Demographically, Reeves and Bennett (2004) reported that in 2000, 15.3% of Thais were under the age of 18, 82.2% were between the ages of 18 and 64, and 2.5% were 65 or older. In addition, 53% reported being married. Thais described themselves as 22.2% American natives, 32.7% foreign-born naturalized citizens, and 45.1% noncitizens. Among the foreign born, 39.1% immigrated to the United States before 1980, 24.7% entered in the 1980s, and 36.2% immigrated between 1990 and 2000. Nearly 47% of Thai families did not speak English at home. Fully 38.6% of Thais in the United States have a bachelor's degree or more advanced degrees, and 23.1% have some college or an associate's degree. It has been estimated that 33.4% of Thais are in management, professional, and related occupations, with many women in the nursing field; 25.9% are employed in the service sector; and 14.4% are at or below the poverty level.

Testing issues

Education in home country

The educational system in Thailand has experienced significant development within the past three decades, which is a ramification of the country's growing economy. Prior to 1980, the average level of formal education was less than nine years.

Resources were limited, and for children of low socioeconomic status, attending school was highly selective and based upon merit (Hyneman & Loxley, 1983). In fact, for many people residing in rural areas, the only education offered was teaching from Buddhist monks at wáts (temple-monasteries) (Cummings & Martin, 2001). Since 1980, expenditures on education increased from 3.42% of the GDP to 5.10% in 2001 (Globalis, n.d.). This increase in monies resulted in the extension of compulsory education to 9 years in 1993, 12 years in 1997 (Cummings & Martin, 2001), and 14 years in 2004, including 2 years of a preprimary education. These infrastructure changes have led to gains in all educational indicators. For example, enrollment in primary school has risen from 75.9% in 1990 to 86.3% in 2001. Literacy rates among youths increased from 96.6% in 1980 to 98% in 2004, while more significant gains were made in adult literacy rates, estimated to be at 87.5% in 1980 and 96% in 2003 (Globalis, n.d.).

Associated with increases in expenditures are improvements in academic achievement. In 1971, science scores for Thai 10- and 14-year-olds on the International Association for the Evaluation of Educational Achievement (IEA) test were about .5 standard deviation lower than U.S. students' scores (Thai, $x = 28.2$, *s.d.* = 6.6; United States, $x = 32.8$, *s.d.* = 9.5) (Hyneman & Loxley, 1983). By contrast, math and sciences scores of 10- and 14-year-olds were more comparable between the two countries in 1994. Thai 10- and 14-year-olds earned mean math scores of 490 and 522, respectively, while U.S. mean students' scores were 545 and 500. In science, scores for Thai 10- and 14-year-olds were 473 and 525, respectively, while for U.S. 14-year-olds the science score was 534 (Lynn, 2006). More recently, Pisa international rankings for reading and mathematics indicated that Thai and U.S. 15-year-olds were below average for mathematics, while Thai students were below average for reading (no data for the United States). Interestingly, other countries that consistently scored below average included Italy, Israel, Spain, and Russia (BBC News, 2007).

Regarding higher education, Thailand has 51 colleges and universities (4International Colleges and Universities, n.d.). According to the Webometrics (n.d.) ranking of world universities, Thailand ranks 29th among all countries, with 3 universities in the top 500. The United States is ranked first. In a similar ranking of 100 top Asian universities, Thailand has 9 schools in the top 100: Prince of Songkla University (19), Chulalongkorn University (27), Kasetsart University (21), Asian Institute of Technology (56), Mahidol University (68), Thammasat University (69), Chiang Mai University (75), Assumption University of Thailand (79), and Khon Kaen University (82).

English skills

English became an important secondary language in Thailand beginning in the 1960s, when America set up military bases in the country (Jones, 2003). Subsequent American tourism and trade also necessitated that Thais speak English, particularly in the major tourist destinations such as Bangkok. Because of efforts for competing in the global economy, starting in 1999 the Thai government mandated English as a foreign language requirement for first graders, the goal being English proficiency in the next generation (Wiriyachitra, 2004).

Although English is taught in Thailand, the majority of Thai immigrants are not proficient in English. In fact, English is not spoken in 47% of the households (Reeves & Bennett, 2004). The Thai language is comprised of 44 consonants, 32 vowels, and 5 tones in Thai pronunciation. Despite the relatively large number of phonemes, there are many sounds in English that Thai-born individuals find difficult to pronounce or hear. Thus, many Thai-born adults experience difficulty learning English.

Generation is a moderating factor in speaking English, as Thai children of immigrant parents may be more exposed to English in everyday life, and thus more fluent in English than in the Thai language, and may use Thai as their second language. Acculturation and primary language spoken in the home are important variables that would affect English proficiency of second-generation Thais.

An issue with intergenerational differences in English proficiency is that it has become conventional for children of immigrant parents to assume the role of interpreter, which can be problematic for some families. Traditionally, Thai children are taught to honor their parents and are grateful for everything their parents have done for them, including giving birth. In many Thai families, it is a duty of good children to serve their parents when they can and to support their parents when they are ill and frail. Thus, being an interpreter for their parents is one of the opportunities to show gratitude to their parents. However, it is also possible that for second-generation Thai children who identify more with the American versus Thai culture, this role reversal may create problems in the family as conflicts and role ambiguity intensify family relationship problems (Bemak, Chung, & Bornemann, 1996).

Religion

About 95% of all Thais are Theravada Buddhists, and almost every aspect of Thais' lives is infused with Buddhist beliefs and practices (Ratner, 2000). Two influential Buddhist beliefs are the Four Noble Truths and the Middle Way. The Four Noble Truths are (1) suffering is part of life, (2) human desires generate suffering, (3) the end of suffering is achieved when all desires are eliminated, and (4) taking the right path will halt all desires. The notion of the Middle Way refers to the harmony between two extremes, the goal of which is to attain synchronization and balance in life (House & Pinyuchon, 1998).

Another central concept in Buddhism is Karma, or *kam* in Thai. The concept of *kam* is found in Buddha's third universal truth. It states that life is determined by the law of cause and effect. Thus, one's thoughts and actions determine the experiences and quality of one's life. If we do good things, good things will happen to us. If we do bad things, bad things will happen to us in this life or the next. This way of thinking helps Thais to recognize that life does not always turn out the way one wants; however, one can learn to understand and live with their situation. This mindset helps Thais be calm and collected in phases of adversity because they "understand" the root of the problems.

House and Pinyuchon (1998) suggested that one implication of *kam* is a resistance to seek help or implement changes to address problems associated with neurological disorders, as suffering is a result of *kam*, and thus the person cannot do anything to change his or her fate. Although some Thais may attribute their poor follow-through on treatment to *kam*, this is actually their own interpretation of Buddhist teaching or rationalization for poor motivation, and not necessarily a true understanding of *kam*. This religious belief does not cause people to have poor motivation. Thais who truly understand the concept of *kam* would try their best to recover from physical illness. However, if their recovery does not meet expectations, they may not experience significant psychological distress due to the belief that their illness is a consequence of past deeds. To improve their health, they may perform good deeds for others, so that good fortune would fall on them within this life or the next.

Pertinent cultural issues

As with most Asian societies, Thai is a collectivist society that emphasizes family obligation over personal needs (House & Pinyuchon, 1998). Family structure is based on paternal authority, and Thais are taught to respect authority figures in general (House & Pinyuchon, 1998). Because of such interdependence within the family, when a person behaves improperly in Thai culture, shame is brought upon the family.

Shame can also extend beyond the immediate family. Unlike Americans, in which many unrelated families share the same last names, Thai last names are specific to one family tree. Thus, people who have the same last name are always relatives. Therefore, it is not uncommon for a person to receive negative reactions from peers if they share the same last name as someone who has engaged in behavior that would shame the Thai community. Likewise, individuals who have the same last name as a prominent person may receive privileged treatment based on their name.

One ramification of family obligation is a reluctance to disclose family problems to nonfamily members. There is a strong stigma associated with mental illness in Thai culture. Thus, Thais are cautious in seeking professional help for mental illness or emotional problems. This concept is captured in the Thai proverb *Fai nai yaa num ok, Fai nok yaa num khao,* which refers to keeping family problems inside and preventing outside problems from coming in (Pratomthong & Baker, 1983).

Another important cultural behavior is a discomfort with expressing feelings and emotions. Some clues to Thai perception of emotion come from their language. The Thai lexicon for emotional states is limited. The Thai word *jai* literally means "heart." When suffixed to another word it becomes a compound word indicating an individual's state of mind or feelings. For example, the word *sook-jai* refers to feeling happy and the word *klum-jai* refers to feeling worried. Sometimes, one word may have subtle differences in meaning depending on the context, such as the word *sia-jai*, which literally means "loss-heart," which can be used to refer to emotional states of being sad, depressed, regretful, and sorry.

Feelings are generally not discussed in everyday Thai conversation. This discomfort is illustrated in common Thai greetings. In America, a common greeting is "How are you?" which elicits the expected answer, "I am fine, thank you." This interactive pattern implies that you may care about how another person might feel. By contrast, common Thai greetings include *Kin-khao-laew-reu-young*, meaning "Have you eaten yet?" or *Pai-nai-ma,* meaning "Where have you been?" or *Pai-yang-rai-ma-yang-rai*, meaning "What brings you here?" These greetings imply concern about the well-being of others that is not related directly to their feelings. For Thais, feelings are considered private and are seldom openly discussed, and definitely not revealed to strangers. In fact, being asked "How are you?" by acquaintances may result in responses such as "I am not fine, thank you" or "Do you really want to know?"

Thais prefer to avoid conflicts and objections and instead embrace nonconfrontational ways of relating to others. It is often difficult to say no; they prefer rather to compromise to keep good relationships. This behavior stems from values of *mai-pen-rai* and *kreng-jai,* which translate to not wanting to inconvenience others. As a result, when Thais do not agree with you or are unhappy about something you did, they will not confront you directly, but may become quiet and avoid meeting with you in the future. As some scholars observed, subservience and silence are valued in Thai culture (House & Pinyuchon, 1998), and Thai children are more overcontrolled than American children (Weisz et al., 1987, 1993).

Difficulties with expressing negative emotions are manifested in several ways. First, negative feelings are generally expressed nonverbally. Body language is an essential way of communication, and in most situations nonverbal communication trumps verbal communication. Another implication is the tendency to somaticize emotional problems. Similar to other Asian cultures, it is likely more acceptable to experience physical ailments than emotional problems (Burnard, Naiyapatana, & Lloyd, 2006).

Third, given the discomfort with the expression of negative emotions, it is not surprising that Thais like to smile. In fact, Thailand has long been called the "Land of the Smiles." However, unlike Western culture, smiling in Thai culture does not always mean being happy. Instead, smiling can have multiple meanings, including nervousness, embarrassment, and being apologetic for interrupting (*kreng-jai*). Sometimes Thais smile in an attempt to comfort another person or to sympathize for another's misfortune. A famous Thai proverb teaching the wisdom of staying calm when facing threat is *yim-dai-mua-pai-ma*, which literally means "can smile when danger comes."

Thus, clinicians working with Thai clients should be aware of their nature of communication and not assume anything until they make sure by observing and collecting more related information about their emotional states. Neuropsychologists should be aware of possible emotional problems even if none are reported, and routinely evaluate clients for internalizing psychopathology, such as depression and anxiety.

Finally, due to differences in traditional Thai and mainstream American culture, generational issues are common as foreign-born parents and U.S.-born children are often at different acculturation levels and have dissimilar inter- and intrafamilial experiences (Ramisetty-Mikler, 1993). Clinicians should also be aware of a self-selection process, as Thais who immigrated to America may have different characteristics from Thais who choose to stay in Thailand.

Neuropsychological norms and literature

The neuropsychology literature on Thais and Thai Americans is sparse. Thai psychologists typically use translated Western tests when conducting neuropsychological evaluations, for example, the Wechsler Intelligence Scales, Raven's Progressive Matrices, the Stanford-Binet Intelligence Scale, and the Wechsler Memory Scale (Ratanadilok, 2010). Some of the translated or adapted tests, such as the Thai Geriatric Depression Scale, the Thai Mental State Examination, the Reitan-Indiana Aphasia Screening Test Battery, and the Continuous Performance Test, have been used in studies to examine Thai populations (Ratanadilok, 2010). The Montreal Cognitive Assessment, a 30-point dementia screen that incorporates tasks such as drawing a clock, verbal fluency, and a mini trailmaking, along with typical orientation, attention, and memory items, also has a Thai translation, which can be accessed at http://www.mocatest.org/ (Nasreddine et al., 2005).

There are a handful of studies reporting neuropsychological norms for Thais or Thai Americans. In an epidemiological study on iron deficiency in Thailand, Pollitt, Hathirat, Kotchabhakdi, Missell, and Valyasevi (1989) reported the mean score on Raven's Standard Progressive for 8- to 10-year-old Thai students was 91 ($n = 2268$). The World Health Organization (WHO) developed several neuropsychological measures, such as the WHO/UCLA Auditory Verbal Learning Test (AVLT) and Color Trails, for use as outcome measures in their international studies on HIV-positive adults (Maj et al., 1993, 1994). Although validated with a Thai population, no specific norms have been published. Currently, the South East Asian Research Collaboration with Hawaii (SEARCH) is collecting age- and education-based norms for healthy Thai controls on the WHO battery (Victor Valcour, personal communication). We compared preliminary findings from subjects in the age groups 20–29 ($n = 25$), 30–39 ($n = 28$), and 40–49 ($n = 19$) with either a high school or associate's/technical vocational certificate with meta-analytic norms from Mitrushina et al. (2005) for the following measures: WHO AVLT Trials 1–5, WHO AVLT Trial 5, Color Trials 1 and 2, Grooved Pegboard dominant and nondominant hands, verbal fluency animals, and Trails A. Norms were almost identical across the three age ranges for the WHO AVLT, animal fluency, and Trails A. Variability was demonstrated on both trials of Color Trails, with some stronger scores for the Thai samples and some stronger for the Mitrushina samples. The 40- to 49-year-old Thai sample also scored .3 standard deviation worse on the nondominant hand for the Grooved Pegboard Test.

Finally, a nonneuropsychological measure of dementia based upon informant report, the Informant Questionnaire on Cognitive Decline in the Elderly (IQCODE) (Jorm & Jacomb, 1989), has been validated on elderly Thai samples. Senanarong et al. (2001) administered the IQCODE in a Thai sample of 87 community elderly and 73 elderly with dementia. The researchers reported good psychometric properties of the test with an area under the receiving operating curve of 0.93. Siri, Okanurak, Chansirikanjana, Kitayaporn, and Jorm (2006) modified the original IQCODE by adding six items. They compared IQCODE scores with *Diagnostic and Statistical Manual of Mental Disorders*, fourth edition (DSM-IV) diagnoses of dementia on 200 elderly subjects visiting a geriatric clinic. Positive predictive and negative predictive values were reported to be 0.94 and 0.90, respectively.

Estimating premorbid IQs

Mechanisms for estimating premorbid IQ in Thais vary depending on level of English proficiency and acculturation. For second-generation Thais whose primary language is English, the standard word recognition reading tests would likely be valid. The possible exception would be for less acculturated Thais living in Thai communities whose primary language is Thai. The biggest challenge would be for first-generation Thais who lack proficient English skills. For these individuals, we recommend examining personal characteristics that have been found to be highly correlated with intelligence, such as years of education, genetic heritability (for a review see Neisser et al., 1996), and occupation (McCall, 1977). When conceptualizing premorbid abilities based upon these qualities, several considerations should be made. First, until recently the mean level of education completed in Thailand was less than nine years, as compulsory education was raised to 9th grade in 1993 and 12th grade in 1997 (Cummings & Martin, 2001). Thus, what is considered average should be based upon these figures. However, quality of education may be more important than the number of years of education because the current education system in Thailand is not well standardized, and it is likely that the schools in rural areas do not hold the same standards as the schools in the urban areas such as Bangkok or other major provinces. This information also holds true for the quality of education in colleges and universities, which can be easily checked from the ranking of the university, mentioned earlier in this chapter. In terms of heritability of intelligence, one manner of estimating intelligence for an immigrant parent would be to determine the educational or occupational achievement of his or her children. When examining occupation as an indicator, occupation in Thailand would be more reflective of abilities, as underemployment is frequent in immigrants, especially those who are not proficient in English.

It is recommended that all of these factors be considered when conceptualizing premorbid intellectual abilities. Clinicians should initially look for consistency of indicators for determining premorbid functioning. If varied, then it is recommended that the highest indicator level should be used, a strategy that is similar to Lezak, Howieson, and Loring's (2004) "best performance(s)" method to estimating baseline cognitive level. It should be emphasized that given the inexactness of the process, only gross level of functioning should be estimated (i.e., about average, low average to average, above average).

Recommendations

There are many general recommendations for neuropsychologists examining ethnic minorities in pertinent areas, such as use of interpreters, test translations, effects of acculturation and English proficiency on test performance, and testing biases. These issues will not be discussed here, as we wish to focus on specific recommendations for working with Thais. For a review of issues in testing ethnic minorities, particularly with Asians, refer to Wong and Fujii (2004).

1. Thais may not readily seek psychological assistance or freely disclose about themselves; thus, neuropsychological evaluations are likely experienced as a stressful situation. To facilitate the therapeutic relationship, House and Pinyuchon (1998) suggested that clinicians should focus on establishing a trusting and welcoming environment. For example, it would be valuable to inquire about the meaning and pronunciation of the client's name, given that most Thai names have personal and cultural meanings. Additionally, during the interview phase, clients might discuss more about their families than themselves because of their sociocultural backgrounds; clinicians should allow the clients to express their thoughts and feelings without rushing to make judgments. Because Thais usually call each other by their first name, calling the Thai client by his or her first name, beginning with the word *khun,* instead of Mr. or Mrs., may help hasten a therapeutic relationship. This practice should be followed only with the permission of the client.
2. The country of Thailand is called the "Land of Smiles," and there is historical significance in Thais' smiles, which often denote their desire to convey friendliness and pleasantness. They often communicate friendliness or a desire to please in order to nourish harmony. Thus, Thais' smiles might not always suggest agreement or comprehension, which could be misinterpreted by Western clinicians. It is a good practice to be extra vigilant in observing their other nonverbal language to convey the meaning of their smiles.
3. Thai clients may not easily volunteer their personal information. Thus, clinicians should take a directive approach. This would entail systematically asking pertinent questions and probing, as the client may not provide or elaborate answers spontaneously. Questions should be balanced with respect for the client's comfort level. Silence and smiles may be a sign of discomfort.
4. Based on their culture, a tendency of Thais is to please others. In addition, Thais generally perceive the clinician as an authority figure who possesses the answers to their problems and someone who would always act in their best interest. Thus, Thais are less likely to question treatments or recommendations that are being offered to them, and therefore could easily be taken advantage of. As a result, it is the clinician's responsibility when working with Thais to ensure that his or her Thai clients truly understand their rights and the application of their consent to assessment and treatment.
5. When working with Thais, it is important to understand the meaning of touching the hand and the head. Ratner (2000) pointed out that Thais do not shake hands for greeting; as an alternative, they salute each other with a prayer-like gesture called *wai,* or they just smile in response. Touching hands is not encouraged because it may lead to misunderstanding in a sexual way, especially between different sexes. In addition, Thais believe that

the head is the highest point of the body and most sacred, so it is forbidden to touch another's head.

6. When working with an interpreter, given the different Thai dialects and the sometimes pronounced differences in Thai dialects, clinicians should be aware of the interpreter's familiarity and ability to meaningfully communicate with the client. Interpreters should always ask the client from which region of Thailand he or she originally comes.
7. For Thai immigrants who are not proficient in English, the vocabulary subtest should not be administered, nor should translations of the words be attempted, as Thai words are frequently literal. For example, the English word *handkerchief* means "a cloth for wiping one's face." In Thai, root words are usually combined to describe many items. *Handkerchief* translates to *pa-ched-na*, which means "cloth-wipe-face." The Thai word for *dinner* is *ahaan-yen*, meaning "meal-eaten-in-the-evening." A test item that asks the meaning of a word whose meaning for an individual is already explicit in its roots may not be interpreted the same way as that same item for an individual whose language is more implicit. Consequently, a Thai person's lexicon may contain fewer words than an American's. Thais would have difficulty conceptualizing abstract English vocabulary such as *handkerchief* and *dinner* because the Thai terms already provide sufficient clarity and concreteness. In many situations, one may be able to provide the same answer on a given test item, but the process in coming up with the solution may not require the same mechanisms of the brain.
8. In testing a first-generation Thai, clinicians should be cognizant that the significance of something may differ from one culture to another, and those differences may affect test results. For instance, the weather forecast is crucial in everyday life in many countries, and even comes up in everyday conversation. In Thailand, weather forecasts are of no significance whatsoever. As a result, a test of memory, in the context of a weather forecast (e.g., Logical Memory story B), would be more difficult for Thai people to remember.
9. Clinicians should bear in mind that not all Thais are the same. The descriptions of Thai culture in this chapter are merely considerations for working with Thais. Clinicians should ultimately learn about the individual from a comprehensive clinical interview with the client.

Case sample

Ms. K is a 71-year-old Thai female who apparently wandered from home and was lost for a day before being found in a neighboring city. She had demonstrated a gradual cognitive decline for the past six years and was referred by her general practitioner to evaluate for dementia. Ms. K was born in Bangkok and received nine years of education. She worked as a nurse in a hospital for a few years before she married an Air Force mechanic and immigrated to the United States when she was 21 years old. Ms. K and her husband divorced a few years later. They had a son, David, who was raised by Ms. K.

Ms. K was not proficient in English, and thus decided to raise her son in "Thai town" in Los Angeles. She worked as a cook at a Thai restaurant. David went on to graduate with a bachelor's degree from Cal-State Northridge and currently works as a realtor. He is married with two children, ages 11 and 9.

Ms. K retired about seven years ago as she was having "difficulties" at work with the new owner. Upon retirement, she moved in with David and his family to help with the kids. About a year after moving in, David reported that his mother demonstrated increased forgetfulness and would repeat herself. Once she left the stove on, almost burning down the house. Since then, he did not allow her to cook. Fortunately, his children attended school around this time, thus reducing her responsibilities. Ms. K's activities progressively lessened as her cognition worsened. One of her favorite activities was walking to a neighborhood park about a block away, where she would take the children. She would walk there daily and sit on a bench for hours and return when her grandchildren passed by on the way home from school. The family knew that she was declining, but attributed it to old age.

Ms. K was accompanied to the interview by her son. Her command of English was poor, and thus an interpreter was used. Being from Bangkok, Ms. K spoke standard Thai. Ms. K was asked about the meaning of her name, which she stated translated to "morning blossom." Ms. K was pleasant and smiled throughout the interview; however, she was a very poor historian. Ms. K was reported to be in good health and not taking any Western medications. She was drinking herbal teas daily for health purposes.

Ms. K was administered the following test instruments, all of which were validated with a Thai population: WHO/UCLA AVLT, Trails A, Color Trails, Grooved Pegboard, Animal Fluency, Montreal Cognitive Assessment (MoCA), and the short form of the Geriatric Depression Scale (GDS). Although these tests have Thai translations, we were not able to obtain the materials, and thus the tests were translated by the interpreter. The IQCODE and the Clinical Dementia Rating (CDR) (Hughes et al., 1982), both informant-based assessment tools, were administered to David, who is fluent in English, and thus did not have to be translated into Thai. David sat in the room during testing to increase the comfort level of his mother.

Test results indicated general impaired level functioning on all cognitive tests with the exception of the Grooved Pegboard, which fell within the low average range. Ms. K's MoCA was 14, which suggested a moderate level of dementia. Scores on the IQCODE and CDR answered by her son also corroborated a moderate level of dementia. Ms. K's GDS score was in the normal range, suggesting that depression was not a factor. Ms. K was diagnosed with a moderate dementia and referred to a geriatrician for a dementia workup.

Ms. K's case is common in Thai families in that families are reluctant to bring in members for mental health purposes until the problem is significant. Thai families like to take care of problems within the family, and Ms. K was only brought for an evaluation after she wandered off and was found a day later by police. In Ms. K's case special care was taken to increase her comfort level, such as asking about the meaning of her name and allowing her son to sit in on the evaluation.

Given Ms. K's place of birth and poor command of English, test selection was based upon tests validated in Thailand. A problem was that translations of these tests were not available, and thus the interpreter had to translate them. Although not an ideal situation, this was noted in the report and the possible negative effects on reliability and validity. A multimethod approach, as recommended by Fujii et al. (2002; Fujii and Wong, 2005), of cognitive functioning was based on history, presentation, collateral information, neuropsychological tests, and informant-based questionnaires. A dilemma in interpretation was whether to use 9th-grade norms or the average (12th grade), given her relatively professional nursing background in Thailand. It was decided that both would be used, and Ms. K still scored within the impaired range.

Acknowledgments

The authors thank Victor Valcour and the South East Asian Research Collaboration with Hawaii (SEARCH) for sharing their preliminary data.

References

4International Colleges and Universities. (n.d.). *Thailand: Colleges and universities by 2007 web popularity ranking*. Retrieved February 25 2008, from http://www.4icu.org/th/

BBC News. (2007). *Pisa international rankings*. Retrieved February 7 2008, from http://news-vote.bbc.co.uk/mpapps/pagetools/print/news.bbc.co.uk/1/hi/education/7126388.stm

Bemak, F., Chung, R. C. Y., & Bornemann, T. H. (1996). Counseling and psychotherapy with refugees. In P. Pedersen, J. Draguns, W. Lonner, & J. Trimble (Eds.), *Counseling across cultures* (pp. 243–265). Thousand Oaks, CA: Sage.

Burnard, P., Naiyapatana, W., & Lloyd, G. (2006). Views of mental illness and mental health care in Thailand: A report of an ethnographic study. *Journal of Psychiatric and Mental Health Nursing, 13*, 742–749.

Central Intelligence Agency. (2007). *2007 the world factbook.* Retrieved August 30, 2007, from http://www.cia.gov/library/publications/the-world-factbook/print/th.html

Cummings, J., & Martin, S. (2001). *Thailand: What to do in the land of wats.* Melbourne, Australia: Lonely Planet Publications.

Fujii, D., Umetsu, D., Schwartz, T., & Hostetter, G. (2002). Culturally sensitive strategies for practicing neuropsychology in Hawaii. *INSNET, 10*(4), 1–2.

Fujii, D. E., & Wong, T. M. (2005). Neuropsychological assessment with Asian-American immigrants: Recommendations for meeting *Daubert* standards. *Journal of Forensic Neuropsychology, 4*, 3–31.

Globalis. (n.d.). *Thailand.* Retrieved March 3, 2008, from http://globalis.gvu.unu.edu/indicator_detail.cfm?country=TH&indicatorid

House, R. M., & Pinyuchon, M. (1998). Counseling Thai Americans: An emerging need. *Journal of Multicultural Counseling and Development, 26*(3), 194–204.

Hughes, C., Berg, L., Danzinger, W., Coben, L., & Martin, R. (1982). A new clinical scale for the staging of dementia. *British Journal of Psychiatry, 140,* 566–572.

Hyneman, S. P., & Loxley, W. A. (1983). The effect of primary-school quality on academic achievement across twenty-nine high- and low-income countries. *American Journal of Sociology, 88*, 1162–1194.

Jones, R. (2003). *Thailand.* London, UK: Bravo Ltd.

Jorm, A. F., & Jacomb, P. A. (1989). The Informant Questionnaire on Cognitive Decline in the Elderly (IQCODE): Socio-demographic correlates, reliability, validity and some norms. *Psychological Medicine, 19*, 1015–1022.

Lezak, M., Howieson, D. B., & Loring, D. W. (2004). *Neuropsychological assessment* (4th ed.). New York, NY: Oxford University Press.

Lynn, R. (2006). *Race differences in intelligence: An evolutionary analysis*. Augusta, GA: Washington Summit Publishers.

Maj, M., D'Elia, L., Satz, P., Janssen, R., et al. (1993). Evaluation of two new neuropsychological tests designed to minimize cultural bias in the assessment of HIV-1 seropositive persons: A WHO study. *Archives of Clinical Neuropsychology, 8*, 123–135.

Maj, M., Satz, P., Janssen, R., Zaudig, M., et al. (1994). WHO neuropsychiatric AIDS study, cross-sectional phase II: Neuropsychological and neurological findings. *Archives of General Psychiatry, 51*, 51–61.

McCall, R. B. (1977). Childhood IQ's as predictors of adult educational and occupational status. *Science, 197*, 482–483.

Mulder, N. (2000). *Inside Thai society: Religion, everyday life, change*. Chiang Mai, Thailand: Silkworm.

Nasreddine, Z., Phillips, N., Bedirian, V., Charbonneau, S., Whitehead, V., Collin, S., … Chertkow, H. (2005). The Montreal Cognitive Assessment, MoCA: A brief screening tool for mild cognitive impairment. *Journal of the American Geriatric Society, 53*, 695–699.

Neisser, U., Boodoo, G., Bouchard, T., Boykin, A. W., et al. (1996). Intelligence: Knowns and unknowns. *American Psychologist, 51*, 77–101.

Osborne, M. (2000). *Southeast Asia: An introductory history* (8th ed.). Crows Nest, Australia: Allen & Unwin.

Pollitt, E., Hathirat, P., Kotchabhakdi, N. J., Missell, L., & Valyasevi, A. (1989). Iron deficiency and educational achievement in Thailand. *American Journal of Clinical Nutrition, 50*, 687–697.

Pratomthong, S. J., & Baker, S. B. (1983). Overcoming obstacles to the growth and development of guidance and counseling in Thailand. *Personnel and Guidance Journal, 67*, 466–469.

Ramisetty-Mikler, S. (1993). Asian Indian immigrants in America and sociocultural issues in counseling. *Journal of Multicultural Counseling and Development, 21*, 36–49.

Ratanadilok, K. (2010). Neuropsychology in Thailand. In D. Fujii (Ed.), *Asian Neuropsychology*. New York, NY: Psychology Press.

Ratner, M. (2000). Thai Americans. In J. Lehman (Ed.), *Gale encyclopedia of multicultural America* (2nd ed., Vol. 3, pp. 1741–1750). Farmington Hills, MI: Gale.

Reeves, T. J., & Bennett, C. E. (2004). *We the people: Asians in the United States*. Washington, DC: U.S. Census Bureau.

Senanarong, V., Assavisaraporn, S., Sivasiriyanonds, N., et al. (2001). The IQCODE: An alternative screening test for dementia for low educated Thai elderly. *Journal of the Medical Association of Thailand, 84*, 648–655.

Siri, S., Okanurak, K., Chansirikanjana, S., Kitayaporn, D., & Jorm, A. F. (2006). Modified Informant Questionnaire on Cognitive Decline in the Elderly (IQCODE) as a screening test for dementia for Thai elderly. *Southeast Asian Journal of Tropical Medicine and Public Health, 37*, 587–594.

U.S. Census Bureau. (2000). *Census*. Retrieved February 29, 2008, from http://www.census.gov/main/www/cen2000.html

Weisz, J. R., Suwanlert, S., Chaiyasit, W., Weiss, B., Achenbach, T. M., & Eastman, K. L. (1993). Behavioral and emotional problems among Thai and American adolescents: Parent reports for ages 12–16. *Journal of Abnormal Psychology, 102*(3), 395–403.

Weisz, J. R., Suwanlert, S., Chaiyasit, W., Weiss, B., Achenbach, T., & Walter, B. (1987). Epidemiology of behavioral and emotional problems among Thai and American children: Parent reports for ages 6–11. *Journal of the American Academy of Child and Adolescent Psychiatry, 26,* 890–897.

Webometrics. (n.d.). *World universities' ranking on the web.* Retrieved March 4, 2008, from http://www.webometrics.info/top4000.sap

Webometrics. (n.d.). *World universities' ranking on the web: Top Asia.* Retrieved March 4, 2008, from http://webometrics.info/top100_continent.asp?cont=asia

Wiriyachitra, A. (2004). *English language teaching and learning in Thailand in this decade.* Retrieved March 10, 2008 from http://www.apecneted.org/knowledgebank

Wong, T. M., & Fujii, D. E. (2004). Neuropsychological assessment of Asian Americans: Demographic factors, cultural diversity, and practical guidelines. *Applied Neuropsychology, 11,* 23–36.

11 Neuropsychology of Vietnamese Americans

Dung Ngo, Minh-Thu Le, and Phuoc Dinh Le

Brief history

Vietnam has a long history that spans over 4000 years (Whitmore, 1986; Vets With a Mission, 2007). According to legend, the Vietnamese people are descendants of the Dragon Prince, Lac Long Quan, and the Immortal Princess of the Mountains, Au Co (Taylor, 1983). However, their union was characterized by irreconcilable cultural differences, as Lac Long Quan was of the dragon descendants and Au Co of the fairy lineage. After Au Co laid a 100-egg pouch producing 100 children, the couple mutually agreed to separate and each took custody of 50 children. Au Co took her children to the mountains and highlands, while Lac Long Quan headed toward the lowland areas—the rivers and seas. King Hung, the eldest son, established the Kingdom of Van Lang, which is present-day North Vietnam and the northern region of Central Vietnam (Vets With a Mission, 2007).

From a more factual perspective, the Vietnamese people are thought to be descendants of people who settled in the Red River Delta thousands of years ago (Microsoft Encarta Online Encyclopedia, n.d.). However, the legend of Lac Long Quan and Au Co has had a profound impact on the ethnic identity of the Vietnamese people. Today, Vietnamese children are still taught about this legend at school and take great pride in their ancestors' origin. Every year, the Vietnamese around the world observe a traditional day in commemoration of their ancestor, King Hung (*Gio To Hung Vuong*). This cultural event is aimed at promoting and preserving Vietnam's traditional values for the next generation of Vietnamese children.

Vietnam's history is also filled with struggles against foreign invasion and dominance. Vietnam was subjected to Chinese occupation for over 1,000 years, spanning, from 111 B.C. to 938 A.D. (Microsoft Encarta Online Encyclopedia, n.d.). During this time, the Vietnamese people resisted tirelessly against the Chinese control. One of the earliest and most notable uprisings in an attempt to regain independence for Vietnam was commenced by the Trung sisters (Trung Trac and Trung Nhi) about 30–40 A.D. Additionally, in the 1880s, France held Vietnam and the neighboring countries of Laos and Cambodia as colonies subjugated to her rules (Bankston, 2000; Ferry, 2004; First Battalion Fiftieth Infantry Association, n.d.). In 1954, following the defeat of the French at Dien Bien Phu, the Geneva Accord stipulated the withdrawal of French troops and the temporary division of the country into North Vietnam and South Vietnam at the 17th parallel, with the Communist North and anti-Communist South. Reunification via national elections was to take place in 1956 but it never occurred (Bankston, 2000; Microsoft Encarta Online Encyclopedia, n.d.).

In the 1960s, with its primary goal of containing international Communism and preserving democracy in the South, the American government became intensely involved in the Vietnam War (Bankston, 2000). In response to the American public's opposition to the war and in accordance with the Paris peace talks in 1973, the United States agreed to a cease-fire agreement and a timetable for the withdrawal of American troops and the turning over of the war to the South Vietnamese army (Bankston, 2000). The Vietnam War (1960s–1975) cost the United States 58,000 lives and 350,000 casualties. It also resulted in approximately 1 to 2 million Vietnamese deaths (Digital History, 2008). In April 1975, the capital of South Vietnam, Saigon (now Ho Chi Minh City), fell to the North Vietnamese Communist invasion and set the stage for the largest exodus in the history of Vietnam.

Present-day Vietnam: The socialist republic of Vietnam

Geography

Vietnam is bordered to the north by China, to the west by Laos and Cambodia, and to the east and south by the Gulf of Tonkin, South China Sea, and Gulf of Thailand. Vietnam is slightly larger than the state of New Mexico. The 2001 Vietnamese census reported a population of over 85 million, with about 5.8% of the population 65 years of age or older (Microsoft Encarta Online Encyclopedia, n.d.). In contrast to the popular belief, Vietnam is quite a multiethnic, multicultural society. It has been documented that Vietnam consists of more than 50 ethnic groups; however, 90% are ethnic Kinh (Vietnamese), 2% are ethnic Chinese, and about 8% are made up of various tribal groups, including the Khmer, Cham, Hmong, Thai, Muong, and others (Microsoft Encarta Online Encyclopedia, n.d.). The majority of these ethnic minorities live in mountain areas and have become increasingly assimilated into the ways of life of the mainstream Vietnamese culture (Ngo, unpublished data).

Language

The Vietnamese language is a tonal language in which the meaning of a word is dependent upon the tone or the pitch with which it is spoken. There are three main regional dialects with subtle variations in vocabulary (local word usage) and differences in pronunciation. For example, northern Vietnamese refer to the "pig" as *con lon,* while southern Vietnamese call it *con heo,* or *cai phanh* and *cai thang* for "the car brake" in the North and South, respectively. Additionally, people from different regions may not be familiar with the local regional dialect. Although subtle, these differences can create troublesome misunderstandings in everyday communication across the three regions of Vietnam.

About the fourteenth century A.D., *Chu Nom* (a form of writing modified from the Chinese *Chu Han*) was developed. By the middle of the seventeenth century, a Jesuit missionary, Alexandre de Rhodes, developed *Quoc Ngu,* a Romanized phonetic script with diacritical marks to help catechize and compile a Vietnamese-Latin-Portuguese dictionary. The French rulers encouraged *Quoc Ngu*, which progressively replaced the Chinese as well as Chu Nom methods of writing. French and Portuguese missionaries are credited for the creation of the current writing system, *Quoc Ngu,* which phonetically transcribes spoken Vietnamese using the Latin alphabet (Bankston, 2000). Although *Quoc Ngu* is considered the official national language of Vietnam, with the increase in Western influences, English has become increasingly popular and is even favored as a second language in educational settings. Other language include French, Chinese, and Khmer. Mountain area languages such as Mon-Khmer and Malayo-Polynesian are also spoken, although they are much less common.

Religion

Common religions in Vietnam include Buddhism, Cao Dai, Catholicism, Confucianism, Taoism, Hoa Hao, Islam, Protestantism, and Animism (Bankston, 2000). The majority of Vietnamese are self-classified as Buddhists, and about 7% are Catholics (Microsoft Encarta Online Encyclopedia, n.d.).

Education

Chinese influence

Historically, Vietnam's educational system was strongly influenced by Chinese and French cultures (Cima, 1987). Under the Chinese control, education was mainly reserved for children of royal backgrounds and other high-ranking officials. During this time, Vietnam's education followed the Mandarin system (or Confucian system) and examinations were highly competitive and used primarily to recruit public officials. The curriculum was based on the philosophies of Confucius and his disciple Mencius, which emphasized Confucianism and the conduct of the civil service (To Thuy Yen, Vietnamese poet, personal communication, 2008). Only scholars well versed in Confucianism could pass the civil service examinations. Learning was based primarily on rote memory, and science and technology were not the main focus under the Confucian system. Opportunities to attend school were strictly reserved for males, and education was the highest cherished ideal. In an agricultural society, such as Vietnam, education was perceived as the only means to advance intellectually and socially. Scholars or the educated were looked up to and highly revered.

Vietnam's first university, the *Quốc Tử Giám* (National University), was established in 1076 to teach Confucianism to children of the royal family and nobility. Vietnamese Mandarins or Confucian scholars, who had passed the examinations, were regarded as social, intellectual, and cultural leaders. Due to the lack of opportunities and resources at the national level, the majority of students received their education at the local levels from small private classes, which were taught by teachers who had been educated. The Confucian school system was administered in Vietnam for approximately 2,000 years (Cima, 1987) and was essential for admission to the ruling class of scholar-officials (To Thuy Yen, renowned Vietnamese poet, personal communication, 2008).

French influence

The French established its colonization in Vietnam in the mid-1900s. During this period, Vietnam's educational system was converted from the old Confucian system into a more Western-oriented one. During the French rule, education was again limited only to members of the elite and the upper class. Poverty was a major obstacle to learning, and secondary and higher education were beyond the reach of many children. The French educational system consisted of 13 years of education: 3 years of elementary school, 3 years of primary education in French, 4 years of vocationally oriented primary superior education in French, and 3 years of French-language secondary education leading to an Indochinese baccalaureate (high school diploma) (Cima, 1987). The content areas did not focus extensively on math and sciences, but rather on the teaching about Vietnam and agricultural life. By this time, the use of Chinese characters in schools was discontinued, and the use of *Quoc Ngu* was included in the curriculum. However, French became the second language of great importance. Many Vietnamese elders who were educated under the French school system may be fluent in both French and Vietnamese.

Current system

As discussed above, the Vietnamese educational system was influenced by the Chinese and French. The current system is now very much affected by the United States and other Western industrialized nations. The current educational levels are very similar to those of the American school system, including preschool, kindergarten, middle school, and high school. Beyond high school education, there are trade or technical schools, as well as universities. Most universities are operated and managed by the government. Although under the Socialist Republic of Vietnam, the current educational system still has some resemblance to the French model; the curriculum was revised to include more emphasis on Vietnamese language, literature, and history, as well as the teaching of revolutionary ethics and ideologies of Marxism-Leninism and Ho Chi Minh.

With the advancement in globalization and high technology, and the increased number of foreign investment companies in Vietnam, the trend to study English has spread rapidly from the city to the countryside. In fact, college graduates must possess a strong command of English in order to find jobs in the cities. Additionally, English proficiency is a prerequisite for studying abroad in English-speaking countries.

Immigration history

From 1951 to 1960, the Vietnamese population in the United States was estimated to be a mere 335 people (Ferry, 2004). However, shortly prior to the fall of Saigon in 1975, President Ford authorized the entry of 125,000 Vietnamese refugees to the United States (Bankston, 2000; Ferry, 2004). These individuals constituted the first wave of Vietnamese immigrants. They were thought to be well educated and among the elite of South Vietnam, with ties to U.S. military personnel or American companies conducting business in Vietnam. Bankston (2000) reported that 30% of the heads of households in the first wave were professionals, 16.9% were in transportation occupations, and 11.7% were in clerical and sales occupations. He also indicated that 70% were from urban areas. Thus, individuals comprising the first wave possessed knowledge and skills that were readily transferable in the host country. They were initially housed at select military camps and departure typically required sponsorship. The sponsor, whether an individual or a group, was expected to assume financial and personal responsibility for the refugee for up to two years and to assist in the procurement of housing, employment, and education (Bankston, 2000; Ferry, 2004).

The second wave of refugees, also known as "the boat people," came between the late 1970s and late 1980s in response to the worsening political and economic conditions in Vietnam. From 1980 to 1981, about 181,300 Vietnamese were admitted to the United States (Bankston, 2000). Many fled in small overcrowded boats to refugee camps in nearby Asian countries prior to secondary relocation to the United States or other host countries. Tales of pirate attacks, drowning, physical and sexual assault, and starvation were plentiful. There were even stories of refugees being chased away by local inhabitants who were ill-equipped to provide for them (Ferry, 2004). This second wave of refugees was said to be less educated, favoring farming and fishing, and coming primarily from rural areas (Bankston, 2000; Ferry, 2004). They were also said to have experienced the most preimmigration trauma.

After 1983, due to an agreement negotiated with the Vietnamese government by the United Nations, Vietnamese entered the United States under the Orderly Departure Program (ODP) (Ferry, 2004). According to Ferry (2004), those who qualified were individuals with close relatives in the United States, individuals who had an established connection to the American government (including being the offspring of a Vietnamese mother and an American soldier), and political detainees in reeducation camps (typically former South Vietnamese government officials and military officers).

Currently, Vietnamese continue to seek entry into the United States at a steady rate through the family reunification program. Statistics from the Department of Homeland Security (n.d.) showed that about 289,000 Vietnamese were admitted to the United States from 1997 to 2006, and that 31,524 Vietnamese immigrants entered the United States in 2004, 32,784 in 2005, and 30,695 in 2006. The number of undocumented immigrants is unknown.

Demographic profile of Vietnamese Americans

According to the 2000 U.S. census (Barnes & Bennett, 2002; Reeves & Bennett, 2004), 11.9 million people in the United States identified themselves as being Asian or of Asian heritage. Among this Asian population, Vietnamese Americans make

Table 11.1 Vietnamese American population in the United States by region

Regions	*Population*
Northeastern states	115,487
Midwestern states	106,938
Southern states	335,679
Western states	564,424
Total	1,122,528

Source: U.S. Census Bureau, 2000.

up 10.9%, or roughly 1.2 million. This includes those who identified themselves as Vietnamese at least in combination with one other race (e.g., Chinese Vietnamese) in the census. From 1990 to 2000, Vietnamese Americans doubled in size, growing from about 614,547 to 1,212,465 (American FactFinder/U.S. Census Bureau, 2007; Reeves & Bennett, 2004). About 76.1% are foreign born and 62.4% speak English less than "very well" (Reeves & Bennett, 2004). The original intent of the immigration program was to disperse Vietnamese refugees throughout the country in order to avoid overburdening a particular community. However, after the initial resettlement period, a secondary migration was observed as Vietnamese started to migrate to more urban areas to be closer to families and fellow Vietnamese (Bankston, 2000; Ferry, 2004). California is said to be the home of about 50% of the Vietnamese American population, and the southern states of Texas, Virginia, Florida, Georgia, and Louisiana account for about 30% (Ferry, 2004). The three largest Vietnamese communities are Little Saigon, a suburb in Orange County, California, with an estimate of 350,000; San Jose, California, with an estimate of 125,000; and Houston, Texas, with an estimate of 100,000 (Ferry, 2004). It is believed that these figures are underestimates.

The 2000 U.S. census (Reeves & Bennett, 2004) reveals that nearly 43% of Vietnamese Americans have at least some college education, with a little over 19% achieving a bachelor's degree or higher. Approximately 56% of Vietnamese American women and 68% of Vietnamese American men participate in the labor force. They are employed in all sectors of the economy, with nearly 27% in management, professionals, and related occupations. About 19% are in the service sector. Another 19% are in sales and clerical positions. Approximately 29% are in production and transportation. The median income of Vietnamese families in 1999 falls below the median income of all families in the United States ($47,103 vs. $50,046) and the median income of Asian families ($47,103 vs. $59,324). The poverty rate in 1999 for Vietnamese Americans is 16%, higher than the rate for the total population (12.4%) and higher than the rate for Asian Americans (12.6%).

With respect to religious affiliations, more than 50% of Vietnamese Americans follow Buddhism, and it is estimated that as many as 40% of Vietnamese in the United States are Roman Catholics (Ferry, 2004). Many Vietnamese Buddhists also adhere to certain beliefs and teachings of Confucianism and Taoism (Ferry, 2004). With the normalization of relations with Vietnam under the Clinton administration,

Vietnamese Americans began to visit their homeland, likely reacquainting themselves with old traditions and learning newly evolved customs.

Trauma and psychiatric disorders

From the clinical perspective, it is important to note that many Vietnamese refugees came to the United States with significant preimmigration traumatic experiences, including war, imprisonment, and torture. The horrific life experiences of Vietnamese refugees who escaped by sea were widely reported in the decade from the late 1970s to the late 1980s. In the early 1980s, the U.S. Committee for Refugees estimated that nearly 80% of the Vietnamese boat people had been brutally attacked by sea pirates. These horrific experiences undoubtedly had long-lasting psychiatric and neuropsychological effects on these individuals.

The amount and types of traumatic experiences that Vietnamese Americans suffered before coming to the United States will likely put these individuals at an increased risk for developing various psychiatric conditions. Vietnamese boat people who escaped in the late 1970s and early 1980s and other newcomers from Vietnam who were detained in reeducation camps are most vulnerable to psychiatric disorders. These individuals reportedly experienced a multitude of traumas, including rape, being lost, hunger, witnessing the death or murder of loved ones, and torture (U.S. Committee for Refugees, 1984; Mollica et al., 1987). Psychiatric disorders such as chronic depression and posttraumatic stress disorder (PTSD) have been documented among the Vietnamese refugees in the United States (Kleinman, 1990; Mollica, Caspi-Yavin, & Bollini, 1992), as well as in Canada, Norway, and Japan (Ebata & Miyake, 1989; Vaglum, 1993). Considerable data have revealed the negative effects of depression on cognitive functioning (Jorm, 2001; Zubenko et al., 2003). Thus, preimmigration trauma and its psychological consequences should be taken into consideration in a standard neuropsychological evaluation among Vietnamese Americans.

Vietnamese who immigrated to the United States were motivated by the hopes of attaining a better life for themselves and their families. However, they continue to face many challenges that can significantly impact mental health in their new country. Racism and prejudice are constant obstacles. It has been reported that only 36% of Americans polled in 1975 favored the admittance of Vietnamese refugees to the United States (Ferry, 2004). The lack of proficiency in English and transferable job skills have limited their job opportunities. Consequently, new immigrants are forced to hold multiple low-paying, menial labor jobs in order to support their families (Nghe, Mahalik, & Lowe, 2003; Ferry, 2004). Economic necessity also propels Vietnamese women into the workforce, thereby altering the family dynamics and traditional gender roles. Differences in the rate of acculturation between parents and children, with parents adhering more closely to traditional values and children quickly adopting more autonomous customs, result in intergenerational conflict.

As illustrated in the previous section, the pattern of immigration within the Vietnamese American population in the United States varied significantly. Each wave of refugees encountered different life experiences; the type and degree of traumatic events among different waves may also be unique. The types and frequency of trauma have also been found to vary between Vietnamese men and women (Ngo, Tran, Gibbons, & Oliver, 2001). Therefore, treating Vietnamese Americans as a homogenous group is likely to threaten external validity. Future studies should attempt to separately examine the psychological well-being of different waves regarding migration of the Vietnamese population.

Posttraumatic stress disorder and cognitive impairments

Studies report that individuals suffering from posttraumatic stress disorder (PTSD) demonstrate impairments across a wide range of cognitive domains, including impaired declarative memory (e.g., Bremner et al., 1995), impaired attention and working memory (e.g., Uddo, Vasterling, Brailey, & Sutker, 1993; Vasterling et al., 1993; Klonoff, McDougall, Clark, Kramer, & Horgan, 1976), and lower intelligence (Buckley, Blanchard, & Neill, 2000). For example, Bremner et al. (1995) found poorer immediate and delayed verbal memory among Vietnam veterans with PTSD than among healthy control subjects. Further, poorer immediate and delayed verbal memory was also reported among survivors of childhood abuse with PTSD, compared to matched controls (Bremner et al., 1995). The authors also reported a significant correlation between trauma severity and verbal memory impairments. Impaired learning, perseverative errors, poorer word fluency, and impaired immediate visual memory have also been documented among Vietnam veterans with PTSD, compared with control subjects (Uddo et al., 1993). Finally, Vasterling, Brailey, Constans, and Sutker (1998) reported impairments in sustained attention, mental manipulation, acquisition of new information, retroactive interference, and errors of commission and intrusion among Gulf War veterans with PTSD, compared with mentally healthy controls. Given the high prevalence rates of PTSD among Vietnamese Americans, it is crucial that neuropsychologists consider the effects of past trauma on cognitive impairments among these individuals. Thus, symptoms associated with past trauma should be investigated and taken into consideration in the assessment and interpretation of the test results.

Conceptualization of mental illness health

An understanding of how Vietnamese Americans view mental illness or neurondegenerative diseases is critical in developing effective assessment, diagnosis, and treatment strategies, as beliefs about the causes of these illnesses may influence how and from whom Vietnamese individuals seek professional services. Significant cross-cultural data are available to suggest that many ethnic minorities have beliefs about illness and treatment that differ significantly from Western scientific medical practices (e.g., Chrisman & Kleinman, 1983; McGoldrick, Pearce, & Giordano, 1982). For example, some Asian cultures perceive the causes of mental illness to be strongly associated with organic factors, with a lack of willpower, and with morbid thinking (i.e., thinking bad thoughts) (Sue, Wagner, Ja, Margullis, & Lew, 1976). Arkoff et al. (1966) reported that in comparison to American students, Asian students were more likely to believe that mental health could be improved through the exercise of willpower and a preoccupation with pleasant thoughts. Similarly, Sue and colleagues (1976) reported that Asian American students were more likely to perceive that the mentally ill look and act different, that willpower is the basis of personal adjustment, that women are more prone to mental disorder than men, that the avoidance of negative thoughts enhances mental health, and that mental disorder is primarily attributed to organic factors.

Different perspectives of deviant behaviors are believed to result from differences in socialization. Asian individuals are generally socialized to exercise greater self-control and conformity to the family or community. Individuals who go against the traditional family system would be considered deviants, lacking strength and character. This clearly contrasts with Western values, which promote and encourage individualism and independence.

Vietnamese perceptions of mental illness are also reflected in their language. Vietnamese laypersons often refer to a person with a psychiatric disorder (e.g., schizophrenia) as "a crazy person." Given this label, in addition to perceptions that those who are mentally ill lack willpower, and the importance of conformity to family and community, it is not surprising that there is a strong stigma associated with mental illness. Consequently, Vietnamese generally do not seek professional help until the condition becomes severe or unbearable.

When seeking treatment, Vietnamese would more likely accept herbal medicine or home remedies to alleviate physical or emotional pain versus psychotherapy or psychotropic medications.

Conceptualization of illness: Alzheimer's disease

Traditional Vietnamese conceptualization of health disorders is illustrated in their beliefs about dementia. In order to understand the perception of and attitudes toward dementia among Vietnamese Americans adults, an author of this chapter (Ngo, unpublished data) conducted a focus group study on these issues among Vietnamese elders in Houston, Texas, during the summer of 2007. The purpose of this study was to explore the perception of Alzheimer's disease and factors that influence treatment issues among Vietnamese American elders. Caring for Vietnamese elders requires an understanding of their specific needs, as well as cultural issues that affect their attitudes and help-seeking behavior on various types of illnesses (Tran, Ngo, & Sung, 2001). The focus group participants were recruited from Lac Hong Day Care Center ($N = 31$). Participation was voluntary. All participants were born in Vietnam, spoke very limited English, and have resided in the United States for an average of 13 years. The average age of the participants was 66 years; no one worked at the time of the study. The average number of years of education in Vietnam was 10th grade for men and 6th grade for women. The qualitative results were systematically coded and summarized according to the methods described by Rosenthal and Rosnow (1991). The results were summarized into two broad categories: "perception of causes of AD" and "assessment, diagnosis, and barriers to treatment."

The vast majority of the participants had not heard of and were not familiar with the English term *Alzheimer's disease* (AD). However, when provided a description of the symptoms, most participants quickly identified AD with a condition called *lu lan* in Vietnamese language, which described a condition of confusion or memory impairment associated with old age. The majority of the participants associated the cognitive impairments of AD with the natural process of aging. The notion that AD may be caused by neurological factors, lifestyle, brain injuries, or genetic factors was never mentioned by any group member. Group members appeared to concur with the comment made by one participant that "memory problem is natural as we grow old, just like a car that has many engine problems as it gets old." Several group members alluded to the relationship between memory loss and mental problems by stating, "When you can't remember, there must be something wrong with your head."

In terms of treatment, most participants did not know that there are specialists for "memory problems" that can evaluate or diagnose dementia. Neuropsychological evaluation remains a foreign concept to all participants. Additionally, the vast majority of the participants did not know that symptoms of AD could be detected early to enhance treatment. None of the focus group participants expressed an awareness of the importance of early detection of symptoms in order to properly diagnose and treat the disease. The vast majority of the focus group participants did not realize that treatment is available for memory-related problems, although over 50% of the group acknowledged experiencing regular mild forgetfulness at the time of the study. Several group members indicated that they knew of someone with severe memory problems but did not seek help and were kept in the home. Several participants indicated that they did not know where to seek help. A few group members indicated that they reported memory problems to their Vietnamese primary care physicians but did not receive any follow-up care. Overall, participants appeared to lack information about the availability of medical care for dementia or cognitive-related problems. Furthermore, it appeared that cultural acceptance of memory loss was a normal part of aging, and this has led to the delay of diagnosis and treatment among Vietnamese American elders.

In summary, the findings from this focus group study suggested that Vietnamese American elders possessed very limited information about the spectrum of symptoms associated with AD, as well as knowledge about the assessment and treatment of this neurodegenerative condition. Further, it was concluded that the cultural perception of memory loss is that it is normal, and consequently contributes to the delay of treatment. Finally, findings from Ngo's study illustrated that the perceptions of AD and knowledge about assessment and treatment of AD varied among various subgroups of Asian Americans. For instance, in Jones et al.'s (2006) study, virtually all participants, regardless of age or experience, had heard, seen, or read about AD. Acculturation appeared to play a powerful role in the perceptions of and attitudes toward AD among subgroups of Asian Americans. These findings attest to the importance of heterogeneity of Asian Americans, and that various cultural factors, as well as levels of acculturation, need to be considered in the assessment and treatment of this population.

Issues in neuropsychological assessment among Vietnamese Americans

In this section we will examine a number of key issues related to conducting a neuropsychological assessment with Vietnamese-speaking patients. Past studies have documented the significant effects of trauma, education, and language on neuropsychological test performance (e.g., Klonoff et al., 1976; Ferraro, 2002; Uzzell, 2007). Accordingly, these cultural factors will be discussed in the sections below.

As mentioned in the previous section, many Vietnamese Americans have undergone horrific trauma prior to coming to the United States. In particular, individuals who escaped by boats or by land and those who were imprisoned after the war (ex–political detainees) are most at risk for various psychiatric disorders. These psychiatric conditions (e.g., depression and PTSD) may confound the results of neuropsychological tests. Additionally, cross-cultural researchers have documented that Asian Americans, including Vietnamese Americans, are prone to somatization due to cultural stigma (Leong & Lau, 2001). Quite often, Vietnamese patients will complain of headaches, sleep disturbances, poor appetite, and dizziness. It is important for the neuropsychologist to assess the underlying cause of these symptoms in order to ascertain if they are organic or psychological in nature.

Formal education has been implicated to have a protective effect on cognitive decline among both healthy and demented individuals (Ostrosky-Solís, 2007). However, past studies that examined the relationship between education and dementia have focused mainly on AD. For instance, it has been postulated that individuals who are highly educated experience a later onset of AD and with a lesser degree of severity (e.g., Katzman, 1993). Education has also been found to affect performance on neuropsychological tests among certain ethnic minority groups. For example, Pontón and colleagues (1996) reported that Hispanic individuals with a sixth-grade education scored two standard deviations below the average norm, compared to individuals with an average of 16 years of formal education. These findings draw attention to the potential of misdiagnosis without appropriate normative data.

Formal education among Vietnamese elders is complex because many of these individuals have endured long decades of war and migration. Our clinical experiences indicated that the majority of Vietnamese elders do not have an educational level higher than the 10th grade. Poverty, migration, and war seemed to be major factors that prevented Vietnamese elders from attaining a higher education. For example, after the French lost their battle at Dien Bien Phu in 1954, more than 1 million Vietnamese migrated from the North to the South (Tarling, 2004). Consequently, their schooling was abruptly ended or interrupted during this chaotic period. The majority of Vietnamese elders who are members of the Vietnamese Seniors Association of Houston classified their educational level as either "elementary" or "high school," equivalent to 1st to 6th grade and 10th to 12th grade levels in the United States, respectively. None of the participants in Ngo's focus group study (n = 31) had additional formal education in the United States. Only 3/31 (9.6%) of the women in this study completed high school in Vietnam, compared to 21/31 of the men (67.7%). Furthermore, elderly individuals who attained higher education during this era likely came from privileged or financially well-off families and represented only a small percentage of the cohort. Another cohort of Vietnamese elders who likely possessed a high school education or specialized training in higher education includes former military officers. This cohort has also been found to experience mass trauma related to combat situations, imprisonment, and torture after the Vietnam War (Mollica et al., 1986). In summary, many Vietnamese elders came to America with very limited formal education due to poverty and the consequences of the war. However, these individuals may develop a broad range of knowledge as a result of continuing their education at home and being self-taught.

English language skills are another important factor that affects neuropsychological test results among Vietnamese Americans. According to the 2000 U.S. census (Reeves & Bennett, 2004), more than 97% of Vietnamese elders were born outside the United States, and the vast majority did not speak English well or at all. Compared with elder Asian Americans from other ethnic backgrounds, Vietnamese elders immigrated to the United States more recently, and more than 75% do not speak fluent English (Reeves & Bennett, 2004). Poor English proficiency has been found to be one of the major obstacles in seeking health and mental health services among Vietnamese Americans (Ngo, 2007), especially if the condition requires a specialist (e.g., neuropsychologist) who is not familiar with the Vietnamese culture or language. For these reasons, Vietnamese neuropsychologists who can speak and are familiar with Vietnamese culture are much needed.

When a culturally and linguistically matched neuropsychologist is unavailable, an interpreter is often used in the evaluation process. One should be very cautious when an interpreter is used. The accuracy and validity of the neuropsychological evaluation may be greatly compromised due to language and cultural factors. For instance, an interpreter who is untrained in the health or mental health profession may lack the knowledge of specialized terminology to interpret. Some experts believe that the accuracy and validity of a neuropsychological evaluation is significantly reduced when using an interpreter (Dr. Robert Kooken, personal communication). In addition, Vietnam is divided into three distinct regions (i.e., North, Central, and South). Locals from each of these regions speak distinct dialects and use terminologies that may be foreign to individuals from a different region. For example, North Vietnamese refer to a funnel as *cái phễu*, whereas Vietnamese from the central region refer to the same object as *cái quăng*; North Vietnamese refer to the car brake as *cai phanh*, whereas South Vietnamese refer to the same object as *cai thang*. Thus, when using an interpreter, it is important to ensure that the individual is well trained in the specialty area, as well as possesses an excellent command of all three regional dialects of the Vietnamese language.

Other cultural factors that may affect the process of a neuropsychological evaluation include communication styles and the hesitancy to reveal personal information among Vietnamese individuals. Psychologists generally are trained to collect as much background information as possible during the initial visit. The authors found that many Vietnamese patients are quite uncomfortable when being asked to provide a detailed family history and personal information on the first visit. A patient once shared his thought with the author (Ngo) that "it makes me uncomfortable when you asked too many personal questions; I don't know what you're going to do with this information." One way to overcome this obstacle is to focus more on the presenting symptoms that the patient is experiencing and provide a medical explanation for these symptoms at the end of the interview. Additional family history and background information can be obtained from the patient, or from another family member, when there is a sense of trust and rapport.

Finally, throughout the process of the evaluation, it is important to be aware that Vietnamese people are socialized to show respect and compliance with authority figures, including individuals from the medical profession. Most Vietnamese would avoid expressing disagreement toward or even asking for clarifications from the psychologist. This cultural behavior would likely affect test results since the vast majority lack knowledge about what a neuropsychological evaluation is. Additionally, from the authors' clinical experiences, Vietnamese patients rarely volunteer to discuss the side effects of their medications, unless asked directly. It is common for Vietnamese patients to discontinue medications when they experience side effects, rather than to discuss the issue with their physician. Also, there are important differences in terms of communication styles. Quite often a "yes" means "I hear you," rather than "I agree with you." The lack of such communication between doctor and patient may lead to the Vietnamese patient discontinuing treatment on his or her own.

Neuropsychological tests

Given the lack of sufficient test norms for use with Vietnamese-speaking adults, the existing norms reported by Dick, Teng, Kempler, Davis, and Taussig (2002) can be helpful when used with caveats. The Cross-Cultural Neuropsychological Test Battery (CCNB) was developed by Dick and colleagues (2002) for the purpose of addressing cultural and linguistic issues associated with diagnosing dementia among diverse populations. Currently, it is the only test with norms for Vietnamese Americans. The CCNB has 11 subtests that assess six cognitive domains typically included in a dementia evaluation. Tests include the Cognitive Abilities Screening Instrument (CASI) (Teng et al., 1994); the Common Objects Memory Test (COMT), a visual memory test presenting pictures of 10 common objects over three trials with immediate, delayed, and recognition recall trials; Body Part Naming; Animal Fluency; Auditory Comprehension; Block Design; CERAD Drawing; Read and Set; Digits forwards and backwards; and Trail Making A. The battery takes about 1 hour 30 minutes to complete.

The standardization sample of the CCNB was based on 336 healthy adults and 90 demented patients from five target groups, including African American, Caucasian, Chinese American, Hispanic American, and Vietnamese American. There were 61 Vietnamese participants in the sample with ages ranging from 62 to 87 years (M = 71.5, SD = 5.8), and their educational level from 0 to 16 years (M = 8.6, SD = 4.1). Furthermore, among the Vietnamese sample, 97% spoke only Vietnamese and 56% did not read English (Dick et al., 2002). For the purpose of this review, we will only provide comparison with the Caucasian group, as most normative data for American neuropsychological tests are based upon predominantly White samples. When compared to the Vietnamese sample, the Caucasian group (n = 70) was significantly older (M = 77.0, SD = 7.4), with a higher level of education (M = 11.4, SD = 3.9).

The Caucasian group scored significantly better than the Vietnamese group on Trails A (Caucasians, M = 51.0, SD = 21.4; Vietnamese, M = 83.9, SD = 58.0), CASI

(Caucasian, *M* = 91.5, *SD* = 5.2; Vietnamese, *M* = 85.7, *SD* = 11.0), and the Modified Picture Completion (Caucasian, *M* = 8.8, *SD* = 1.1; Vietnamese, *M* = 6.6, *SD* = 2.7). The Vietnamese group (*M* = 17.3, *SD* = 5.2) produced significantly more animal names than the Caucasian group (*M* = 16.3, *SD* = 4) (Kempler, Teng, Dick, Taussig, & Davis, 1998). No differences were found on the remainder of the tests.

Although the CCNB is currently the only dementia battery that assesses cognitive function among a diverse ethnic population, clinicians should use it with caution. It is important for the clinician to consider the effects of age and education on test results. As reported by the test's authors, education affected performance on nearly every test and accounted for about 15% of the variance in scores. Besides the Hispanic American subsample, Vietnamese Americans had lower educational attainment than other target groups in the standardization sample. Despite the lower level of education, except for the aforementioned tests, the Vietnamese sample scored comparably to the older, but more highly educated Caucasian sample, and even performed better on animal fluency. These comparative test results may guide clinicians in test selection and interpretation with elderly Vietnamese clients and can particularly guard against false positives in diagnosing dementia.

Other Western neuropsychological tests have been translated into Vietnamese, which may facilitate administration to a primarily Vietnamese-speaking client. However, these tests do not have norms for a strictly Vietnamese sample, and thus test scores would have to be interpreted with caution. The Montreal Cognitive Assessment (MoCA; Nasreddine et al., 2005) is a 30-point dementia screen that incorporates tasks such as draw a clock, verbal fluency, and a mini trail making, along with typical orientation, attention, and memory items. The MoCA and its Vietnamese translation are available online at http://www.mocatest.org/.

The Bilingual Verbal Abilities Test (BVAT) (Munoz-Sandoval, Cummins, Alvarado, & Ruef, 1998) evaluates language skills in both English and Vietnamese, which may provide useful information for interpreting neuropsychological test scores on Western tests with a strong language component. The BVAT consists of three subtests from the Woodcock-Johnson Revised Tests of Cognitive Ability and Language Proficiency Battery–Revised: Picture Vocabulary (58 items), Oral Vocabulary Synonyms (20 items) and Antonyms (20 items), and Verbal Analogies (35 items). The test requires a bilingual administrator or interpreter and takes approximately 30 minutes to complete. Items are administered in English, and missed items are then administered in the client's native language. Norms range from 5 to 90.

Recommendations

1. Vietnamese patients may not readily volunteer personal, family, and medical information at the initial meeting. It is recommended that the neuropsychologist maintains a close communication with the patient's primary care physician and other family members. Also refrain from an extensive clinical interview during the first session. It is best to obtain information over a couple of sessions and from different informants. The patient's report

should be corroborated with an observer's report (e.g., spouse or other family member).

2. Since the vast majority of Vietnamese are unfamiliar with the procedures and contents of a neuropsychological assessment, it is critical to spend sufficient time to educate the patient and his or her significant other about the procedures, the assessment process, and how the results are used clinically.
3. Due to the high prevalence rates of PTSD and depression in this population, it is important for neuropsychologists to routinely assess for these potential confounding factors, as they may affect test results.
4. Levels of formal education are not always an accurate indicator of IQ or a good estimate of premorbid functioning. General intellectual functioning or premorbid functioning should be assessed within the context of cultural expectations and environmental demands. For instance, how did the patient overcome the economic hardships in his or her native country, endure the acculturative stress in the host country, or endure the political persecutions back in Vietnam.
5. When an interpreter must be used, the neuropsychologist should be aware of the following:
   a. The interpreter's formal training and qualifications
   b. The interpreter's native language skills and dialects, as well as English proficiency
   c. The interpreter's knowledge of Vietnamese culture
   d. The interpreter's familiarity with medical, psychological, and psychiatric terminologies

Case sample

CT is a 20-year-old, left-handed male who has been living in the United States for 2 years. Although CT was born and raised in Vietnam, he speaks both Vietnamese and Chinese. CT has a long-standing history of intractable seizure disorder. He experienced febrile convulsions at age 5 months and also has a history of meningitis in infancy. Nonetheless, he reportedly achieved the appropriate developmental milestones within the same time frame as his three healthy older sisters. It was not until the age of 5 years that he began experiencing recurring seizure activities with episodes during which he feels fearful and his vision is gradually obscured by an approaching and expanding shadow. At age 12 years, he began having secondarily generalized tonic-clonic seizures. Despite trials of multiple anticonvulsants, good seizure control has not been achieved. According to his mother, his schooling has been limited to home tutoring due to his seizures. Social interaction has also been restricted to the immediate family, not an uncommon way for his family to cope with the stigma of epilepsy.

Given the medically intractable nature of his seizure disorder, he and his family have been exploring possible surgical intervention through a local epilepsy surgery program in California. Presurgical workup thus far has included an MRI scan showing post-traumatic or post-ischemic changes within the left posterior parietal and occipital cortex. A small focal area of gliosis was also observed within the right occipital subcortical white matter. An interictal SPECT study demonstrated mild decreased activity in the left temporal tip. EEG revealed frequent interictal spikes arising from the right occipital-parietal region.

To complete the first phase of the presurgical evaluation, CT will also be undergoing an extended inpatient video and EEG recording (through scalp electrodes) of seizure activities, and he has been referred for a neuropsychological assessment to obtain baseline cognitive status and to provide collateral data for the lateralization and localization of the seizure focus. The initial referral was made to the program's neuropsychologist. However, due to his very limited English, he was then secondarily referred to the second author, who is a Vietnamese-speaking neuropsychologist with specific training in epilepsy surgical workup.

CT came to his appointment accompanied by his mother and his sister. He was somewhat shy, and the above history was obtained through his medical records and an interview with his mother and his sister. He spoke Vietnamese with the dialect of people from the South, which is coincidentally familiar to the examiner.

As it was a surgical workup, a comprehensive test battery was employed. Test selection needed to take into consideration language and cultural factors while at the same time maintaining as much uniformity as possible with the standard surgical test battery. Consequently, the tests administered included TONI-3, WAIS-III selected subtests (Digit Span, Digit Symbol–Coding, Picture Completion, and Block Design), WMS-R (Visual Reproductions I and II and Mental Control), RAVLT (translated into Vietnamese), Color Trails 1 and 2, Boston Naming Test, Controlled Oral Word Association, Categorical Fluency (Animals), Judgment of Line Orientation, Rey-Osterrieth Complex Figure (Copy and Recall), Ruff Figural Fluency Test, Grooved Pegboard, and Wisconsin Card Sorting Test. The battery was overall weighted in favor of nonverbal tests to minimize language biases. It was believed that the TONI-3, as a nonverbal measure of intelligence, would provide a more valid estimate of his intellectual abilities than the WAIS-III, as some of the verbal subtests contain items that cannot be easily or appropriately translated into Vietnamese. Subtests such as Information and Comprehension contain culturally incompatible items. Although Vietnam adopted the Latin alphabet many years ago, there are differences between the English and the Vietnamese alphabet. Thus, Color Trails was chosen over the Halstead-Reitan Trail Making Test. In addition, with Controlled Oral Word Association, the letter F was substituted with the letter M, as F is not part of the Vietnamese alphabet. Logical Memory and Verbal Paired Associates from the WMS-R, standard memory tasks of the surgical testing protocol, were omitted, as neither could be reliably translated nor could substitution be made with retention of all test characteristics. While not ideal, the Boston Naming Test and Controlled Oral Word Association were included because lateralization and localization cannot be determined without assessment of language. However, interpretation will be tempered with qualitative analyses. As a general rule, interpretation will take into account potential confounds associated with the translation of test material and the lack of available normative data that are representative of CT's cultural, linguistic, and educational background.

The assessment yielded the following impressions:

1. Generally impaired executive functioning and select deficits in attention, which suggest dysfunction of the frontal lobe or its subcortical projections.
2. The presence of visuospatial difficulties and overall better recall of verbal information than the recollection of visual data support the relative involvement of the nondominant hemisphere.
3. Involvement of the dominant neocortex cannot be entirely ruled out in view of impairment in naming and phonemic verbal fluency. However, categorical verbal fluency, which is a more appropriate measure, linguistically and culturally, was intact. Further, with naming, CT correctly named 20 out of the first 30 "easier" items. Five of the items he was not able to name either did not exist naturally or were not common in Vietnam. The second half contained many items that did not have equivalent terminology in Vietnamese. Thus, language impairment may have been reflective of flawed instrumentation.

Subsequent to the completion of the first phase of CT's presurgical workup, the decision was made to proceed to the second phase of investigation rather than resective surgery, as both the imaging studies and the neuropsychological profile provided discordant data regarding a possible seizure focus. The patient was required to undergo an invasive study with implantation intracranial depth electrodes to record seizure activities during another hospital stay. Unfortunately, he became oppositional and combative and posed a danger to himself such that the study was necessarily aborted for the time being.

The ideal neuropsychological assessment of a minority non-English-speaking individual is to have the evaluation conducted by a well-trained neuropsychologist who speaks the same language and using tests developed specifically for that minority population. Of course, the ideal does not yet exist for Vietnamese patients. Nonetheless, despite the complexity of the situation, a reasonable evaluation providing clinically relevant information can be performed if care is taken to minimize language and cultural confounds. In this case, communication barriers as well as the potential pitfalls of testing via an interpreter were eliminated with the referral to the second author, who was familiar with the patient's dialect and was able to administer the tests in Vietnamese. (When there is no option other than the use of an interpreter, then recommendations mentioned above should be followed.) Further, to ensure the validity and reliability of the findings, tests given were carefully selected, keeping in mind possible cultural biases and omitting and substituting tests as necessary. Lastly, interpretation of the results took into consideration the cultural strengths and weaknesses of the testing instruments, qualifying outcomes to render more accurate conclusions.

Summary

With the continued increase in the Vietnamese American population, the need for cross-cultural neuropsychology remains imminent. This chapter addressed a number of important issues that may affect the integrity of neuropsychological assessment results among Vietnamese Americans. We also examined the potential effects of PTSD on neuropsychological results among Vietnamese refugees who have undergone mass trauma. We discussed several important cultural factors, such as conceptualization of health and perception about the causes of dementia that may influence the assessment, diagnosis, and treatment for neurodegenerative diseases such as Alzheimer's. Finally, we investigated other factors that may affect neuropsychological assessment results, including the complexity of the Vietnamese language (i.e., regional dialects), the low levels of formal education among Vietnamese elders, and the use of an interpreter for non-English-speaking patients. All of these factors must be considered by those who conduct neuropsychological assessment among Vietnamese Americans. As the Vietnamese American population continues to increase steadily, we argue that experts should focus on the development of culturally and linguistically appropriate neuropsychological assessment instruments to meet the high demands of this growing population.

References

Arkoff, A., Thaver, F., & Elkind, L. (1966). Mental health and counseling ideas of Asian and American students. *Journal of Counseling Psychology, 13*, 219–223.

Bankston, C. L., III. (2000). Vietnamese Americans. In J. Lehman (Ed.), *Gale encyclopedia of multicultural America, 1847–1862*. Detroit, MI: Gale.

Barnes, J. S., & Bennett, C. E. (2002). *The Asian population: 2000*. Retrieved January 20, 2009, from http://www.census.gov/prod/2002pubs/c2kbr01-16.pdf

Bremner, J. D., Randall, P., Scott, T. M., Bronen, R. A., Seibyl, J. P., Southwick, S. M., … Innis, R. B. (1995). MRI-based measurement of hippocampal volume in patients with combat-related posttraumatic stress disorder. *American Journal of Psychiatry, 152,* 973–981.

Buckley, T. C., Blanchard, E. B., & Neill, W. T. (2000). Information processing and PTSD: A review of the empirical literature. *Clinical Psychology Review, 20,* 1041–1065.

Cima, R. J. (1987). *Vietnam: A country study*. Washington, DC: GPO for the Library of Congress.

Department of Homeland Security (n.d.). *Persons obtaining legal permanent resident status by region and country of birth: Fiscal years 1997 to 2006* (Table 3). Retrieved September 26, 2007, from http://www.dhs.gov/xlibrary/assets/statistics/yearbook/2006/table03d.xls

Dick, M. B., Teng, E. L., Kempler, D., Davis, D. S., & Taussig, I. M. (2002). The cross-cultural neuropsychological test battery (CCNB): Effects of age, education, ethnicity, and cognitive status on performance. In F. R. Ferraro (Ed.), *Minority and cross-cultural aspects of neuropsychological assessment* (pp. 17–41). Lisse, Netherlands: Swets & Zeitlinger.

Digital History. (2008). *A succinct history of the Vietnam War*. Retrieved November 15, 2008, from http://www.digitalhistory.uh.edu/database/subtitles.cfm?titleID=71

Ebata, K., & Miyake, Y. (1989). A mental health survey of the Vietnamese refugee in Japan. *International Journal of Social Psychiatry, 35*, 164–172.

Ferraro, F. R (Ed.). (2002). *Minority and cross-cultural aspects of neuropsychological assessment*. Lisse, The Netherlands: Swets & Zeitlinger Publishers.

Ferry, J. (2004). *The changing face of North America: Immigration since 1965*. Stockton, NJ: Mason Crest Publishers.

First Battalion Fiftieth Infantry Association. (n.d.). *Ancient Vietnam 12,000 BC–1845*. Retrieved September 30, 2007, from http://www.ichiban1.org/html/history/bc_1964_prewar/chinese_invasions_500bc_1427.html

Hauff, E., & Vaglum, P. (1993). Vietnamese boat refugees: The influence of war and flight traumatization on mental health on arrival in the country of resettlement: A community cohort study of Vietnamese refugees in Norway. *Acta Psychiatrica Scandinavica, 88*, 162–168.

Jones, R. S., Chow, T. W., & Gatz, M. (2006). Asian Americans and Alzheimer's disease: Assimilation, culture, and beliefs. *Journal of Aging Studies, 20,* 11–25.

Jorm, A. F. (2001). History of depression as a risk factor for dementia: An updated review. *Australian and New Zealand Journal of Psychiatry, 35,* 776–781.

Katzman, R. (1993). Education and the prevalence of dementia and Alzheimer's disease. *Neurology, 43,* 13–20.

Kempler, D., Teng, E. L., Dick, M., Taussig, I. M., & Davis, D. S. (1998). The effects of age, education and ethnicity on verbal fluency. *Journal of the International Neuropsychological Society, 4,* 531–538.

Kleinman, S. (1990). Terror at sea: Vietnamese victims of piracy. *The American Journal of Psychoanalysis, 50,* 351–362.

Klonoff, H., McDougall, G., Clark, C., Kramer, P., & Horgan, J. (1976). The neuropsychological, psychiatric, and physical effects of prolonged and severe stress: 30 years later. *Journal of Nervous and Mental Disease, 163,* 246–252.

Leong, F., & Lau, A. (2001). Barriers to providing effective mental health services to Asian Americans. *Mental Health Services Research, 3,* 201–214.

Microsoft Encarta Online Encyclopedia. (n.d.). *Vietnam*. Retrieved September 30, 2007, from http://encarta.msn.com/text_761552648__0/Vietnam.html

Mollica, R., Caspi-Yavin, Y., Bollini, P., & Truong, T. (1992). The Harvard Trauma Questionnaire: Validating a cross-cultural instrument for measuring torture, trauma, and posttraumatic stress disorder in Indochinese refugees. *Journal of Nervous and Mental Disease, 180,* 111–116.

Mollica RF, Wyshak G, Lavelle J. (1987). The Psychosocial Impact of War Trauma and Torture on Southeast Asian Refugees. *American Journal of Psychiatry, 144,* 1567–1572.

Munoz-Sandoval, A. F., Cummins, J., Alvarado, C. G., & Ruef, M. L. (1998). *Bilingual Verbal Ability Tests*. Itasca, IL: Riverside Publishing.

Nasreddine, Z., Phillips, N., Bedirian, V., Charbonneau, S., Whitehead, V., Collin, S., … Chertkow, H. (2005). The Montreal Cognitive Assessment, MoCA: A brief screening tool for mild cognitive impairment. *Journal of the American Geriatric Society, 53,* 695–699. http://www.mocatest.org/

Nghe, L. T., Mahalik, J. R., & Lowe, S. M. (2003). Influences on Vietnamese men: Examining traditional gender roles, the refugee experience, acculturation, and racism in the United States. *Journal of Multicultural Counseling and Development, 31,* 245–261.

Ngo, D. (2007). *Attitudes toward seeking professional psychological help among Vietnamese-Americans*. Paper presentation at the World Federation for Mental Health Conference: Transcultural Mental Health in a Changing World, Minneapolis, MN.

Ngo, D., Tran, T. V., Gibbons, J. L., & Oliver, J. M. (2001). Acculturation, premigration traumatic experiences and depression among Vietnamese Americans. In N. G. Choi (Eds.), *Psychosocial aspects of the Asian American experience: Diversity within diversity* (pp. 225–242). Binghamton, NY: The Haworth Press, Inc.

Ostrosky-Solís, F. (2007). Educational effects on cognitive functions: Brain reserve, compensation, or testing bias? In B. P. Uzzell, M. Pontón, & A. Ardila (Eds.), *International handbook of cross-cultural neuropsychology* (pp. 215–225). Mahwah, NJ: Lawrence Erlbaum Associates.

Pontón, M. O., Satz, P., Herrera, L., Urrutia, C. P., Ortiz, F., Young, R., … Namerow, N. (1996). Normative data stratified by age and education for the Neuropsychological Screening Battery for Hispanics (NesSB-HIS): A standardization report. *Journal of the International Neuropsychological Society*, 2, 96–104.

Reeves, T. J., & Bennett, C. E. (2004). *We the people: Asians in the United States*. Retrieved February 26, 2009, from http://www.census.gov/prod/2004pubs/censr-17.pdf

Rosenthal, R., & Rosnow, R. L. (1991). *Essentials of behavioral research: Methods and data analysis* (2nd ed.). Boston, MA: McGraw-Hill.

Sue, S., Wagner, N., Ja, D., Margullis, C., & Lew, L. (1976). Conceptions of mental illness among Asian and White-American students. *Psychological Reports, 38*, 703–708.

Tarling, N. (2004). *Cambridge history of Southeast Asia*. Cambridge, UK: Cambridge University Press.

Taylor, K. W. (1983). *The birth of Vietnam*. Berkeley, CA: University of California Press.

Teng, E. L., Hasegawa, K., Homma, A., Imai, Y., Larson, E., Graves, A., … White L. R. (1994). The Cognitive Abilities Screening Instrument (CASI): A practical test for cross-cultural epidemiological studies of dementia. *International Psychogeriatrics, 6,* 45–58.

Tran, T. V., Ngo, D., & Sung, T. H. (2001). Caring for elderly Vietnamese Americans. In L. K. Olson (Ed.), *Age through ethnic lenses: Caring for the elderly in a multicultural society* (pp. 59–70). Lanham, MD: Rowman & Littlefield Publishers, Inc.

Uddo, M., Vasterling, J. J., Brailey, K., & Sutker, P. B. (1993). Memory and attention in combat-related posttraumatic stress disorder, PTSD. *Journal of Psychopathology and Behavioral Assessment, 15*, 43–52.

U.S. Census Bureau. (n.d.). Retrieved October 1, 2007, from http://factfinder.census.gov/servlet/DTTable?_bm=y&-geo_id=01000US&-ds_name=DEC_1990_STF1_&-_lang=en&-mt_name=DEC_1990_STF1_P007&-format=&-CONTEXT=dt (HELP

U.S. Committee for Refugees. (1984). *Vietnamese boat people: Pirates' vulnerable prey*. Washington, D.C.: American Council for Nationalities Service.

Uzzell, P. (2007). Grasping the cross-cultural reality. In B. P. Uzzell, M. Pontón, & A. Ardila (Eds.), *International handbook of cross-cultural neuropsychology* (pp. 1–22). Mahwah, NJ: Lawrence Erlbaum Associates.

Vasterling, J. J., Brailey, K., Constans, J. I., & Sutker, P. B. (1998). Attention and memory dysfunction in posttraumatic stress disorder. *Neuropsychology, 12,* 125–133.

Vasterling, J., Jenkins, R., Tope, D., & Burish, T. (1993). Cognitive distraction and relaxation training for the control of side effects due to cancer chemotherapy. *Journal of Behavioral Medicine, 16*, 65–80.

Vets With a Mission (2007). *History of Vietnam—Origin of Vietnam*. Retrieved September 30, 2007, from http://www.vwam.com/vets/history/vietnam.html

Whitmore, J. K. (1986). An outline of Vietnamese history before French conquest. *The Vietnam Forum, 8,* 1–9.

Zubenko, G. S., Zubenko, W. N., McPherson, S., Spoor, E., Marin, D. B., & Farlow, M. R., et al. (2003). A collaborative study of the emergence and clinical features of the major depressive syndrome of Alzheimer's disease. *American Journal of Psychiatry, 160,* 857–866.

12 Neuropsychology in China

Agnes S. Chan, Winnie W. Leung, and Mei-Chun Cheung

Brief description of country

China, officially known as the People's Republic of China, is located in eastern Asia. The country is bordered on the north by Mongolia, Russia, and Korea, on the south by Burma, Laos, and Vietnam, on the west by Nepal, India, and Kazakhstan, and on the east by the Pacific Ocean. With a landmass of 9.6 million square kilometers, it is the third largest country in the world, second only to Russia and Canada.

China is also the most populous country in the world, with approximately 1.3 billion people (Chinese Government, 2008). There are 56 ethnic groups residing in China. The overwhelming majority (91.6%) are Han, whereas the other 55 ethnic groups account for the remaining 8.4% of the population. A total of 54 languages are spoken in the country, with Putonghua being the official national language.

Although considered ethnically Chinese, Taiwan has been an independent territory for about 50 years, while Hong Kong and Macao have developed independently for 150 years. Hong Kong and Macao recently reunited with the Mainland in 1997 and 1999, respectively, becoming Special Administrative Regions (SARs). Despite unification, both still retain a high degree of autonomy from the Mainland in terms of political and economic systems, language, and culture. Similarly, developments in education, science, and technology also evolved differently from the Mainland. This includes the field of neuropsychology. Therefore, in the remainder of this chapter, references will be made to Hong Kong (and Macao) and Taiwan independently of Mainland China where appropriate.

Brief history of neuropsychology

China

Neuropsychology is a relatively young science in Mainland China with a history of about 20 years. The beginnings can be dated to 1987, when the Chinese Neuropsychology Association was founded and the first national neuropsychology conference was held. These two events signified the establishment of neuropsychology as an independent field of study in Mainland China. Since inception, the Chinese

Neuropsychology Association has hosted biennial national neuropsychology conferences, with about 80 participants at each meeting and about 50 presentations.

Early neuropsychological studies in Mainland China were primarily descriptive in nature and clinical driven. Aphasia and dementia, the latter including dementia of the Alzheimer's type and vascular dementia, were among the first brain disorders to be extensively researched during the 1980s. Studies examining characteristics, subtypes, deficits, diagnostic criteria, and neuropsychological profiles of these two disorders generated useful clinical knowledge and resulted in the development of assessment instruments (Gao, 2003; Wang & Wang, 2005). Since 2000, research focus has shifted from dementia to mild cognitive impairment (MCI), with the goal of early identification of dementia through ecologically valid diagnostic criteria and neuroimaging studies and laboratory tests (see Gao, 2003).

Other areas of research include amnesia, neglect, agnosia, and apraxia in adult populations (Wang & Wang, 2005), and childhood disorders such as mental retardation, developmental dyslexia (see Wang & Li, 2006), learning disorders, and attention deficit/hyperactivity disorder (see Hu & Yu, 1999). In addition, considerable efforts have also been made to adapt Western tests such as the Wechsler Adult Intelligence Scales, Wechsler Memory Tests, and the Halstead-Reitan Neuropsychological Battery for clinical use in Mainland China (see Yuan, 2000).

Neuropsychological studies conducted in Mainland China are primarily published in national journals written in Chinese. The major journals include the *Chinese Mental Health Journal*, *Chinese Journal of Clinical Psychology*, *Chinese Behavioral Medicine* (Hong, 2003), and *Chinese Journal of Neurology*. Because the journals are written in Chinese, these studies are not readily accessible to audiences outside of China. Hence, development in the field remains contained within the country and rather isolated from the rest of the world.

Hong Kong

Development of neuropsychology in Hong Kong followed a different path from the Mainland. Instead of developing from within, most of the pioneering young scholars from Hong Kong trained in the United States in the 1990s. They returned with a strong foundation in assessment, scientific methods, and brain behavioral relationships. The formation of the Hong Kong Neuropsychological Association in 1998 marked the firm establishment of the field in the territory.

Neuropsychology in Hong Kong has enjoyed rapid and fruitful development in the past 10 years in both research and clinical practice. Modern technologies such as functional magnetic resonance imaging (fMRI) and quantitative electroencephalography (qEEG) are commonly used to study attention, language, memory, and executive functioning in normal and clinical samples. In terms of clinical practice, much effort has been expended in adapting Western neuropsychological instruments for use in Hong Kong, as well as developing indigenous assessment tools that are ecologically valid for the local population.

Due to their training abroad, neuropsychologists in Hong Kong developed collegial relationships with clinicians and researchers in the United States. These relationships fostered a strong exchange of information between countries. With their easy access to the most updated knowledge, research skills, and technologies, Hong Kong neuropsychologists have spearheaded efforts to develop the field in the SAR and the Mainland. Continuous efforts are being made to organize training programs and courses in the Mainland by Hong Kong neuropsychologists, and collaborative research is also being actively forged. For example, in 2003 an international conference was held in Hong Kong with the goal of bringing Western knowledge to China. In 2004, the Chinese Board of Neuropsychology was founded with the aim of advancing both training and registration of Chinese neuropsychologists in research and clinical practice.

Taiwan

Neuropsychology is a relatively new science in Taiwan, as very few neuropsychologists are engaged in research and teaching. Most Taiwanese neuropsychologists are either clinical psychologists or behavioral neurologists involved in clinical practice. Taiwan does not have an independent neuropsychological association. The academic societies most closely related to neuropsychology are the Taiwan Association of Clinical Psychology and the Taiwan Neurological Society (Hua & Lu, 2003). Since the science of neuropsychology is still in its infancy and clinicians have not established their own identity, development in the field lags far behind the Mainland and Hong Kong.

Current practices: Who practices

Unlike the United States, where neuropsychology is a board-certified specialization, specialized training such as coursework or supervised internships are not required for clinical practice in the three Chinese societies. To redress this situation, the Chinese Board of Neuropsychology (CBN) was established in 2004 to promote professionalization in neuropsychology through the development of training standards. The board provides registration for clinicians and researchers in neuropsychology who fulfill minimal requirements in training and practical work experience. At present, the registration system is not mandatory for neuropsychological practice.

China

Mainland China has formal master's and doctoral level neuropsychological training programs that are offered by medical schools. Despite the availability of these programs, most professionals practicing neuropsychology lack adequate training. Clinicians are generally neurologists and middle-level medical professionals who practice without a solid foundation in neuropsychology. Similarly, research psychometrists frequently receive only cursory training. This practice may pose a significant threat to the validity of the testing. A more systematic and regulated manner of training is needed to ensure competency in both clinical and research settings (Yuan, 2000).

Hong Kong

Neuropsychologists are generally clinical psychologists practicing in hospital settings (Chan, 2003). Most receive training at two Hong Kong universities where modules in clinical neuropsychology are part of the clinical psychology curriculum. Neuropsychological training is also periodically offered by the Hong Kong Neuropsychological Association.

Taiwan

As mentioned previously, most practicing Taiwanese neuropsychologists are clinical psychologists belonging to the Taiwan Association of Clinical Psychology, and behavioral neurologists belonging to the Taiwan Neurological Society (Hua & Lu, 2003).

Test development

The maturation of neuropsychology in China is evidenced by a growing number of assessment instruments developed and normed on Chinese populations. During the early stage of test development, instruments were mainly translated and adapted from Western tests (Chan, Shum, & Cheung, 2003). This practice, however, is problematic due to difficulties with equivalent translations of words and concepts between Western and Eastern cultures (Tamayo, 1987). This problem is compounded given the substantive cultural and language differences of Mainland China, Hong Kong, and Taiwan, as tests in one population are not readily usable in the other two. Problems in test translation are clearly demonstrated in the adaptation of the Wechsler Intelligence Tests for adults and children. While Mainland China has developed its own Chinese version of the adult scale (WAIS-R; Dai, Gong, & Zhong, 1990; Gong, 1989), Hong Kong (WAIS-R-HK; Hong Kong Psychological Society, 1989) and Taiwan (WAIS-III; Chen & Chen, 2002) also have their own adapted versions of the test. More recently, test construction has focused on developing indigenous tests with local norms (Chan, Shum, & Cheung, 2003).

Chan, Shum, & Cheung (2003) reviewed studies on neuropsychological assessment tools in Asian regions that included Mainland China, Hong Kong, and Taiwan over the past 20 years (Japan, India, Korea, Singapore, and Thailand were also included). The researchers found the greatest number of instruments was used for dementia screening, followed by tests of memory and learning, language, and executive functions. Aside from dementia, other common clinical populations receiving neuropsychological testing include temporal lobe damage, stroke, and schizophrenia. The number of adapted tests to developed tests was 30:6. There was also a higher percentage of tests for older adults (95%) than for other age groups.

Chan, Shum, & Cheung (2003) also examined the clinical validity of each Asian-developed neuropsychological test by analyzing validation studies based upon the following five criteria: (1) proper documentation of test development procedures, (2) sound design of validation studies, (3) the availability of normative data based upon a reasonable sample, (4) the use of translation and back-translation for adaptation of

Western tests, and (5) cross-cultural comparisons between Western and local norms. The authors reported that only 8 of the 36 instruments met these stringent criteria for test validity. Three were indigenous tests and five were adaptations of Western tests. Of the latter, two were from Mainland China and three from Hong Kong (the other three tests came from Korea and Japan). The following are brief descriptions of the clinically valid Chinese tests (see Table 12.1).

Adaptation of Western tests

The *Chinese version of the Category Fluency Test (CCFT)* was developed in Hong Kong by Chan and Poon (1999) and uses the categories of animals and transportation. Normative data were based on 316 Hong Kong Chinese aged 7 to 95. Test scores are consistent with those of Western populations. Another set of normative data is provided by Chiu et al. (1997) on older adults in Hong Kong (see Chan, Shum, & Cheung, 2003).

The *Chinese version of the Mattis Dementia Rating Scale (CDRS)* (Chan, Choi, Chiu, & Lam, 2003; Chan, Poon, Choi, & Cheung, 2001) was developed in Hong Kong. It was adapted from the original Mattis Dementia Rating Scale (Mattis, 1988) with cultural modification on four items. Normative data were based on 83 healthy older adults and 40 adults with Alzheimer's disease. A cutoff score of 112 yielded a sensitivity of 80.0% and specificity of 91.6%. A comparison of Hong Kong and American older adults reported differences in the pattern of subscale scores and overall lower mean DRS scores in the Hong Kong sample (see Chan, Shum, & Cheung, 2003).

The *Chinese Mini-Mental State Examination (CMMS)* (Katzman et al., 1988) is an adaptation of the Mini-Mental State Examination (MMSE) (Folstein, Folstein, & McHugh, 1975) that was developed in Mainland China. Sensitivity and specificity for diagnosing dementia in a sample of Shanghai adults were 69.5% and 90.2%, respectively. Cross-cultural comparisons with samples of older Finnish and U.S. adults demonstrated similar predictive validity when scores were corrected for education (see Chan, Shum, & Cheung, 2003). A Cantonese version of the MMSE was later developed in Hong Kong with a recommended cutoff score of 19 as an indication for further evaluation of the possibility of dementia (Chiu, Lee, Chung, & Kwong, 1994).

Indigenous test development

The *Hong Kong List Learning Test (HKLLT)* (Chan, 2006) is a verbal learning test developed in Hong Kong for assessing memory functions. Normative data were based on 394 Hong Kong Chinese aged 6 to 95. The test has also been validated on clinical populations including schizophrenia (Chan et al., 2000), temporal lobe damage due to necrosis (Cheung, Chan, Law, Chan, & Tse, 2000, 2003; Cheung & Chan, 2003) or epilepsy (Cheung, Chan, Chan, & Lam, 2006; Cheung, Chan, Chan, Lam, & Lam, 2006), and patients with Alzheimer's disease (Au, Chan, & Chiu, 2003). The HKLLT differs from some common Western list learning tests such as the California Verbal Learning Test (CVLT; Delis, Kramer, Kaplan, & Ober, 1987) and the Rey Auditory Verbal Learning Test (RAVLT; Rey, 1964; see Lezak, Howeison, & Loring, 2004) in

Table 12.1 Neuropsychological assessment tools adapted or developed in Mainland China, Hong Kong, and Taiwan in the past 20 years

Mainland China		*Hong Kong*	*Taiwan*
Alzheimer's Disease Assessment Scale (Chinese version)	Hiscock's Forced-Choice Digit Memory Test	Blessed-Roth Dementia Scale	Mini-Mental Status Examination
Aphasia Test	Halstead-Reitan Neuropsychological Test Battery (HRNB) (Chinese revision)	Cantonese Aphasia Test Battery	Neuropsychiatric Inventory Scale (Chinese version)
Auditory Verbal Memory Test	Language Ability Test	Category Fluency Test (Chinese version)	Random Chinese Word Cancellation Test
Bender Visual Motor Gestalt Test	Luria-Nebraska Neuropsychological Battery	Chinese Anomalous Sentence Test	
Benton Line Orientation Test	Mini-Mental Status Examination	Chinese version of Alzheimer's Disease Behavioral Pathology Rating Scale	
Blessed-Roth's Alzheimer's Disease Scale	Chinese MMSE	Chinese version of Mattis Dementia Rating Scale	
Benton Visual Retention Test	Revised Chinese edition of the HRNB for younger children	Clock Drawing Test	
Chinese Neurobehavioral Evaluation 2	Senile Cognitive Function Scale	Color Trails Test	
Chinese Standard Aphasia Scale	Sorting Test	Hong Kong List Learning Test	
Chinese Version Expansive Scale of Dementia	The Clinical Memory Test	Neuropsychiatric Inventory (Chinese version)	
Cognitive Abilities Screening Instrument 2.0	Trail Making Test	Olfactory Identification Test	
Cognitive Abilities Screening Instrument (for cross-cultural studies)	Verbal and Visuospatial Speed of Processing and Working Memory	Trail Making Test	
Computer Neurobehavioral Test System	Visual Space Test		
Digit Symbol	Wechsler Adult Intelligence Scale–Revised (WAIS-R)		
Finger Tapping Test	Wisconsin Card Sorting Test (WCST)		
Grooved Pegboard	Western Aphasia Battery		
Handed Test	Wechsler Memory Scale (WMS)		

Source: Adapted from Chan, A. S., et al., *Psychological Assessment, 15*, 261, 2003.

that both random and blocked lists are included to discriminate between frontal and temporal forms of memory problems (Chan, 2006).

The *Clinical Memory Test (CMT)* (Xu & Wu, 1986) was developed for assessing memory in Mainland China. The test has two alternate forms and consists of five subtests, including paired-associate learning, directed memory, picture recall, recognition of meaningless figures, and recall of portraits and their characteristics. Construct validity was established by differential test performances between patients with unilateral brain damage.

The remaining Asian-developed neuropsychology tests only partially fulfilled the validity criteria. For example, a number of Chinese-adapted tests, such as the Chinese version of the Alzheimer's Disease Behavioral Pathology Rating Scale from Hong Kong (Lam, Tang, Leung, & Chiu, 2001) and the Chinese revision of the Halstead-Reitan Neuropsychological Test Battery for Adults from Mainland China (Gong, 1986), fulfilled all criteria except for cross-cultural comparison. Others, such as the Cantonese version of the Western Aphasia Battery from Hong Kong (Yiu, 1992), the Olfactory Identification Test from Hong Kong (Chan, Tam, Murphy, Chiu, & Lam, 2002), and the Computerized Neurobehavioral Test System from China (Li et al., 2000), lacked an adequate sample.

Overview of literature: Children

Learning disorders

According to the *Diagnostic and Statistical Manual of Mental Disorders*, fourth edition (DSM-IV; American Psychiatric Association, 2000), learning disorders (LDs) are diagnosed when an individual's achievement on standardized tests in reading, mathematics, or written expression is substantially below that expected for age, schooling, and level of intelligence. LD in the three Chinese societies, however, is not as clearly defined.

Mainland China

There is no standard definition of LD in the Mainland. Researchers use different terms to describe LD, such as "poor learning," "poor academic achievement," "learning difficulties," and "learning disabilities" (see Chen & Xiang, 2005). Practitioners vary in their basis for diagnosis, with some using academic performance, some using teacher ratings, some using adapted and developed assessment scales, and some using cognitive impairments such as reading, mathematics, writing, memory, and cognition (see Chen & Xian, 2005). Prevalence rates of LD in Mainland China range from 6.5% to 17.8% (Jing & Yu, 1995; Cheng, Cui, & Wu, 1999; Yao & Wu, 2003). About 80% of children diagnosed with a LD are reported to have dyslexia (see Dou, 2003). Interestingly, studies reported a significantly lower prevalence rate of dyslexia in Chinese children than in Western children and suggested that differences are due to the Chinese logographic writing system, which is qualitatively different from the alphabetic system of Western languages (Tzeng, 2007).

Hong Kong

LD, known as specific learning disabilities (SpLDs) in Hong Kong, was defined in 2005 as "a group of disorders manifested as significant difficulties in the acquisition and use of listening, speaking, reading, writing or mathematical abilities, despite access to conventional teaching. These disorders are intrinsic to the individual and neurobiological in origin, with onset in childhood and extending beyond it" (Hong Kong Society of Child Neurology and Developmental Pediatrics, 2005, p. 2). According to the territory's government statistics, the incidence of SpLD in primary school children in Hong Kong from 2002 to 2005 ranged between 0.22% and 0.43% (Office of the Ombudsman, 2007). The assessment of SpLD in Hong Kong is based on the locally developed Test of Specific Learning Disabilities, for primary (Ho, Chan, Tsang, & Lee, 2000) and secondary (Chan, Ho, Tsang, Lee, & Chung, 2007) school children.

As with the Mainland, dyslexia (reading disorder) is the most highly documented and studied SpLD in Hong Kong. Hong Kong adopts the definition proposed by the International Dyslexia Association of the National Institutes of Health (NIH) in the United States (see Mak, Lam, Ho, & Wong, 2006). While there are no population-based statistics on dyslexia, local research showed that the prevalence ranges from 9.7% to 12.6% (Chan, Ho, et al., 2007), with a ratio of boys to girls at about 2.8 to 1, according to the Department of Health statistics.

Recent studies have reported a differential pattern of cognitive deficits in dyslexic Chinese children in comparison with children from Western countries. The major impairments of Hong Kong Chinese children with dyslexia were naming speed, orthographic awareness (Chan, Ho, Tsang, Lee, & Chung, 2006, 2007), and morphological awareness (Shu, McBride-Chang, Wu, & Liu, 2006). By contrast, children in Western countries were most prominently impaired in phonological awareness (Ziegler & Goswami, 2005). It is believed that these discrepant findings are due to differences in the language systems. The Chinese writing system is more logographic, thus relying heavily on visual processing, while English and other alphabetic written languages are more phonological, thereby making sound identification salient for reading (Chan, Ho, et al., 2006, 2007; Ziegler & Goswami, 2005).

Taiwan

LD is a disputable term in Taiwan, with definitions changing from time to time. According to the National Taiwan Normal University (NTNU, 2007), there are currently three commonly used definitions of LD. The most popular definition of LD is "significant disorders in attention, memory, comprehension, reasoning, expression, perception, or perceptual-motor coordination caused by neuropsychological dysfunctions which results in significant difficulties on listening, speaking, reading, writing, and calculating. The disability is neither directly caused by disability factors such as sensory, intellectual, emotional impairments, nor by environmental factors such as lacking of cultural stimuli and inadequate instruction" (see Tzeng, 2007, p. 171). Diagnostic criteria include (1) normal or above normal intelligence, (2) significant intraindividual competence discrepancy, and (3) significant difficulties in any one of the following abilities: attention, memory, listening comprehension, oral expression, basic reading skills, reading comprehension, handwriting, mathematical calculation, reasoning, or perceptual-motor coordination (see Tzeng, 2007). According to the Ministry of Education statistics (2006), the prevalence of LD in school children is less than 1.0%, which is much lower than the 5.5% reported in the United States (Hallahan, Lloyd, Kauffman, Weiss, & Martinez, 2005). It is believed that this low rate is due to either Chinese parents' reluctance to label their children or misconceptions about LD (Tzeng, 2007). LDs are identified with both adapted Western tests, such as Chinese versions of the Wechsler Intelligence Scale for Children and the Peabody Picture Vocabulary Test, and locally developed tools that consider China's orthographic writing system (see Tzeng, 2007).

Mental retardation

Similar to LD, the three Chinese societies differ in their definition of mental retardation (MR). The State Department of Mainland China adopts the AAMR international definition (Luckasson et al., 2002; see Xu, Wang, Xiang, & Hu, 2005). The Taiwan definition is based on the 1998 *Principles and Criteria of Diagnosis for Children With Disabilities and Giftedness*, which defines MR using a functional point of view as "occurring during developmental ages, developmental delays in general intelligence leading to difficulties in adaptive behaviors" (NTNU, 2007). Under this definition, there are five IQ-based categories: borderline (IQ 68–83), mild (52–67), moderate (36–51), severe (20–35), and profound (below 20). Hong Kong adopts the DSM-IV four-tier classification of mild (IQ 50–69), moderate (35–49), severe (20–34), and profound (below 20). Reported prevalences of MR in the three societies are 2% in children under 14 in China (Sonnander & Claesson, 1997), 0.9% to 1.3% in Hong Kong (Census & Statistics Department, 2009), and 0.88% in Taiwan (NTNU, 2007).

Autism spectrum disorder (ASD)

Recent statistics from the National Autism Association (2007) in the United States reported a prevalence rate of ASD at 1 in 150 children. There has been an increasing trend in the prevalence of ASD worldwide (Bertrand et al., 2001; Chakrabarti & Fombonne, 2001), likely as a result of changes in diagnostic criteria (Baird, Cass, & Slonims, 2003; Wing & Potter, 2002). The figures for the three Chinese societies appear to be lower. A recent study reported a prevalence rate of 1.10 cases per 1000 for children aged 2 to 6 in China (Zhang & Ji, 2005). While there is no prevalence data for Hong Kong (Wong & Hui, 2007), statistics at the Child Assessment Centers in Hong Kong reported 658 diagnoses in 2004 (Mak et al., 2006). A search in the literature did not turn up any information on prevalence of ASD in Taiwan.

Hong Kong adopts the ICD-10 or the DSM-IV criteria in diagnosing ASD (Mak et al., 2006), supplemented by the use of common observational scales translated from the United States, including the Childhood Autism Rating Scale (CARS; Schopler, Reichler, & Renner, 1986), ADOS (Lord et al., 1989), and ADI-R (Le Couteur et al., 1989). Similar to other parts of the world, an increasing trend of ASD has been observed in Hong Kong, where the number of children with ASD diagnosed at the Child Assessment Centers in Hong Kong has increased from 198 cases in 1995 to 658 in 2004 (Mak et al., 2006). ASD has traditionally been diagnosed based on these diagnostic criteria, but there have been recent efforts to develop objective measures of ASD in Hong Kong. Chan and colleagues (Chan & Leung, 2006; Chan, Sze, & Cheung, 2007) have studied the applicability of using quantitative EEG in the differentiation of ASD from normal children. Their results suggested that children with ASD have qEEG profiles that are significantly different from those of normal children, particularly in the alpha and delta bands (Chan, Sze, et al., 2007). Further research is being conducted in this area. In addition, their studies on language deficits of ASD children have suggested that tests of expressive language are more sensitive than those of comprehension in differentiating Chinese children with autism from normal age-matched children (Chan, Cheung, Leung, Cheung, & Cheung, 2005).

Overview of the literature: Adults

Head injury

Similar to most industrialized countries, the leading cause of traumatic brain injuries in the three Chinese societies is traffic-related events, which account for approximately 54.4% of all head injuries in Mainland China (see Hao, Zhao, & Guo, 1988), over 50% of injuries in Hong Kong (Hsiang et al., 1996), and 69.4% in Taiwan. Interestingly, the vehicles most commonly involved in traffic accidents are bicycles in Mainland China and Hong Kong, and motorcycles in Taiwan. While both Taiwan and Hong Kong use the Glasgow Coma Scale (Teasdale & Jennet, 1974) to classify the severity level of a brain injury, Mainland China developed its own classification system (see Duan, 1989).

Temporal lobe damage

Exciting research on language and memory functions is being conducted in China on persons sustaining damage to the temporal lobes, which adds to our understanding of brain–behavior relationships. It is well known that populations in southern China have a high rate of nasopharyngeal carcinoma (NPC). Increased morbidity for NPC is assumed to result from the unique diet of these people. Persons with NPC are commonly treated with radiation therapy, which frequently damages the temporal lobes. These persons typically demonstrate memory impairments that are proportional to lesion volume (Cheung et al., 2000, 2003). An interesting subgroup of radiation-treated NPC patients are those with intact hippocampi but temporal damage to lateral areas. Studies indicate that bilateral damage of the lateral temporal lobes in this population is associated with both verbal and visual memory impairments (Chan et al., 2003; Cheung & Chan, 2003).

Another interesting finding comes from fMRI studies in patients with temporal lobe epilepsy. Researchers found that memory deficits were associated with duration of illness and were limited to the side of seizure, but were also observed in the contralateral hemisphere (Cheung et al., 2006b).

Language

Studies on the language lateralization in Chinese patients with temporal lobe damage have provided interesting findings concerning cross-cultural issues in language mediation by the brain (Cheung et al., 2006a; Cheung, Cheung, & Chan, 2004). While it has been well established in Western studies that language is mediated by the left hemisphere, studies in Hong Kong have provided evidence indicating that the neural basis of processing Chinese language is different from that for English (Cheung et al., 2006a). Patients with temporal lobe epilepsy (TLE) in Hong Kong, who are Chinese-English bilinguals (which makes up the great majority of the Hong Kong population), demonstrate the usual left lateralization in reading English words, but utilize bi-hemispheric activation in reading Chinese characters. In addition, when reading English words, left-TLE patients were more likely than right-TLE patients to demonstrate bilateral activation. This difference is interpreted as an example of plasticity where the right hemisphere takes up some of the language mediation function of the left hemisphere. By contrast, when reading Chinese words, both left- and right-TLE patients were as likely to demonstrate bilateral activation, suggesting that Chinese is mediated by both hemispheres. In another study (Cheung et al., 2004), Chinese patients with temporal lobe damage in the left and right hemispheres demonstrated similar levels of naming impairments. These studies have provided important information for clinicians when assessing the language functions of Chinese patients and support conceptualization of the hemispheres as mediating specific processes versus complex skills (Mesulam, 2000).

Dementia

Dementia studies in China also provide contrasts to findings in the West with both epidemiological and testing differences. For example, studies in the West typically report that AD is the most common cause of dementia. By contrast, earlier studies from Mainland China and Taiwan reported a higher incidence of vascular dementia (VD) versus AD (see review by Chiu & Zhang, 2000). More recent studies, however, indicate a higher prevalence of AD than VD in Mainland China (Liu et al., 1995; Zhou et al., 2006). Similar findings have been shown in Hong Kong, where AD accounts for as much as 80% of dementia cases (Lam, 2004).

In spite of its current predominance, the prevalence rates of AD have been reported to be lower in Chinese societies than the West (Chiu et al., 1998; Liu et al., 1995; Zhou et al., 2006). A recent study conducted in the United States (Plassman et al., 2007) reported a prevalence of dementia among individuals aged 71 and older at 13.9% with 9.7% being dementia of the Alzheimer's type (AD). Dementia prevalence increases with age, from 5.0% of those aged 71–79 years to 37.4% of those aged 90 and older. By contrast, adjusted prevalence rates of dementia in rural Mainland China were 0.33% for age group 50–54, 0.89% for 55–64, 3.43% for 65–74, and

8.19% for 75 and above (Zhou et al., 2006). Dementia prevalence rates in Hong Kong were 1.7% for age 70–74, 4.7% for 75–79, 10.7% for 80–84, 18.8% for 85–89, and 25.8% for 90 and older (Chiu et al., 1998). The age-specific prevalence for dementia in Taiwan was 0.21% for age 60–69, 2.67% for 70–79, and 5.98% for 80–88 (Liu et al., 1995). These rates are much lower than those reported in the West, with Taiwan having the lowest and Hong Kong the highest among the three societies.

Diagnosis of dementia in these Chinese societies is usually based on Western instruments such as the Mini-Mental State Examination (MMSE; Folstein et al., 1975), Clock Drawing Test (Critchley, 1953), Dementia Rating Scale (DRS; Mattis, 1988), and the Blessed Dementia Scale (Blessed, Tomlinson, & Roth, 1968). Some of these scales have been used in Chinese populations (Lam, Chiu, Ng, & Chan, 1998; Chan et al., 2001, 2003; Chiu et al., 1994), and Chinese versions developed, such as the CDS (Lam et al., 1997), CMMSE (Chiu et al., 1994; Katzman et al., 1988), and CDRS (Chan et al., 2003), have local norms.

Studies examining performance patterns on dementia tests have reported differences between elderly in China and the United States. On the Mattis Dementia Rating Scale (Mattis, 1988), Chan and colleagues (Chan, Choi, & Salmon, 2001) found that Hong Kong elderly scored significantly higher than elderly from the United States on the Construction subscale, while U.S. elderly scored higher on the Initiation/Perseveration and Memory subscales. No differences were found in total score. The same study also found stronger educational effects on the DRS score for the Hong Kong sample.

These findings highlight the important issue of cultural effects on test performance. For example, it is highly likely that stronger educational effects for elderly Chinese are due to their generally lower educational level, which was affected by political reasons. Similarly, China's logographic written language may have resulted in stronger construction skills in comparison with Western populations. Differences in test performance underscore that caution is needed when adapting neuropsychological tests from the West.

Although clinical neuropsychology has enjoyed a brief history in China, this chapter shows that the impressive growth of the field during the short period of a little more than 10 years has been truly remarkable.

References

American Psychiatric Association. (2000). *Diagnostic and statistical manual of mental disorders* (4th ed., text rev.). Washington, DC: Author.

Au, A., Chan, A. S., & Chiu, H. (2003). Verbal learning in Alzheimer's dementia. *Journal of the International Neuropsychological Society, 9*, 363–375.

Baird, G., Cass, H., & Slonims, V. (2003). Diagnosis of autism. *British Medical Journal, 327*, 488–493.

Bertrand, J., Mars, A., Boyle, C., Bove, F., Yeargin-Allsopp, M., & Decoufle, P. (2001). Prevalence of autism in a United States population: The Brick Township, New Jersey, investigation. *Pediatrics, 108,* 1155–1161.

Blessed, G., Tomlinson, B. E., & Roth, M. (1968). The association between quantitative measures of dementia and of senile change in the cerebral grey matter of elderly subjects. *British Journal of Psychiatry, 114*, 797–811.

Census and Statistics Department, Hong Kong Government (2009). Hong Kong monthly digest of statistics. Feature articles: Persons with disabilities and chronic diseases in Hong Kong. Government Printer: Author.

Chakrabarti, S., & Fombonne, E. (2001). Pervasive developmental disorders in preschool children. *Journal of the American Medical Association, 285*, 3093–3099.

Chan, A. (2003, December). *Recent development of neuropsychology in Hong Kong*. Paper presented at the International Conference on Neuropsychology, Hong Kong.

Chan, A. S. (2006). *Hong Kong List Learning Test* (2nd ed.). Hong Kong: Department of Psychology and Clinical Psychology Centre, Chinese University of Hong Kong.

Chan, A. S., Cheung, J., Leung, W. W. M., Cheung, R., & Cheung, M. (2005). Verbal expression and comprehension deficits in young children with autism. *Focus on Autism and other Developmental Disorders, 20*(2), 117–124.

Chan, A., Choi, A., Chiu, H., & Lam, L. (2003a). Clinical validity of the Chinese version of Mattis Dementia Rating Scale in differentiating dementia of Alzheimer's type in Hong Kong. *Journal of the International Neuropsychological Society, 9*, 45–55.

Chan, A. S., Choi, M., & Salmon, D. P. (2001). The effects of age, education, and gender on the Mattis Dementia Rating Scale performance of elderly Chinese and American individuals. *Journal of Gerontology, 56*, 356–363.

Chan, A. S., Kwok, I. C., Chiu, H., Lam, L., Pang, A., & Chow, L. (2000). Memory and organizational strategies in chronic and acute schizophrenic patients. *Schizophrenia Research, 41*, 431–445.

Chan, A. S., & Leung, W. W. M. (2006). Differentiating autistic children with quantitative encephalography: A three-month longitudinal study. *Journal of Child Neurology, 21*(5), 391–399.

Chan, A. S., & Poon, M. W. (1999). Performance of 7- to 95-year-old individuals in a Chinese version of the category fluency test. *Journal of the International Neuropsychof logical Society, 5*, 525–533.

Chan, A. S., Poon, M. W., Choi, A., & Cheung, M. C. (2001). *Dementia Rating Scale* [in Chinese]. Hong Kong: Chinese University of Hong Kong.

Chan, A. S., Shum, D., & Cheung, R. W. Y. (2003b). Recent development of cognitive and neuropsychological assessment in Asian countries. *Psychological Assessment, 15*, 257–267.

Chan, A. S., Sze, S. L., & Cheung, M. (2007). Quantitative electroencephalographic profiles for children with autistic spectrum disorder. *Neuropsychology, 21*, 74–81.

Chan, A. S., Tam, J., Murphy, C., Chiu, H., & Lam, L. (2002). Utility of Olfactory Identification Test for diagnosing Chinese patients with Alzheimer's disease. *Journal of Clinical and Experimental Neuropsychology, 24*, 251–259.

Chan, D. W., Ho, C. S. H., Tsang, S. M., Lee, S. H., & Chung, K. K. H. (2006). Exploring the reading–writing connection in Chinese children with dyslexia in Hong Kong. *Reading and Writing, 19*, 543–561.

Chan, D. W., Ho, C. S. H., Tsang, S. M., Lee, S. H., & Chung, K. K. H. (2007). Prevalence, gender ratio and gender differences in reading-related cognitive abilities among Chinese children with dyslexia in Hong Kong. *Educational Studies, 33*, 249–265.

Chen, H., & Xiang, W. (2005). Discussions and suppositions on the issues of learning disability researches in China [in Chinese]. *Journal of Mianyang Normal University, 24*, 75–79.

Chen, Y. H., & Chen, X. Y. (2002). *Wechsler Adult Intelligence Scale-III (Chinese)* [in Chinese]. Taipei, Taiwan: Chinese Behavioral Science Corporation.

Cheng, Y., Cui, Y., & Wu, H. (1999). Psychological characteristics of learning disabled children [in Chinese]. *Chinese Journal of Mental Health, 13*, 215–217.

Cheung, M. C., & Chan, A. S. (2003). Memory impairment in humans after bilateral damage to lateral temporal neocortex. *NeuroReport, 14*, 371–374.

Cheung, M. C., Chan, A. S., Chan, Y. L., & Lam, J. M. K. (2006a). Language lateralization of Chinese-English bilingual patients with temporal lobe epilepsy: A functional MRI study. *Neuropsychology, 20*, 589–597.

Cheung, M. C., Chan, A. S., Chan, Y. L., Lam, J. M. K., & Lam, W. (2006b). Effects of illness duration on memory processing of patients with temporal lobe epilepsy. *Epilepsia, 47*, 1320–1328.

Cheung, M. C., Chan, A. S., Law, S. C., Chan, J. H., & Tse, V. K. (2000). Cognitive function of patients with nasopharyngeal carcinoma with and without temporal lobe radionecrosis. *Archives of Neurology, 57*, 1347–1352.

Cheung, M. C., Chan, A. S., Law, S. C., Chan, J. H., & Tse, V. K. (2003). Impact of radionecrosis on cognitive dysfunction in patients after radiotherapy for nasopharyngeal carcinoma. *Cancer, 97*, 2019–2026.

Cheung, R. W., Cheung, M. C., & Chan, A. S. (2004). Confrontation naming in Chinese patients with left, right or bilateral brain damage. *Journal of the International Neuropsychological Society, 10*, 46–53.

Chinese Government. (2008). *China: Quick facts*. Retrieved May 27, 2008, from the official Chinese Government Web site: http://www.china.org.cn/e-changshi/index.htm on

Chiu, H. F. K., Lam, L. C. W., Chi, I., Leung, T., Li, S. W., Law, W. T., … Lau, J. (1998). Prevalence of dementia in Chinese elderly in Hong Kong. *Neurology, 50*, 1002–1009.

Chiu, H. F. K., Lee, H. C., Chung, W. S., & Kwong, P. K. (1994). Reliability and validity of the Cantonese version of Mini-Mential State Examination—A preliminary study. *Journal of Hong Kong College of Psychiatrists, 4* (Suppl. 2), 25–28.

Chiu, H. F. K., & Zhang, M. (2000). Dementia research in China. *International Journal of Geriatric Psychiatry, 15*, 947–953.

Chiu, W. T., Yeh, K. H., Li, Y. C., Gan, Y. H., Chen, H. Y., & Hung, C. C. (1997). Traumatic brain injury registry in Taiwan. *Neurology Research, 19*, 261–264.

Critchley, M. (1953). *The parietal lobes*. New York, NY: Hafner.

Dai, X. Y., Gong, Y. X., & Zhong, L. P. (1990). Factor analysis of the Mainland Chinese version of the Wechsler Adult Intelligence Scale. *Psychological Assessment, 2*(1), 31–34.

Delis, D. C., Kramer, J. H., Kaplan, E., & Ober, B. A. (1987). *California Verbal Learning Test*. New York, NY: Psychological Corporation.

Dou, B. (2003). Brief analysis of the impediment in study [in Chinese]. *Journal of Luoyang University, 18*, 117–119.

Duan, X. (1989). International and Chinese classification systems of severity of traumatic brain injury [in Chinese]. *Chinese Journal of Neurosurgery, 5*, 71–72.

Folstein, M. F., Folstein, S. E., & McHugh, P. R. (1975). Mini-Mental State: A practical method for grading the cognitive state of patients for the clinician. *Journal of Psychiatric Research, 12*, 189–198.

Gao, X. (2003). Review of neuropsychology in China [in Chinese]. *Journal of Postgraduates of Medicine, 26*, 1–3.

Gong, Y. X. (1986). The Chinese revision of the Halstead-Reitan Neuropsychological Test Battery for Adults [in Chinese]. *Acta Psychologica Sinica, 18*, 433–442.

Gong, Y. X. (1989). *Manual for the Wechsler Adult Intelligence Scale: Revised in China* [in Chinese]. Changsha, Hunan, China: Hunan Medical University.

Hallahan, D. P., Lloyd, J. W., Kauffman, J. M., Weiss, M., & Martinez, E. A (2005). *Learning disabilities: Foundations, characteristics, and effective teaching (3rd ed.)*. Boston, Massachusetts: Allyn & Bacon.

Hao, W., Zhao, M., & Guo, Z. (1988). Important issues in examining the causes of death from traumatic brain injury [in Chinese]. *Chinese Emergency Medicine, 2*, 9–12.

Ho, C. S. H., Chan, D. W. O., Tsang, S. M., & Lee, S. H. (2000). *The Hong Kong Test of Specific Learning Difficulties in Reading and Writing*. Hong Kong: Hong Kong Specific Learning Difficulties Research Team.

Hong Kong Psychological Society. (1989). *Wechsler Adult Intelligence Scales–Hong Kong* (rev. ed.). Hong Kong: Author.

Hong Kong Society of Child Neurology and Developmental Pediatrics. (2005, July). *Specific learning disabilities and dyslexia in Hong Kong: Position paper on future directions*. Forum on Specific Learning Disabilities of the Hong Kong Society of Child Neurology and Developmental Pediatrics, Hong Kong.

Hong, Z. (2003, December). *Brief history of Chinese neuropsychology*. Paper presented at the International Conference on Neuropsychology, Hong Kong.

Hsiang, J. N. K., Cheung, T. K. W., Goh, K. Y. C., Lam, J. M. K., Zhu, X., & Poon, W. S. (1996). Features of head injury at Prince of Wales Hospital, Hong Kong, from 1989 to 1993. *Hong Kong Medical Journal, 2*, 141–145.

Hu, Y., & Yu, J. (1999). Research on children with attention deficit/hyperactivity disorder [in Chinese]. *International Social Medicine, 16*, 62–66.

Hua, M. S., & Lu, L. H. J. (2003, December). *Neuropsychology in Taiwan: The present and the future*. Paper presented at the International Conference on Neuropsychology, Hong Kong.

Jing, J., & Yu, M. (1995). Revision of a childhood scale of learning disability and its use on primary students [in Chinese]. *Psychological Development and Education, 3*, 65.

Katzman, R., Zhang, M. Y., Qu, O. Y., Want, Z. Y., Liu W. T., Yu, E., et al. (1988). A Chinese version of the Mini-Mental State Examination: Impact of illiteracy in a Shanghai dementia survey. *Journal of Clinical Epidemiology, 10*, 971–978.

Lam, L. C. W., Chiu, H. F. K., Li, S. W., Chan, W. F., Chan, C. K. Y., Wong, M., & Ng, K. O. (1997). Screening for dementia: A preliminary study on the validity of the Chinese version of the Blessed-Roth Dementia Scale. *International Psychogeriatrics, 9*, 39–46.

Lam, L. C. W., Chiu, H. F. K., Ng, K. O., & Chan, C. (1998). Clock-face drawing, reading and setting tests in the screening of dementia in Chinese elderly adults. *Journal of Gerontology: Psychological Sciences, 53*, 353–357.

Lam, L. C. W., Tang, W. K., Leung, V., & Chiu, H. F. K. (2001). Behavioral profile of Alzheimer's disease in Chinese elderly: A validation study of the Chinese version of the Alzheimer's Disease Behavioral Pathology Rating Scale. *International Journal of Geriatric Psychology, 16*, 368–373.

Lam, T. C. P. (2004, June). Update on dementia. *HKMA CME Bulletin*, 1–5.

Le Couteur, A., Rutter, M., Lord, C., Rios, P., Robertson, S., Holdgrafer, M., et al. (1989). Autism Diagnostic Interview: A standardized investigator-based instrument. *Journal of Autism and Developmental Disorders, 19*, 363–387.

Lezak, M. D., Howieson, D. B., & Loring, D. W. (2004). *Neuropsychologicla assessment* (4th ed.). New York, NY: Oxford University Press.

Li, X., Wu, X., Han, L., Wang, J., Want, T., Zhuang, Y., et al. (2000). A computerized neurobehavioral test system [in Chinese]. *Chinese Mental Health Journal, 14*, 309–311.

Liu, H., Lin, K., Teng, E. L., Wang, S., Fuh, J., Guo, N., … Chiang, B. N. (1995). Prevalence and subtypes of dementia in Taiwan: A community survey of 5297 individuals. *Journal of the American Geriatrics Society, 43*, 144–149.

Lord, C., Rutter, M., Goode, S., Heemsbergen, J., Jordan, H., Mawhood, L., et al. (1989). Autism diagnostic observation schedule: A standardized observation of communicative and social behavior. *Journal of Autism and Developmental Disorders, 19*, 182–212.

Luckasson, R., Borthwick-Duffy, S., Buntinx, W. H. E., Coulter, D. L., Craig, E. M., Reeve, A., … Tasse, M. (2002). *Mental retardation: Definition, classification, and systems of supports*. Washington, DC: American Association on Mental Retardation.

Mak, R. H. L., Lam, C. C. C., Ho, C. C. Y., & Wong, M. M. Y. (2006). *A primer in common developmental disabilities: Experience a Child Assessment Service, Hong Kong*. Hong Kong: Child Assessment Service, Department of Health.

Mattis, S. (1988). *Dementia Rating Scale professional manual*. Odessa, FL: Psychological Assessment Resources.

Mesulam, M. (2000). *Principles of behavioral and cognitive neurology* (2nd ed.). New York, NY: Oxford University Press.

Ministry of Education. (2006). *Annual statistics of special education in 2005* [in Chinese]. Taipei, China: Author.

National Autism Association. (2007). Retrieved October 31, 2007, from the NAA Web site: http://www.nationalautismassociation.org/definitions.php)

National Taiwan Normal University. (2007). *Learning disabilities*. Retrieved September 26, 2007, from http://www.spc.ntnu.edu.tw/english/index.htm

Office of the Ombudsman, Hong Kong. (2007). *Direct investigation on assessment of children with specific learning difficulties by the Education and Manpower Bureau and Department of Health* (Issue 6 of Reporting Year 2006/2007). Hong Kong: Author.

Plassman, B. L., Langa, K. M., Fisher, G. G., Heeringa, S. G., Weir, D. R., Ofstedal, M. B., et al. (2007). Prevalence of dementia in the United States: The aging, demographics, and memory study. *Neuroepidemiology, 29*, 125–132.

Rey, A. (1964). *L'examen clinique en psychologie*. Paris: Presses Universitaires de France.

Schopler, E., Reichler, R. J., & Renner, B. R. (1986). *The Childhood Autism Rating Scale (CARS)*. New York, NY: Irvington.

Shu, H., McBride-Chang, C., Wu, S., & Liu, H. (2006). Understanding Chinese developmental dyslexia: Morphological awareness as a core cognitive construct. *Journal of Educational Psychology, 98*, 122–133.

Sonnander, K., & Claesson M. (1997). Classification, prevalence, prevention and rehabilitation of intellectual disability: An overview of research in the People's Republic of China. *Journal of Intellectual Disability Research, 41*(2), 180–192.

Tamayo, J. M. (1987). Frequency of use as a measure of word difficulty in bilingual vocabulary test construction and translation. *Educational and Psychological Measurement, 47*, 893–902.

Teasdale, G. M., & Jennett, B. (1974). Assessment of coma and impaired consciousness: A practical scale. *Lancet, 2*, 81–84.

Tzeng, S.-J. (2007). Learning disabilities in Taiwan: A case of cultural constraints on the education of students with disabilities. *Learning Disabilities Research & Practice, 22*, 170–175.

Wang, H., & Li, X. (2006). Reason and essence of developmental dyslexia [in Chinese]. *Chinese Journal of Clinical Rehabilitation, 10*, 138–140.

Wang, S., & Wang, Y. (2005). Retrospect and prospect of neuropsychology in China [in Chinese]. *Chinese Journal of Neurology, 38*, 151–153.

Wing, L., & Potter, D. (2002). The epidemiology of autism spectrum disorders: Is the prevalence rising? *Mental Retardation and Developmental Disabilities Research Reviews, 8*, 151–161.

Wong, V. C. N., & Hui, S. L. H. (2007). Brief report: Emerging services for children with autism spectrum disorders in Hong Kong (1960–2004). *Journal of Autism and Developmental Disorders, 38*(2), 383–389.

Xu, J., Wang, M., Xiang, Y., & Hu, X. (2005). Quality of life for people with intellectual disabilities in China: A cross-culture perspectives study. *Journal of Intellectual Disability Research, 49*, 745–749.

Xu, S., & Wu, Z. (1986). The construction of "The Clinical Memory Test" [in Chinese]. *Acta Psychologica Sinica, 18*, 100–108.

Yao, B., & Wu, H. R. (2003). Risk factors of learning disabilities in Chinese children in Wuhan. *Biomedical & Environmental Sciences, 16*, 392–397.

Yiu, E. M. L. (1992). Linguistic assessment of Chinese-speaking aphasics: Development of a Cantonese aphasia battery. *Journal of Neurolinguistics, 7*, 379–424.

Yuan, G. (2000). Improving the development of neuropsychology in China [in Chinese]. *Chinese Journal of Neurology, 33*, 133–134.

Zhang, X., & Ji, C. (2005). Autism and mental retardation of young children in China. *Biomedical & Environmental Sciences, 18*, 334–340.

Zhou, D. F., Wu, C. S., Qi, H., Fan, J. H., Sun, X. D., Como, P., … Kieburtz, K. (2006). Prevalence of dementia in rural China: Impact of age, gender and education. *Acta Neurologica Scandinavica, 114*, 273–280.

Ziegler, J. C., & Goswami, U. (2005). Reading acquisition, developmental dyslexia, and skilled reading across languages: A psycholinguistic grain size theory. *Psychological Bulletin, 131*, 3–29.

13 Neuropsychology in India

J. Keshav Kumar

Demographics

India is one of the oldest civilizations in the world, with a rich cultural heritage dating back about 9,000 years. Geographically, it is the seventh largest country in the world, covering an area of 3,287,263 km^2. India is the second most populous country, with a population of 1.028 billion people. Although the population density is one of the highest in the world (16.7% of the world population within 2.4% of the world's surface area), an overwhelming majority of Indians (72.2%) live in rural areas (Ministry of Information and Broadcasting, Government of India, 2008). Males outnumber females 532.1 million to 496.4 million, while the life expectancy is very similar: 63.7 for males and 60.9 to 66.9 for females.

India has 28 states and 7 federally governed union territories, each with their own elected government. There are 22 official languages with about 1,652 dialects. Hindi is the national language and is spoken primarily in northern India. By contrast, most of the southern states have their own regional language. English is widely spoken and is considered to be the link between northern and southern India (Manorama Year Book, 2007). The literacy rate is 64.84%, with a higher rate of literacy among males (75.26) than females (53.67).

India has one of the fastest-growing economies with a per capita income of about US$820. Agriculture is the mainstay of the economy, with 60% to 70% of the population dependent on agriculture. More recently, other industries, such as iron and steel, tourism, tobacco, cotton, wool, silk, jute and textile, leather, chemicals, rubber, plastic, petroleum, automobile, machinery, movies, and technology, are flourishing. Although there has been a steady growth in the economy during the past two decades, the growth and development has been uneven among various social, economic, and geographic regions, resulting in an inequality of income.

History of neuropsychology

Clinical psychology and neuropsychology originated at the National Institute of Mental Health and Neurosciences (NIMHANS), Bangalore, in 1957. A clinical neuropsychology unit was established to provide services to and research persons with neurological and psychiatric disorders. Research initially focused on assessing cognitive functioning in psychiatric populations (Bhattacharya & Sen, 1957; Kapur & Sen, 1957; Rao & Sen, 1957; Vardachar & Gopalswamy, 1957). New developments in the 1970s included development of a comprehensive Indian neuropsychological test battery (Mukundan & Murthy, 1979) and a research laboratory incorporating electrophysiological measures such as EEG and event-related potentials (ERPs). This lab has been one of the most prolific in India, examining various populations over the years. Research topics have included arousal mechanism of attention and EEG in schizophrenia (Joseph & Mukundan, 1983), psychophysiological correlates of attention in frontal lobe patients using auditory evoked potential (AEP) (Sujatha & Mukundan, 1985), P300 in schizophrenia (Gonsalvez & Mukundan, 1990), ERP and related neuropsychological deficits in head injury (Easvaradoss & Mukundan, 1983), recovery in head injury (Thakur & Mukundan, 1990), alteration in visual attention (Dwivedi & Mukundan, 1994), frontal lobe contribution to memory (George, Mukundan, & Nagaraja, 1997), physiological correlates of hypnosis in mental disorders (Kamarajan, Mukundan, Ramachandra, & Chaturvedi, 2000), and electrophysiological study of working memory components in mild head injury (Kumar et al., 2005). Currently, the lab is equipped with a 128-channel neuroscan system.

Today, the NIMHANS is the premier research and clinical training institute in India, with about 21 departments in mental health and neurosciences. It is still the only center that provides clinical services as well as supervised training in clinical neuropsychology and neuropsychological research.

Education and training programs in psychology

Clinical psychologists in India receive their training from graduate-level programs modeled after the British postgraduate system. Students initially earn a master's degree, known as MPhil (clinical psychology). There are two types of MPhil degrees in clinical psychology. The one-year degree is university based, focusing on research methodology and theoretical aspects of clinical psychology with minimal or no patient contact. Students enrolled in the two-year MPhil clinical psychology program are trained in an interdisciplinary clinical setting. Only two-year MPhil students can become practitioners upon graduation.

Each year, students in the two-year MPhil program undergo about three postings, or rotations, of three months' duration. An example of a typical posting is the adult psychiatry unit, which consists of a multidisciplinary team including consultants from the departments of psychiatry, clinical psychology, and psychiatric social work. In addition, post-MD senior residents, MD and DPM psychiatry residents, and PhD clinical psychology scholars function as junior consultants for the clinical team. The team as a whole provides supervision to both MPhil scholars and psychiatry residents.

The primary areas of study in the first year are assessment and psychiatric diagnosis. Students receive supervised training in the administration, scoring, and interpretation of psychometric tests such as intelligence tests, memory assessments, adjustment inventories, personality tests including structured, semistructured, and projective tests, and psychotherapy. The second-year MPhil scholars are posted in specialty areas with three months' posting in child mental health services, behavior therapy and biofeedback, neuropsychology, and family therapy, and one month's posting each in de-addiction, psychiatric and neurological rehabilitation, and general hospital psychiatry. Supervised training in psychotherapies for adult and child populations, and cognitive and behavioral interventions, are provided during the second year. Specializations in clinical psychology include child psychology, counseling psychology, organizational and industrial psychology, and clinical psychology programs. Training programs vary according to the specialization offered.

Most practicing neuropsychologists in the country are clinical psychologists with specialization in neuropsychology. The curriculum includes a series of lectures on the biological basis of neurological and psychiatric disorders, including formal lectures in neurochemistry, neurophysiology, and neuropsychology. Clinical supervision in assessment and remediation occurs within the clinical neuropsychological unit during a three-month clinical posting. Supervision is provided by neuropsychology consultants and students pursuing PhDs in neuropsychology. Students are required to conduct a minimum of 50 to 60 neuropsychological assessments on child, adult, and geriatric populations with neurological, neurosurgical, and psychiatric conditions. In addition to assessments, the scholars are trained in neuropsychological rehabilitation for various conditions under the supervision of senior neuropsychology consultants.

At present, the neuropsychology unit at the Department of Mental Health and Social Psychology (NIMHANS) is the only unit in the country providing specialized clinical training in neuropsychology. However, due to the increasing demand for psychological services in India, psychological services across the country employ clinical psychologists to carry out neuropsychological services (assessment and rehabilitation) for the respective communities. The neuropsychology unit at NIMHANS continues to be the nodal training center providing theoretical and supervised clinical inputs for clinical psychologists all over the country when required. For example, other training institutes in clinical psychology can request one- to three-month postings for their students. Short-term training is also provided to clinical psychologists working in the community or professional psychologists desiring to specialize in neuropsychology or when required to work with neurological, neurosurgical, or neuropsychiatric clientele. In addition, the neuropsychology unit conducts annual continuing education programs in neuropsychological assessment and rehabilitation that are open to clinical psychologists practicing in the community.

The minimum training requirement for practicing clinical psychology in India is a two-year MPhil degree in clinical psychology from teaching hospitals. However, many students (with either hospital-based or university-based training) earn a PhD before they begin practicing professionally. PhDs are offered at universities as well as teaching hospitals.

Given the enormous Indian population, opportunities for training psychologists are limited. The MPhil degree in clinical psychology was initially offered only at two institutes: National Institute of Mental Health and Neurosciences (NIMHANS), Bangalore, and Central Institute of Psychiatry (CPI), Ranchi. The number of clinical programs has recently increased to 10.

At NIMHANS, the admission process for the MPhil program is fairly competitive. Approximately 200 students take the entrance exam, with the top scorers invited for personal interviews conducted by clinicians within the institution. NIMHANS has typically funded 12 students per year, which increased to 18 students in 2008.

About 60 students per year apply and take the entrance exam for the NIMHANS PhD program. The top 10 students are interviewed and four are selected for the PhD program. These students are supported by an institutional fellowship. Other universities and teaching hospitals around the country attempt to use the NIMHANS model while recruiting students into a clinical psychology doctoral program, though some enroll students without entrance exams. Funding for these students is also available from several external governmental funding agencies.

Licensing of clinical psychologists

Currently, India has no licensure in clinical psychology. This lack of a credentialing process exists despite the existence of the Mental Health Act (Prabhu, 1998) and Rehabilitation Council of India Act (1992, 2000). Thus, many practicing clinical psychologists are not adequately trained, and there is inconsistency in the quality of psychological services across the country (Prabhu, 1998). To address this problem, several psychological organizations, such as the Indian Association of Clinical Psychologists (IACP) and the Indian Psychological Council (IPC), conduct continuing educational programs and conferences. These training opportunities allow professionals across the country to exchange/share information about research and other academic activities happening across the country. Efforts to introduce a licensing process are being undertaken by IACP and IPC by setting up task forces in various subspecialties of clinical psychology.

Neuropsychological test batteries used in India

There are three types of neuropsychological tests used in India: (1) Western neuropsychological test batteries translated and adapted for Indian culture, (2) individual Western neuropsychological tests translated and adapted for Indian culture, and (3) indigenous tests. The vast majority of Indian neuropsychological tests have been adapted from the West.

NIMHANS neuropsychological battery (Mukundan & Murthy, 1979)

The earliest Western neuropsychological battery adapted for Indians is the NIMHANS Neuropsychological Battery (Mukundan & Murthy, 1979). This battery is based on Luria's principles of cerebral localization and lateralization of higher mental functions and is one of the most extensively used instruments in India. Consistent with Luria's theory of brain functioning and neuropsychological practices of the time, one of the primary uses of the NIMHANS battery is to identify cerebral localization and lateralization of neurological disorders. This battery consists of several Western tests and a few indigenous tests standardized on the

Indian population (Mukundan & Murthy, 1979) and validated against radiological CT findings by neuropsychologists performing "blind" interpretations consistent with the approach of Ralph Reitan (Mukundan, Rao, Jain, Jayakumar, & Shailaja, 1991). The battery provided good lateralization and localization with 70% accuracy for right hemispheric lesions and 67% accuracy for left hemispheric lesions (Mukundan et al., 1991). The details of functions assessed and tests used to assess these functions are mentioned in Table 13.1.

PGI battery of brain dysfunction (PGI-BBD; Pershad & Verma, 1990)

The PGI Battery of Brain Dysfunction (PGI-BBD) was developed at the Post-Graduate Institute of Medical and Education Research (PGI). The PGI-BBD is a compilation of individual tests of memory, intelligence, and visual perception that was standardized on the Indian population. The battery consists of the following scales: (1) PGI Memory Scale (Pershad & Wig, 1976, 1988), (2) Bhatia's Short Battery of Performance–Revised (Murthy, 1966), (3) Verbal Adult Intelligence (VAIS), (4) Bender-Gestalt Test (BGT), and (5) Nahor-Benson Test (Nahor & Benson, 1970).

1. PGI Memory Scale: This scale consists of 10 subtests, including verbal and nonverbal memory, remote memory, recent memory, short-term memory, and long-term memory. The test was standardized on 360 subjects between the ages of 20 and 45 years. Test-retest reliability for the 10 subtests ranged from 0.69 to 0.85 ($n = 45$). Construct validity was established by correlating the test with the Boston Memory Scale (0.71) and the Wechsler Memory Scale (0.85).
2. Bhatia's Short Battery of Performance–Revised (BSBPR) (Murthy, 1966): This battery of nonverbal visual-processing subtests, including Koh's Block Design and Pass Along Test, was originally designed in 1955 (Bhatia, 1955). Scores from each subtest are calculated into a composite score that yields an intelligence quotient. The BSBPR was standardized on a healthy Indian population in the age range of 20 to 59 years. Norms were developed for four age groups and three educational levels for both males and females. The intelligence quotient correlated significantly with the Wechsler Adult Intelligence Scale (WAIS) Performance IQ and Raven's Progressive Matrices (Mahajan, Pershad, & Verma, 1988; Verma, Pershad, Malhotra, & Arunima, 1988).
3. The Verbal Adult Intelligence Scale (VAIS) includes subtests of Information, Digit Span, Arithmetic, and Comprehension, which are adapted from the Wechsler Adult Intelligence Scale (WAIS). The VAIS was standardized on 3,600 Hindi-speaking males and females ages 20–69 years from different states of India.
4. The Bender Visual Motor Gestalt Test (Bender-Gestalt Test) is the Western screen for organicity. It consists of nine simple geometric designs that are copied by the subject.

Table 13.1 NIMHANS neuropsychological test batteries

Function/test	*NIMHANS battery (Mukundan & Murthy, 1979)*	*NIMHANS neurospychological battery (Rao et al., 2004)*	*NIMHANS neuropsychological battery for children (Kar, Rao, Chandramouli, & Thennarasu, 2004)*
Visual scanning			
Picture/Number Scanning	Yes	X	X
Colour Cancellation	X	Yes	Yes
Colour Trails	X	Yes	Yes
Motor functions			
Continuous Drawing	Yes	X	X
Optic Spatial Organization/Relation	Yes	X	X
Kinetic Melody	Yes	X	X
Psychomotor Perseveration	Yes	X	X
Hand Tapping	X	Yes	X
Finger Tapping	X	Yes	Yes
Expressive speech			
Animal Naming	X	Yes	X
Cowa/Verbal Fluency	X	Yes	Yes
Category Fluency	Yes	X	X
Design Fluency	X	Yes	Yes
Delayed Response Learning	Yes	X	X
Digit Span	X	Yes	Yes
N-Back	X	Yes	Yes
Stroop Colour Word Test	X	Yes	Yes
Abstraction/Similarity	Yes	X	X

Planning			
Tower of London	X	Yes	X
Maze Test	X	X	Yes
Bender-Gestalt Test	Yes	X	X
Complex Figure Test	Yes	Yes	X
Block Design	Yes	Yes	Yes
Spatial Relation Test	Yes	X	X
Object Assembly	Yes	X	X
Motor Free Visual Perception Test	X	X	
Focal signs (agnosia, apraxia, alexia, agraphia, acalculia, right-left orientation)	Yes	Yes	X
Logical Memory Passage	Yes	X	X
Verbal Learning	X	Yes	Yes
Memory for Designs	X	X	
Benton Visual Retention Test		X	X
Academic Function Tests	X	X	Yes
Raven's Progressive Matrices	Yes	Yes	Yes

Note: Yes = test included in the battery; X = test not included.

5. Nahor-Benson Test (NBT) (Nahor & Benson, 1970): The NBT was developed as a quick and simple screening test for organic brain pathology. The test discriminated between individuals with and without brain damage with 99% sensitivity and 75% specificity using a cutoff score of 2 (Pershad & Verma, 1978). Test performance is not affected by age, whereas a negative correlation was found between the number of errors made and the VAIS (–0.45).

The scoring of the PGI-BBD is very similar to the Halstead-Reitan Neuropsychological Battery, where each test is scored on a 0–3 rating scale, with 0–1 indicating no deviation, 2 is a deviation, and 3 a great deviation. The sum of the deviation score yields a Brain Damage Score (BDS). The BDS cutoff scores are based upon a retrospective chart review of 180 patients referred to the PGI Center between 1976 and 1980 who were administered at least two of the three tests of cognitive functions (intelligence, memory, and perceptual-motor). Cutoff scores were cross-validated in a prospective study on 28 patients with brain damage who were administered the PGI-BBD.

NIMHANS neuropsychological battery for adults (Rao et al., 2004)

A second NIMHANS Neuropsychological Battery, comprised of contemporary Western tests, was developed by Rao et al. (2004) (Table 13.1). Unlike the original NIMHANS battery, which emphasized localization, the emphasis of the new battery is the evaluation of strengths and weakness in different domains of cognition. Thus, scores are reported in percentiles versus cutoff. Normative data were collected on 540 healthy volunteers from the community with demographic categorization into three age groups (16–30, 31–50, 51–65 years), two education levels (school and college education), and gender. Normative data were also collected on an illiterate sample. This version of the NIMHANS was validated on clinical groups with focal lesions, head injury, movement disorders, and refractory epilepsy.

NIMHANS Neuropsychological battery for children (Kar, Rao, & Thennarasu, 2004)

The NIMHANS Neuropsychological Battery for Children (NBC) was developed by Kar et al. in 2004. Similar to the revised NIMHANS, the child version consists of Western tests to evaluate different domains of cognitive functions, including attention, executive functions, memory, comprehension, and visual-spatial skills. The test battery includes Color Cancellation, Trail Making Test, Phonemic Fluency, Design Fluency (Jones-Gotman, 1986), Visual-Spatial Working Memory (Milner, 1971), Porteus Maze (Porteus, 1950), Motor Free Visual Perception Test (Colarusso & Hammill, 1972), Picture Completion, Block Design (Malin, 1969), Token Test (De Renzi & Vignolo, 1962), Rey Auditory Verbal Learning Test (RAVLT) (Maj, D'Elia, Satz, & Janssen, 1993), and Memory for Design (Jones-Gotman, 1986). The battery was normed on 400 healthy school children aged between 5 and 15 years, with a sample of 33 children in each age group. Test-retest reliability ranged from 0.59 to 0.92. The battery has been validated against 16 brain-damaged children.

Additional tests have been adopted from Western tests for research on executive functioning as well as decision making for individuals with brain lesion, head injury, obsessive compulsive disorder, affective disorder, and schizophrenia. These tests include Iowa Gambling Task (IGT) and Object Alternation Test (OAT), as well as computerized versions of the IGT and OAT, Corsi Block Tapping Test for visuospatial working memory, and N-Back Test for verbal working memory (Ray, Kumar, & Pillai, 2008).

Indigenously developed tests

Very few indigenous tests have been developed in India. Among the indigenously developed tests, most are based on existing neuropsychological tests found in the West, but with different stimuli and instructions. Some of the indigenous tests are as follows.

Delayed response test (DRT) (Mukundan & Murthy, 1979; Mukundan et al., 1991)

This is a working memory test similar to the Paced Auditory Serial Addition Test (PASAT) that requires the subject to perform simple mental operations like addition, multiplication, and division. The answer of the first problem (4 + 3) is held online, while the second mental operation (6 + 5) is performed. The subject is required to add or subtract the answer of the first problem to the answer of the second problem. Subjects with working memory deficits experience difficulty in remembering the answer of the first problem while working on the second problem. Therefore, they often ask for the repetition of the first part. The test consists of 20 items divided into three sections. The first two sections consist of statement problems, and the third section consists of numerical problems. Acalculia is ruled out before the onset of this test.

Ideational fluency test

This is a word generation test similar to the Control Oral Word Association Test. In the Indian version, the subject is given two minutes to generate as many items as possible for two categories: things made out of "wood" and "round" objects. The number of items generated in each category forms the score.

Verbal learning and memory

The Indian version of Logical Memory is the Verbal Learning and Memory Functions Test. In this test, the administrator reads a logical passage and the subject is asked to recall the material immediately after presentation. There are three immediate recall trials and a 20-minute delayed recall trial. A comparison of the three immediate recall trials provides a learning curve with repetition, while the difference between the third trial and the delayed trial indicates the amount of information forgotten after the delay.

Visual learning and memory

In the Visual Learning and Memory Functions Test, a complex pattern similar to the Rey Complex Figure Test is exposed to the subject for 15 seconds and he or she must draw the pattern from memory. The design consists of 23 facts and is presented on a 6 × 4 inch card. Similar to the verbal learning test, there are three immediate recall trials, and the subject is asked to draw the design from memory after a 10-minute delay. A fifth trial asks the subject to copy the design, thus assessing visuospatial skills. Similar to the verbal passage, the amount of information learned across trials and the amount forgotten after a delay can be obtained for the visual pattern.

Comprehensive neuropsychological battery (Gupta et al., 2000)

The All India Institute of Medical Sciences Comprehensive Neuropsychological Battery (AAIMS) is the only indigenous Indian test battery. It was developed in Hindi (Gupta et al., 2000). The AIIMS is based on Luria's functional approach and consists of 160 items subdivided into 10 basic scales and four secondary scales, including Motor, Tactile, Visual, Receptive Speech, Expressive Speech, Reading, Writing, Arithmetic, Memory, and Intellectual Process. Additional scales include the Pathognomic Scale, Left Hemisphere Scale, Right Hemisphere Scale, and Total Scale. Each scale is rated on a 5-point system from 0–4 with 0 indicating no deficits and a score of 4 indicating severe impairment. Each item is scored for accuracy, speed, frequency, quality, and appropriateness. The test-retest reliability for the 10 basic scales of the AIIMS ranges from 0.79 to 0.98, with a high interrater reliability of 0.98. Validity was established on 175 normal controls, 70 schizophrenics, and 160 brain-damaged individuals. The hit rates ranged from 66.6% to 89.62% (Gupta et al., 2000).

Challenges in Indian neuropsychology

The major challenges for providing neuropsychological services in India include testing persons with low levels of or no education, testing persons who are illiterate, and providing services to a population where over 1,600 dialects are spoken. Similar to studies in Mexico, we have found that Indians with low educational levels demonstrate significant problems on tests evaluating for construction ability (copying of figures), language functions such as comprehension, phonological verbal fluency, conceptual functions such as similarities, calculation abilities, and sequencing (Ardila, 1995; Ardila, Ostrosky-Solis, Rosselli, & Gomez, 2000; Ostrosky-Solis, Ardila, & Rosselli, 1998). The greatest difficulty seen in Indian illiterates is on tests of visuoconstructive ability that requires the subject to draw or copy figures. This deficit is most likely due to a complete lack of exposure to writing with a pencil or a pen. It is not uncommon to find subjects in rural areas reporting holding pencils for the first time in their lives during testing. Another contributing factor to the poor test performance of Indian illiterates is poor motivation, test anxiety, and perceptions of irrelevancy, due to their lack of exposure to testing situations (Ardila, 1995). Most of the patients with low education levels from rural areas may not be exposed to formal education.

One manner of addressing performance problems of illiterates due to lack of exposure to writing with pencils is to use rangoli, a chalk-like material that rural persons use to draw designs or create artwork. When administering a construction task, the illiterate person is told that the purpose of the test is to see if they can copy a picture instead of evaluating their artwork. The examinee is also given constant encouragement to overcome the anxieties related to this novel situation.

The other significant challenge for Indian neuropsychologists is testing individuals in a country where there are 22 official languages and 1,652 dialects. Because it would be impossible to translate and standardize tests in all the official languages or dialects, tests developed are judiciously translated into some of the regional official languages (such as Kannada, Malayalam, Tamil, Telugu, and Marathi), Hindi (the national language), and English (the medium of instruction in most of the urban and some of the rural schools). Normative data are collected on rural and urban populations across different ages and education levels, including the illiterate population.

Current practices

The neuropsychology program at NIMHANS provides services to a wide variety of patients, including those with neurological and psychiatric disorders, as well as those who will be undergoing neurosurgery. Geriatric patients, epileptics, patients with head injuries, and children are the most common populations receiving neuropsychological services.

Geriatrics

Neuropsychological consultation is provided in the NIMHANS geriatric clinic, which runs once a week. These patients are primarily referred for an evaluation of cognitive strengths and weaknesses, baseline assessment, and diagnostic clarification for patients in the early stages of the disease process. Common diagnoses include cortical and subcortical dementias such as Alzheimer's disease, Pick's disease, fronto-temporal dementia, dementia with Lewy bodies, vascular dementias, Wilson's disease, Parkinson's disease, and progressive supranuclear palsy. Attempts to develop simple and culture-specific tests, as well as intervention programs to enhance overall cognitive functions and quality of life, are currently underway.

Epilepsy

Clinical services for individuals with epilepsy have been provided from the time of inception of the neuropsychology unit at NIMHANS. In addition, cognition in epileptic patients has been extensively studied. Studies on epileptic patients have examined attention, perception, and intelligence (Sheela & Rao, 1962); executive, and sensory and motor functioning in posttraumatic syndrome and epilepsy (Mukundan & Murthy, 1979); cognitive functions and adjustments (George & Murthy, 1976); memory and information processing (Prasada, Rao, & Rao, 1987); automatic and effortful processing (Saraswathy & Rao, 1987); and divided attention in epilepsy (Chandiramani & Rao, 1992). Neuropsychological rehabilitation of cognitive deficits associated with epilepsy was administered to 28 patients compared to a control group consisting of 28 patients who were placed on a wait list for treatment. This intervention resulted in significant improvements on neuropsychological tests as well as psychosocial functioning (Bharathy & Rao, 1998). More recently, a sensitive and specific test battery for epilepsy (Kavitha, Rao, Satish Chandra, & Jayakumar, 2004) was developed for patients undergoing surgery for temporal lobe epilepsy. The authors found good lateralization and localization prior to the surgery on neuropsychological assessment.

Head injury

Extensive research and clinical services have been conducted and developed in the area of head injury at NIMHANS. Early studies focused on establishing profiles of cognitive deficits in head-injured individuals, such as deficits in information processing, serial processing, parallel processing, and reaction time (Gangadhar, Rao, & Hegde, 1985; Nayak & Rao, 1984; Rao, Gangadhar, & Hegde, 1985; Uma & Rao, 1987); visual information processing (Mariadas, Rao, Gangadhar, & Hegde, 1989); ideational fluency and visual scanning (Rao, 1998); long-term memory associated with difficulty in depth of processing (Menon & Rao, 1997); and divided attention (Misra & Rao, 1994). Deficits such as visual scanning, visual learning and memory, mental arithmetic, social adjustment, and emotional problems were found to persist one year after injury (Mukundan, Narayana Reddy, Hedge, Shankar, & Kaliaperumal, 1987).

Neuropsychology in children

Neuropsychological studies in children have generally focused on cognitive remediation. Successful programs have been developed for both reading disabilities (Sadasivan & Rao, 1997) and arithmetic disorder (Bhasi, Rao, & Ooman, 2003). Similarly, neuropsychological rehabilitation administered to children with head injury demonstrated improvements on neuropsychological tests and also resulted in symptom reduction (Ajayan & Rao, 1998).

Neuropsychological rehabilitation

Cognitive rehabilitation is an important service provided by the NIMHANS neuropsychology unit. The first neuropsychological rehabilitation program was developed by Rao et al. (1985) with interdisciplinary support from the departments of neurosurgery, neurology, and psychiatry. Originally developed for head injury patients, neuropsychological rehabilitation has subsequently been extended to other neurological conditions, such as epilepsy and cerebral vascular accidents. Efficacy of this intervention has been supported by several studies reporting symptomatic improvement and improvement in cognitive functions (Mishra & Rao, 1994; Nag-Arulmani, & Rao, 1999; Bharathi & Rao, 1998; Kumar, Rao, & Chandramouli, 2000; Kumari & Mukundan, 2000).

A major challenge in developing neuropsychological rehabilitation programs was to ensure cost-effectiveness so that programs are available to the entire spectrum of the Indian population, including the low socioeconomic strata. Unlike other industrialized countries, India has no social security or government-sponsored health insurance. Thus, the vast majority of the population cannot afford health care services. To address this problem, three sets of rehabilitation programs have been developed at NIMHANS: a hospital-based rehabilitation program (Kumar, Rao, & Chandramouli, 2000), a home-based program (Rao, Nair, et al., 2004), and a computerized rehabilitation program (Kumar & Mukundan, 2000).

Hospital-based rehabilitation is a one-month program administered to hospital inpatients by professional staff. It is comprised of tasks to enhance attention, memory, executive function, and response inhibition (Kumar, 2007; Kumar, Rao, & Chandramouli, 2000, 2005). The sustained-attention module includes tasks such as grain sorting, letter cancellation, and shading/coloring. The grain-sorting task is a timed exercise in which the patient is given a mixture of three grains that he or she must sort into different piles as quickly as possible. On the letter-cancellation task, the patient is required to cancel two letters from a sheet of a magazine. Performance is based on time and number of errors. Feedback is given intermittently. The shading/coloring task consists of geometric designs drawn on a sheet of paper. The patient is required to color/shade within the boundaries of the design. Neatness and consistency are emphasized. Task assignments are based on the nature and the severity of the attention deficit, which is determined by the initial neuropsychological assessment. Often, patients may complete these tasks with ease, and may require a more complex task, such as divided attention.

Rehabilitation for memory deficits involves training on verbal and visual encoding techniques. Patients are taught and encouraged to use organizational strategies such as chunking and rehearsal. Typically, patients are presented with a list of six words, divided into three segments. Patients are encouraged to organize each segment into a meaningful statement, rehearse, and recall. A second segment is presented upon completion of the first segment, and patients are requested to apply a similar learning strategy, while holding the first set of words in working memory. The same procedure is repeated for the third set of words, while holding the first two sets online. This technique improves not only organizing, encoding, rehearsal, and recall, but also working memory and executive functions.

Spatial encoding tasks are used to train visual memory. Six to 15 objects, depending on severity of deficit, are placed on a table. Objects are exposed for about 10 seconds and then covered with a board. The patient is required to name as well as identify the location of the objects hidden under the board. The number of objects used is based on severity of memory deficit, and the level of difficulty is increased by adding more objects to the task.

Executive functioning is rehabilitated through several activities. Essay writing requires a patient to write a short 100-word essay on a specific topic. This exercise develops not only writing skills, but also skills in problem solving, organizing, and generating ideas. Divided attention tasks such as sorting grain while simultaneously generating as many words as possible starting with a designated letter develop multitasking skills. As mentioned previously, organizational strategies are also taught for improving memory.

The hospital-based intervention program was simplified and instructions adopted for a home-based program that could be administered by family members of the patients. Family members such as spouses, parents, or an educated relative are trained to carry out the rehabilitation program, record performance scores, and discuss progress or lack thereof with the treating team. Difficulty levels are adjusted based on the improvements noticed on the recorded data. The rehabilitation program typically consists of four modules focusing on information processing, sustained attention, spatial working memory, and verbal long-term memory. Modules run for about a week; however, they can be extended or tasks staggered if the patient has severe cognitive deficits. Upon successful completion and satisfactory gains on the task set for the target week, as well as demonstration of generalization to other situations, the patient is graduated to modules of increasing complexity. Rehabilitation is terminated when the patient improves symptomatically based on self-report and reports of the trainers. If no changes are perceived by the patient or the family members, then a hospital-based rehabilitation program may be warranted.

Brain Function Therapy (BFT) is a computerized rehabilitation program developed for retraining various cognitive functions, such as visual attention, visual perception, working memory, mental control, verbal processing, and response inhibition. The program involves presentation of stimulus material on a computer monitor with increasing levels of difficulty. Exposure time, intertrial duration, and complexity of the stimuli are controlled, and increased in a graded manner. Performance is evaluated by response accuracy. This computerized program has been found to be efficacious in rehabilitation of cognitive deficits following head injury (Kumar & Mukundan, 2000).

Future challenges

From the establishment of a neuropsychology unit and lab, to the adaptation of several neuropsychological batteries and tests in Indian languages, to the development of rehabilitation programs that can service the masses, Indian neuropsychology has made significant progress in servicing an ethnically, linguistically, and educationally diverse people. Still, many challenges exist for the field of neuropsychology to continue or improve services to the people of India. First, more training centers are needed to address the shortage of neuropsychologists. Currently, NIMHANS is the only institute providing training in neuropsychology. With a graduating class of less than 20 a year, NIMHANS alone cannot train enough neuropsychologists to service over a billion people. Second, government regulation of the practice of clinical psychology and neuropsychology is needed to develop minimum training and competency standards to ensure quality services for the Indian population. Third, advancements in neuropsychological test development are needed with an increase in indigenous culture-specific tests, as well as translations and norms for more languages to increase the capacity to provide assessments to the diverse population. Fourth, more research is needed to develop the knowledge base required to provide competent services and to better understand brain–behavior relationships. Currently, research in neuropsychology is primarily conducted by students fulfilling requirements for their MPhil and PhD degrees. A major problem is the dearth of funding available for research in neuropsychology.

Acknowledgments

The author is grateful to Ms. Renu George, PhD scholar, Neuropsychology Unit, NIMHANS, and Mrs. Akila Sadasivan, PhD scholar, Department of Psychology, Canterbury University, New Zealand, for editing, as well as Dr. Manoj Kumar Sharma, Assistant Professor, National Institute of Mental Health and Neurosciences, and Dr. Masroor Jahan, Assistant Professor, RINPAS, Ranchi, for providing information regarding existing tools and practices in their domains.

References

Ajayan, P., & Rao, S. L. (1998). *Neuropsychological rehabilitation in head injured children.* Bangalore, India: National Institute of Mental Health and Neurosciences (NIMHANS).

Ardila, A. (1995). Directions of research in cross-cultural neuropsychology. *Journal of Clinical and Experimental Neuropsychology, 17*, 143–150.

Ardila, A., Ostrosky-Solis, F., Rosselli, M., & Gomez, C. (2000). Age-related cognitive decline during normal aging: The complex effect of education. *Archives of Clinical Neuropsychology, 15*, 495–513.

Bharathy, B. K., & Rao, S. L. (1998). *Neuropsychological rehabilitation in epilepsy.* Unpublished PhD thesis, National Institute of Mental Health and Neurosciences (NIMHANS), Bangalore, India.

Bhasi, S., Rao, S. L., & Ooman, A. (2003). *Neuropsychological remediation for children with specific learning disorder of arithmetic*. Bangalore, India: National Institute of Mental Health and Neurosciences (NIMHANS).

Bhatia, C. M.(1955). *Performance tests of intelligence under Indian conditions.* Bombay, India: Oxford University Press.

Bhattacharya, & Sen, N. N. (1957). *Comparative study of motor ability and variability in schizophrenia and normals*. Bangalore, India: National Institute of Mental Health and Neurosciences (NIMHANS).

Chandiramani, R., & Rao, S. L. (1992). *Divided attention in epilepsy.* Unpublished MPhil dissertation, National Institute of Mental Health and Neurosciences (NIMHANS), Bangalore, India.

Colarusso, R. P., & Hammill, D. D. (1972). *Motor-free visual perception test.* Novato, CA: Academic Therapy Publications.

De Renzi, E., & Vignolo, L. (1962). The token test: A sensitive test to detect receptive disturbances in aphasics. *Brain, 85*, 665–678.

Dwivedi, P., & Mukundan, C. R. (1994). *Lateralization of visual attention*. Bangalore, India: National Institute of Mental Health and Neurosciences (NIMHANS).

Easvaradoss, & Mukundan, C. R. (1983). *Deficits of attention in head trauma. An event-related potential study*. Bangalore, India: National Institute of Mental Health and Neurosciences (NIMHANS).

Gangadhar, B. N., Rao, S. L., & Hegde, A. S. (1985). Information-processing deficits and post-concussion syndrome: Role of symptoms. *NIMHANS Journal, 3*, 147–150.

George, R. M., Mukundan, C. R., & Nagaraja, D. (1997). *Frontal contribution to memory*. Bangalore, India: National Institute of Mental Health and Neurosciences (NIMHANS).

George, V. C., & Murthy, V. N. (1976). *Cognitive function and adjustment in epileptics in response to treatment: A follow-up study*. Bangalore, India: National Institute of Mental Health and Neurosciences (NIMHANS).

Gonsalvez, C., & Mukundan, C. R. (1990). *A study of the P300 component of evoked potential in schizophrenia*. Bangalore, India: National Institute of Mental Health and Neurosciences (NIMHANS).

Gupta, S., Khandelwal, S. K., Tandon, P. N., Maheshwari, M. C., Mehta, V. S., Sundaram, K. S., et al. (2000). The development and standardization of the comprehensive neuropsychological battery in Hindi (adult form). *Journal of Personality and Clinical Studies, 16,* 75–109.

Jones-Gotman, M. (1986). Memory for designs: The hippocampal continuation. *Neuropsychologia, 24*, 193–203.

Joseph, C., & Mukundan, C. R. (1983). *An experimental study of arousal mechanisms in schizophrenia*. Bangalore, India: National Institute of Mental Health and Neurosciences (NIMHANS).

Kamarajan, C. K., Mukundan, C. R., Ramachandra, S., & Chaturvedi, S. K. (2000). *Psychophysiological correlates of hypnosis in functional mental disorders*. Bangalore, India: National Institute of Mental Health and Neurosciences (NIMHANS).

Kapur, R. L., & Sen, N. N. (1957). *A study of intellectual impairments in schizophrenia by psychodiagnostic tests*. Bangalore, India: National Institute of Mental Health and Neurosciences (NIMHANS).

Kar, B. R., Rao, S. L., Chandramouli, B. A. & Thennarasu, K. (2004). *NIMHANS neuropsychological battery for children manual*. Bangalore, India : NIMHANS Publications.

Kavitha, P. R., Rao, S. L., Satish Chandra, P., & Jayakumar, P. N. (2004). *Development of neuropsychological battery for evaluation of mesial temporal epilepsy*. Bangalore, India: National Institute of Mental Health and Neurosciences (NIMHANS).

Kumar, K. J. (2007). *Neuropsychological rehabilitation: A functional neural network approach*. Paper presented at the Continuing Neuropsychological Education (CEN), NIMHANS, Bangalore, India.

Kumar, K. J., Rao, S. L., & Chandramouli, B. A. (2000). *Neuropsychological rehabilitation in head injury*. Unpublished PhD thesis, National Institute of Mental Health and Neurosciences (NIMHANS), Bangalore, India.

Kumar, K. J., Rao, S. L., & Chandramouli, B. A. (2005). *Innovative methods of rehabilitation in head injury*. Paper presented at the World Congress on Brain Injury, Melbourne, Australia.

Kumar, S., Rao, S. L. Nair, R. G., Chandramouli, B. A. & Subbakrishna, D. K. (2005). Sensory gating impairment in development of post concussion symptoms in mild head injury. *Psychiatry and Clinical Neurosciences, 59,* 466–472.

Kumar, S., & Mukundan, C. R. (2000). *Computer-aided cognitive retraining for head injury patients*. Unpublished MPhil dissertation, National Institute of Mental Health and Neurosciences (NIMHANS), Bangalore, India.

Mahajan, A., Pershad, D., & Verma, S. K. (1988). Influence of age, education and sex on performance test of intelligence. *Indian Journal of Psychometry and Education, 19*, 65–71.

Maj, M., D'Elia, L., Satz, P., & Janssen, R. (1993). Evaluation of two neuropsychological tests designed to minimize cultural bias in the assessment of HIV-1 seropositive persons: A WHO study. *Archives of Clinical Neuropsychology, 8*, 123–135.

Malin, A. J. (1969). Malin's intelligence scale for Indian children. *Indian Journal of Mental Retardation, 4*, 15–25.

Manorama. (2008): *Manorama year book 2008*. Ernakulam, India: Malayala Manorama Co. Ltd.

Mariadas, C. A., Rao, S. L., Gangadhar, B. N., & Hegde, A. S. (1989). Neuropsychological functioning in post-concussion syndrome. *NIMHANS Journal, 7*, 37–41.

Menon, P., & Rao, S. L. (1997). Memory storage and encoding in patients with memory deficits after closed head injury. *NIMHANS Journal, 15*, 83–92.

Milner, B. (1971). Interhemispheric differences in the localization of psychological processes in man. *British Medical Bulletin, 27*, 272–277.

Ministry of Information and Broadcasting, Government of India, (2008): *India 2008: A reference annual year book*. New Delhi, India: Publication Division, Ministry of Information & Broadcasting, Government of India .

Mishra, S., & Rao, S. L. (1994). Divided attention in head injury. *NIMHANS Journal, 12*, 156–162.

Mukundan, C. R., & Murthy, V. N. (1979). *Lateralization and localizing cerebral lesions by a battery of neuropsychological tests*. Paper presented at the Joint Conference of Neurology, Psychiatry, Clinical Psychology and Psychiatric Social Work Societies of India, NIMHANS, Bangalore, India.

Mukundan, C. R., Narayana Reddy, G. N., Hedge, A. S., Shankar, J., & Kaliaperumal, V. G. (1987). Neuropsychological and clinical recovery in patients with head trauma. *NIMHANS Journal, 5*, 23–32.

Mukundan, C. R., Rao, S. L., Jain, V. K., Jayakumar, P. N., & Shailaja, K. (1991). Neuropsychological assessment: A cross validation study with neuroradiological/operative findings in patients with cerebral hemisphere lesions. *Pharmacopsychologia, 4*, 33–39.

Murthy,H.N. (1966) A short scale of Bhatias's performance test. *Indian Psychological Review, 2*, 133–134.

Nag-Arulmani, S. & Rao, S.L. (1999) Remediation of attention deficits in head injury *Neurology India, 47*, 32–39.

Nahor, A., & Benson, D. F. (1970). A screening test for organic brain disease in emergency psychiatric evaluation. *Behavioural Neuro-Psychiatry, 2*, 23–26.

Nayak, N. P., & Rao, S. L. (1984). *Attentional and informational processing defects in post-traumatic syndrome*. Unpublished MPhil dissertation, National Institute of Mental Health and Neurosciences (NIMHANS), Bangalore, India.

Ostrosky-Solis, F., Ardila, A., Rosselli, M. N., Lopez-Arango, G., & Uriel-Mendoza, V. (1998). Neuropsychological test performance in illiterate subjects. *Archives of Clinical Neuropsychology, 13*, 645–660.

Pershad, D., & Verma, S. K. (1978). A preliminary report on the adaptation of Wechsler's Adult Intelligence Scale (verbal section) in Hindi. *ISPT Journal of Research, 2*, 81–91.

Pershad, D. & Verma, S. K. (1990): *Handbook of PGI battery of brain dysfunction (PGI-BBD)*. Agra, India: National Psychological Corporation.

Pershad, D. & Wig, N. (1988).*Handbook for PGI memory scale clinical test*. Agra: Nat Psych Corp.

Porteus, S. (1950). *The Porteus maze test and intelligence*. Oxford, England: Pacific Books.
Prabhu, G. G. (1998). Progress of the clinical psychology in India. In Q. Hasan (Ed.), *Applied psychology: Indian perspective* (pp. 47–64). New Delhi, India: Gyan Publishing House.
Prasada Rao, P. S. D. V., & Rao, S. L. (1987). *A study of memory deficits in epilepsy through automatic and effortful processing*. Unpublished MPhil dissertation, National Institute of Mental Health and Neurosciences (NIMHANS), Bangalore, India.
Rao, M. P., & Sen, N. N. (1957). *The effect of electrical convulsion therapy on attention, memory, and motor functions in psychiatric patients*. National Institute of Mental Health and Neurosciences (NIMHANS), Bangalore, India:.
Rao, S. L. (1998). Neuropsychological sequelae after head injury and its treatment. *Quarterly Journal of Surgical Sciences, 34*, 47–57.
Rao, S. L., Gangadhar, B. N., & Hegde, A. S. (1985). Remedying information-processing deficits in post-concussion syndrome through cognitive retraining: A case study. *NIMHANS Journal, 3*, 151–153.
Rao, S. L., Nair, R. G., Kumar, S., Chandramouli, B. A., Pillai, S. & Subbakrishna, D. K. (2004). Efficacy of cognitive retraining. Paper presented at the Continuing Neuropsychological Education (CEN), NIMHANS, Bangalore, India.
Rao, S. L., Subbakrishna, D. K. & Gopukumar, K. (2004). *NIMHANS neuropsychological battery manual*. Bangalore, India: NIMHANS Publications.
Ray, S., Kumar, K. J., & Pillai, S. (2008). *Mental flexibility, working memory and planning in decision-making ability in head injury*. Unpublished MPhil dissertation, National Institute of Mental Health and Neurosciences (NIMHANS), Bangalore, India.
Rehabilitation Counsel of India Act (1992 and Amendment, 2000). Rehabilitation Council of India. Retrieved March 18, 2009 from http:// rehabcouncil.nic.in/council/acts_amend.htm
Sadasivan, A., & Rao, S. L. (1997). *Neuropsychological remediation of adolescents with reading disability*. Unpublished MPhil dissertation, National Institute of Mental Health and Neurosciences (NIMHANS), Bangalore, India.
Saraswathy, N. E., & Rao, S. L. (1987). *A study of memory deficits in epilepsy through automatic and effortful processing*. Unpublished MPhil dissertation, National Institute of Mental Health and Neurosciences (NIMHANS), Bangalore, India.
Sheela, N., & Rao, R. S. K. (1962). *A study of attention, perception and intelligence in a group of epileptics*. Unpublished MPhil dissertation, National Institute of Mental Health and Neurosciences (NIMHANS), Bangalore, India.
Sujatha, D., & Mukundan, C. R. (1985). A *neuropsychological study of cognitive deficits in schizophrenia*. Unpublished PhD thesis, National Institute of Mental Health and Neurosciences (NIMHANS), Bangalore, India.
Thakur, D., & Mukundan, C. R. (1990). *Pattern of neuropsychological recovery in head injury: A psychophysiology study*. Bangalore, India: National Institute of Mental Health and Neurosciences (NIMHANS).
Uma, H., & Rao, S. L. (1987). Information processing in patients with closed head injury. *Journal of Psychological Researches, 31*, 70–76.
Vardachar, & Gopalswamy, M. V. (1957). *A study of personality profile of clinical and non-clinical groups*. Unpublished MPhil dissertation, National Institute of Mental Health and Neurosciences (NIMHANS), Bangalore, India.
Verma, S. K., Pershad, D., Malhotra, A., & Arunima. (1988). *The revised Bhatia Short Battery of Performance test of intelligence for adults*. Agra, India: National Psychological Corporation.

14 Neuropsychology in Japan

Angelica Isomura-Motoki and Masaru Mimura

Sociodemographics

Japan is an archipelago in Far East Asia consisting of over 3,000 islands. The largest four islands are Honshu, Hokkaido, Kyushu, and Shikoku, which account for 97% of the country's land mass. Japan's current population is estimated to be 127.4 million, the 10th largest in the world. The greater Tokyo area is the largest metropolitan area in the world, with over 30 million residents. Japanese society is linguistically and culturally homogeneous. Over 95% of the population is ethnically Japanese, with only a small population of foreigners, including Koreans, Chinese, Filipinos, and Brazilian Japanese. Ninety-nine percent of the people speak Japanese as their first language. The two major religions, Buddhism and Shintoism (ancestor worship), are practiced by 84% to 96% of the Japanese population.

Japanese government is a constitutional monarchy run by an elected prime minister and parliament. Similar to Great Britain, Japan also has a royal family with more symbolic versus political power. The national government is located in Tokyo. Japan is a modern society that boasts the world's second largest economy based upon nominal GDP at about US$4.5 trillion. The economic clout of Japanese society is illustrated in several areas. Japan has one of the most competitive educational systems, with approximately 75% of high school graduates continuing at universities or junior colleges. There is an excellent health care system, as evidenced by Japan having one of the highest life expectancy rates in the world, at 86.0 (female) and 79.2 (male) years of age. Japan is also a leader in scientific research, particularly in the areas of technology, machinery, and biomedicine.

Medical insurance system in Japan

The medical insurance and reimbursement system for clinical services in Japan is quite different from that in other countries, such as the United States. Payment for personal medical services is offered through a universal health care insurance system that provides relative equality of access, with fees set by a governmental committee. There are three kinds of health insurance in Japan: employer-based insurance, national health insurance administered by local governments for persons without employer-based insurance, and government-sponsored health insurance for the elderly. Therefore, medical services are delivered based on medical policy at the national level, and all medical services are reimbursed by the Japanese government. In general, all Japanese are provided with relative equality of access to the medical services and are also free to select physicians or facilities of their choice.

Japanese medical insurance is physician driven, and only services ordered by physicians can be reimbursed. Reimbursement is based upon a point system where each service is assigned a point that has been fixed at the national level.

Psychological practice

Clinical psychology is a relatively new discipline in Japan. As with many new developing professions, there are struggles with determining and regulating minimum qualifications for education, training, and credentialing.

Psychology began as an academic discipline focusing on research and theory. The first discipline-specific organization, the Japanese Psychological Association, was established in 1972 as a forum for academic psychologists. The subspecialty of clinical psychology is of more recent origin, but with different roots. It developed to meet the growing needs of persons with emotional problems who would benefit from psychotherapy and counseling. The predominant psychotherapeutic orientations of Japanese clinical psychologists are traditional psychoanalysis or Jungian analytical psychology, which have more of a philosophical versus research base in understandings of the human mind. In fact, clinical psychology as a field is not recognized as a science. The majority of clinical psychology graduate programs continue to be a part of literature departments, and some still consider the field to be a nonscience. Given its philosophical foundation, the scientific approach is frequently ignored, and discussions derived from philosophical ideas continue to exist today.

Although Western-based psychoanalysis has been the predominant form of therapy, a small number of professionals continue to utilize nonpsychological indigenous approaches, such as Morita therapy and Naikan therapy. Morita therapy is a treatment for neurosis that uses lifestyle change as a way of reducing obsessive thoughts. Naikan therapy emphasizes introspection to treat patients with neurosis and personality disorders. Both Morita and Naikan therapies reflect cultural values and are accepted by the professional community despite little support for the efficacy of treatment.

Given that clinical psychology is in its nascent stages in Japan, with ambiguity of whether it is a philosophy or science, it is not too surprising that there is a wide range of educational background among psychologists. The majority of older-generation clinical psychologists hold bachelor's degrees in psychology or related fields. Many of them have taken counseling courses/classes at private professional schools or workshops and have been supervised by experienced psychologists or psychiatrists who have been trained in psychoanalysis and the analytical psychology approach (Jungian approach). There are also clinicians who do not have degrees in psychology or related fields, but have had opportunities for training and currently work as psychological professionals in clinical settings. The trend, however, particularly for younger clinical psychologists, is to obtain a master's degree in clinical psychology or related fields; thus, educational expectations are becoming more standardized. Doctoral-level clinical psychologists are few, as most doctoral-level psychologists are academic researchers.

Unlike educational qualifications, training standards for Japanese clinical psychologists have been much more problematic, as expectations of clinical experiences for graduate students have not been defined. The majority of clinical psychology trainees do not receive much hands-on experience during practicum or internship, and many of them only have opportunities to observe clinical practice performed by medical professionals, including physicians, nurses, clinical psychologists, social workers, and case workers. This problem exists because psychology trainees are not generally considered to be "professionals in training" whose work can be beneficial to clinical training sites, and thus only small numbers of professionals are committed to train psychology students and interns. Instead, psychology trainees are generally perceived as a burden for professional clinicians due to the amount of time it requires for supervision. The end result is that the majority of psychologists lack solid clinical skills upon completion of their training and when beginning their professional careers. Inadequate training is a major hurdle for clinical psychologists to obtain credibility as an independent profession.

Given the state of education and training in Japanese clinical psychology, it is not surprising that a professional licensing system does not exist for clinical psychology.

Any individual can identify herself or himself as a psychologist, and clinicians who provide psychological services vary in their professional titles. Some examples of titles include counselor, psychotherapist, psychological consultant, mental health counselor, and clinical counselor.

For the last decade, a private organization known as the Japanese Certification Board for Clinical Psychologists has attempted to develop minimum standards for a certification process for professionals, educational programs, and training programs. The board has certified professionals meeting minimum educational and training criteria as clinical psychologists. This certification has become a standard for professionals who practice clinical psychology; however, it is not regulated by the legal system. Thus, noncertified psychology professionals can still practice psychology without legal restrictions. The board has also developed academic and practicum guidelines for clinical psychology graduate programs and issued accreditation for graduate programs that meet its standards. However, the monitoring system is still immature and the quality of training at a given clinical site is generally not reviewed or evaluated by the board. Thus, although the efforts of the Japanese Certification Board for Clinical Psychologists are a step in the right direction, there is still much to accomplish in the way of regulation for clinical psychology.

Clinical neuropsychology

Neuropsychology in Japan is primarily practiced in rehabilitation hospitals and clinics. The process is insurance, hence physician, driven, as they are the only ones who can technically be reimbursed for services by health insurance. In a typical referral, a physician will order the specific tests to be administered for a patient. For reimbursement,

Table 14.1 Three categories of psychological/neuropsychological tests

Easy to administer	*Difficult to administer*	*Extremely difficult to administer and analyze*
(80 points)	(280 points)	(450 points)
Raven's Colored	WAIS-III	Rorshach
Progressive Matrices	Bender Gestalt	WISC-IV
TAT	CLAC-II	SLTA (language)

he or she should theoretically administer the tests. However, in reality, other professionals, such as speech pathologists, occupational therapists, and psychologists, who are considered to be paraprofessionals, act as psychometrists for the treating physician. Historically, speech pathologists would be the discipline responsible for administering neuropsychological tests. Psychologists are relatively new to this field.

Psychological/neuropsychological tests are categorized into three levels depending on the complexity of administration and interpretation. Categories include (1) easy to administer (administration and interpretation take 40–60 minutes), (2) difficult to administer (administration and interpretation take 60–90 minutes), and (3) extremely difficult to administer and analyze (administration and interpretation take more than 90 minutes). Tests in category 1 can be reimbursed for 800 Japanese yen (approximately $6.70), tests in category 2 can be reimbursed for 2800 Japanese yen (approximately $24.30), and tests in category 3 can be reimbursed for 4500 Japanese yen (approximately $39.20). Moreover, psychological and neuropsychological services are only claimed and reimbursed once a month. Examples of tests that are listed in each category are presented in Table 14.1.

Once the test data are collected, the raw data are reported to the physician who will interpret the data and formulate diagnoses. No other discipline can perform this higher-level task, as the insurance companies will not pay for this service. Given these conditions, neuropsychological services delivered by speech pathologists, occupational therapists, and psychologists are not reasonably reimbursed for the time and labor spent for delivery of neuropsychology services.

Similar to clinical psychology, education and training issues exist in the subspecialty of neuropsychology. Currently, there is no undergraduate or graduate program that offers a comprehensive curriculum in neuropsychology, and thus clinicians must acquire their knowledge base and clinical skills through work experience and individual study. Unfortunately, training and supervision are limited and extremely varied. Many training sites do not even provide neuropsychological testing. The lack of adequate training for clinical neuropsychologists is problematic, as neuropsychological services are not available for all patients requiring services, and many do not even know that these options (i.e., neuropsychological services and cognitive rehabilitations) exist.

Neuropsychological tests

Neuropsychological tests include both adaptation of Western tests and indigenous developed instruments. There are only a few Western neuropsychological tests that are standardized and normed with the Japanese population; these include the Wechsler Intelligence Tests (WAIS, Fujita, Maekawa, Ohroku, & Yamanaka, 2006; WISC, Azuma et al., 1991), the Wechsler Memory Scale–Revised (WMS-R, Sugishita, 2000), and the Raven's Colored Progressive Matrices (Sugishita & Yamazaki, 1992). Many more Western assessment materials have been translated, with modifications for both clinical and research purposes; however, they have not been standardized or normed with the Japanese population. These tests include the Mini-Mental Status Examination, Trail Making Test Parts A and B, the Rey Auditory Verbal Learning Test (AVLT), the Wisconsin Card Sorting Test (WCST), and the Behavioral Assessment of the Dysexecutive Syndrome (BADS) (Kashima, 2003). Clinically, nonstandardization and lack of norms are problematic and result in numerous versions of the same test with different instructions and test materials. Clinicians thus are often required to qualitatively interpret the data or only report raw scores.

Since neuropsychology in Japan has roots in neurology and tests are interpreted by physicians, it is not surprising that indigenous tests are based upon neurological conceptualizations of abnormal brain functioning and use neurological terminology.

The first standardized indigenous test published in Japan was the Standard Language Test of Aphasia (SLTA, second revision; Japan Society for Higher Brain Dysfunction, 1997a). This comprehensive language battery was initially developed for speech pathologists evaluating language impairment in patients with cerebrovascular disease.

The test battery consists of many subtests evaluating listening, speaking, reading, writing, and calculation. The SLTA has undergone minor revisions over the years, and the SLTA together with SLTA supplementary tests (SLTA-ST) (Japan Society for Higher Brain Dysfunction, 1999a) continue to be the most frequently used by professionals in this field.

Another test developed by the Society for Higher Brain Dysfunction is the Standard Performance Test of Apraxia (SPTA; originally developed in 1975; revised by the Brain Function Test Committee of the Japan Society for Higher Brain Dysfunction, 1999). The SPTA is intended to systematically examine apraxia and related movement problems. Normative data allow an examiner to compare the profile of apraxic patients with that of healthy individuals and nonapraxic patients.

The Visual Perception Test for Agnosia (VPTA) was published in 1977 (revised by the Brain Function Test Committee of the Japan Society for Higher Brain Dysfunction, 1997b) to comprehensively evaluate visual agnosia and related perceptual problems. The VPTA test battery consists of six subtests and provides a systematical profile of visual perception by examining various visual perceptual domains.

The two most recently developed tests by the Brain Function Test Committee of the Society for Higher Brain Dysfunction are the Clinical Assessment for Attention (CAT) and the Clinical Assessment for Spontaneity (CAS) (Japan Society for Higher Brain Dysfunction, 2006). The CAT consists of seven subtests to capture different aspects of attention and concentration. The CAS consists of five different questionnaires, which can be completed by an examiner, an examinee, and a caregiver to provide perspective from different sources. The CAS allows the professional to qualify and quantify spontaneity of the patient.

History of neuropsychology research in Japan

During the Meiji Restoration in the late 1800s, Japan had been heavily influenced by Western ideas and technology, which was instrumental in developing the country into a modern technological society. Thus, the history of neuropsychological research has generally mirrored that of the West. The term *aphasia* was first introduced into Japanese medical journals in 1875, and in the next several decades, other terms of neurological symptoms, such as *apraxia* and *agnosia*, were translated to Japanese (Yamadori, 2004). Early Japanese researchers include Onishi, who in 1893 attempted to systematically map the pathology of aphasia. In the same year, Watanabe presented a case study of a patient with amyotrophic lateral sclerosis and its neuropsychological symptoms, focusing on dysarthria and inability of spontaneously expressive written language (Hamanaka, 2002).

During the 1930s, the interest of neurological and neuropsychological symptoms spread beyond language disorders. However, these reviews were neither systematically examined nor comprehensively operationalized. A seminal study was conducted by Imura (1943), who defined semantic dementia, or Gogi aphasia, in Japanese-speaking patients. This study piqued the interest of Western researchers and clinicians who had great interest in cases with language impairments that were unique to Japanese-speaking individuals and theoretical explanations of these cases.

The first comprehensive textbooks of neuropsychology were written by Hiroshi Ohashi in the 1960s: *Aphasia, Apraxia, Agnosia* (Ohashi, 1960) and *Clinical Neuropsychology* (Ohashi, 1965). The latter was the first book focusing on the clinical practice of neuropsychology and was highly influential in directing the future pathways of clinical neuropsychology in Japan. In the 1970s, three of Japan's oldest professional organizations were established: the Japanese Society of Aphasiology, which later changed its name to the Japan Society for Higher Brain Dysfunction (http://www.higherbrain.gr.jp); the Japanese Society of Neurology; and the Neuropsychology Association of Japan (http://www.neuropsychology.gr.jp) (Torii & Oyama, 2003). These societies continue to grow with annual meetings that provide neuropsychological researchers opportunities to present their research findings and exchange information among them. Both the Japan Society for Higher Brain Dysfunction and the Neuropsychology Association of Japan have good relations with the International Neuropsychological Society.

Specific contemporary neuropsychological research topics in Japan

Adult research

Traumatic brain injury (TBI) is a significant problem in Japan's industrialized society that has been receiving much media coverage. Over the past 10 years, the Japanese government has conducted systematic research on determining the extent of the problem and services required to treat this epidemic. The initial phase of the project was collecting epidemiological data of TBI at 10 different clinical sites, which was compiled into the Kumamoto Traumatic Coma Data Bank (K-TCDB) (Ishida, 2005).

Following the K-TCDB, the Ministry of Health, Labor, and Welfare conducted a five-year project from 2001 to 2006 with the goals of defining higher brain dysfunction, clarifying its diagnosis, and determining service needs for patients and families. The overall objective of the project was to develop nationwide welfare system services for facilitating independence and social participation of persons with cognitive/behavioral impairments. Based on these data, programs for medical rehabilitation and support systems by various communities have been developed. The effectiveness of these programs and support systems has also been evaluated, and evidence-based procedures introduced to various clinical settings to help the patients and their families. Another aspect of the project involved educating the public about TBI and higher brain dysfunction to facilitate identification and referral for treatment.

Geriatric research

Similar to other countries around the world, there has been an explosion of interest in geriatric neuropsychological research. This topic is of particular interest to Japanese researchers, as Japan's geriatric population, estimated to be 21%, is reported to be the highest in the world. The aging population has become one of the major problems in society because of its effects on the workforce and cost of medical care.

The leading geriatric research organization is the Japanese Psychogeriatric Society, which focuses on dementia research, including neuroimaging, cognitive rehabilitation, and patient care. Currently, mild cognitive impairment (MCI) has been receiving increased interest among researchers in this field. Longitudinal and community-based studies on MCI have been conducted in several regions in Japan, such as Miyagi, Ehime, and Ibaragi. The most well-known study is the Osaki-Tajiri Project conducted in Miyagi (Meguro, 2004; Meguro, Ishii, & Yamaguchi, 2006). This project has been evaluating cognitive changes of the participants and conversion from MCI to dementia since 1988. In addition, the Osaka-Tajiri Project has also provided comprehensive medical care and social support to the community.

Child research

Historically, children with developmental disabilities were assessed by speech pathologists to identify special needs children and make plans for cognitive rehabilitation. These evaluations, however, were problematic due to the lack of universal diagnostic criteria and sensitivity of testing for identifying cognitive deficits. In addition, services for identified special needs children were not provided on a systematic basis.

To address these problems, in 2005 the Ministry of Health, Labor, and Welfare issued an assistance act for children receiving special education and their families. It was the first law to clarify responsibilities of local government to provide services for people with special needs and assist them for independent living. Since this law was issued, research on developmental disabilities has drawn attention to identify specific needs and interventions for these children and clarify diagnoses of various developmental disabilities (Koeda, 2002; Oishi, 2002).

Summary

Psychology/neuropsychology is a nascent discipline within Japanese society with its own unique and interesting history and challenges to ensure growth, development, and respect among other health care professions. One of the major issues in clinical neuropsychology is the fact that there is no unified training model or guideline for trainees. Consequently, clinical skills of neuropsychology professionals vary, and one cannot expect a high quality of practice for all institutions. Further, a licensing system for clinical neuropsychologists does not exist. The field has been a multidisciplinary one, and roles of professionals who conduct neuropsychological assessment are undefined. This leads to the problem of neuropsychologists being unable to acquire credentials as an independent profession. Considering these challenges, it is critical for future neuropsychologists in Japan to establish a unique identity as an independent profession. In order to achieve this goal, it is necessary for the field to develop a training model for a clinical neuropsychologist, which includes not only academic courses but also a high standard of clinical training. Neuropsychology professionals must prove the importance of neuropsychological assessment in the process of treating patients with brain damage. Finally, the field of neuropsychology needs to be recognized not only by other medical professionals, but also by law and government, people, and society in general, that such services are useful and necessary for individuals with brain damage.

References

Azuma, H., Ueno, K., Fujita, K., Maekawa, H., Ishiguma, T., & Sano, H. (1991). *Wechsler Intelligence Scale for Children* (3rd ed.). Tokyo, Japan: Nihon Bunka Kagakusha.

Fujita, K., Maekawa, H., Ohroku, K., & Yamanaka, K., (Eds.). (2006). *Wechsler Adult Intelligence Scale* (3rd ed.). Tokyo, Japan: Nihon Bunka Kagakusha.

Hamanaka, T. (2002). Acceptance of Western neuropsychology of the 19th century in Japan. *Seishin-Igaku, 44*, 1119–1130.

Imura, T. (1943). Aphasia: Characteristics observed in Japanese. *Seishin-Shinkeigaku Zasshi, 47*, 196–218.

Ishida, A. (2005). *A practical guide to understanding traumatic brain injury and overcoming the resultant disabilities*. Tokyo, Japan: Ishiyaku Shuppan.

Japan Society for Higher Brain Dysfunction (Ed.). (1997a). *Standard Language Test of Aphasia: SLTA* (2nd rev.). Tokyo, Japan: Shinkoh Igaku Shuppan.

Japan Society for Higher Brain Dysfunction (Ed.). (1997b). *Visual Perception Test for Agnosia: VPTA*. Tokyo, Japan: Shinkoh Igaku Shuppan.

Japan Society for Higher Brain Dysfunction (Ed.). (1999a). *Supplementary Test for Standard Language Test of Aphasia: SLTA-ST*. Tokyo, Japan: Shinkoh Igaku Shuppan.

Japan Society for Higher Brain Dysfunction (Ed.). (1999b). *Standard Performance Test for Apraxia*. Tokyo, Japan: Shinkoh Igaku Shuppan.

Japan Society for Higher Brain Dysfunction (Ed.). (2006). *Clinical Assessment for Attention (CAT), Clinical Assessment for Spontaneity (CAS)*. Tokyo, Japan: Shinkoh Igaku Shuppan.

Kashima, H. (Supervisor of translation). (2003). *Behavioural Assessment of the Dysexecutive Syndrome* (Jpn. ed.). Tokyo, Japan: Shinkoh Igaku Shuppan.

Koeda, T. (2002). Language impairments in children: Current problems and situation. *Higher Brain Function Research*, *22*, 108–113.
Meguro, K. (2004). Comprehensive intervention for dementia: Possibility of cognitive rehabilitation. *Higher Brain Function Research*, *24*, 176–183.
Meguro, K., Ishii, H., & Yamaguchi, S. (2006). Community approach for mild cognitive impairment. *Japanese Journal of Geriatric Psychiatry*, *17*, 67–72.
Ohashi, H. (1960). *Aphasia, apraxia, agnosia*. Tokyo, Japan: Igaku-Shoin.
Ohashi, H. (1965). *Clinical neuropsychology*. Tokyo, Japan: Igaku-Shoin.
Oishi, N. (2002). Intervention for developmental dyslexia. *Higher Brain Function Research*, *21*, 185–193.
Onishi, T. (1893). About aphasia. *Japanese Journal of Geriatric Psychiatry*, *50*, 10–13.
Sugishita, M. (2000). *Wechsler Memory Scale* (rev.). Tokyo, Japan: Nihon Bunka Kagakusha.
Sugishita, M., & Yamazaki, K. (1992). *Raven's Colored Progressive Matrices*. Tokyo, Japan: Nihon Bunka Kagakusha.
Torii, H., & Oyama, Y. (2003). Neuropsychology Association of Japan. *Seishinigaku*, *102*, 706–711.
Yamadori, A. (2004). A very brief history of the Neuropsychological Association of Japan. *Japanese Journal of Neuropsychology*, *20*, 157–163.

15 Neuropsychology in Korea

Jeanyung Chey and Heyeon Park

Long and dynamic history of Korea

Korea is located in the northeast region of Asia in the Korean peninsula (see Figure 15.1). It borders China and Russia and is less than 200 miles from Japan across the East Sea. Koreans are generally very proud of their 4,000-year history, which began with the prehistoric kingdom of Gojoseon, followed by four periods of historic kingdoms: the three kingdoms period (B.C. 57~A.D. 676), the Unified Silla and Balhae period (A.D. 675~935), the Goryeo dynasty (A.D. 918~1392), and the Joseon dynasty (A.D. 1392~1910). In 1945, modern Korea was established after 35 years of Japanese colonial rule. The modern nation, however, was quickly divided into the South and the North, each endorsing capitalism and Communism, respectively. In 1950, the conflict resulted in a bitter war that lasted three years, and the two states have remained antagonistic with virtually no communication and mobility between the states until very recently. This chapter will focus on the neuropsychology of South Korea since no data on North Korean neuropsychology are available to date.

With a population of 48 million people, South Korea evolved into a dynamic and prosperous capitalistic society since the devastating Korean War, which ended in 1953. Despite periodic political or economic hardship during the past half century, it successfully joined the OECD in 1996, and its citizens have enjoyed political freedom since the early 1990s. The GDP of the nation is $1,201 billion, the fourteenth biggest economy in the world, and its per capita income is $24,801 (OECD, 2007).

Partly due to the expeditious growth in economy since the early 1960s, South Korea has experienced dynamic and rapid social change. Therefore, the psychological gap between the younger and the older generations is significantly greater than that in societies with more gradual change. For example, the elderly population of Korea was born in a mainly agricultural society that experienced frequent economic hardship. They experienced the difficult transition from a traditional Confusionist society to a modern nation that was fraught with colonial exploitation, war, poverty, and political upheaval. Since the modern education system was only in its infancy during their youth, a significant portion of the elderly population did not receive formal education, especially women. This is in sharp contrast to younger-generation Koreans, most of whom have received a high school education, and many college

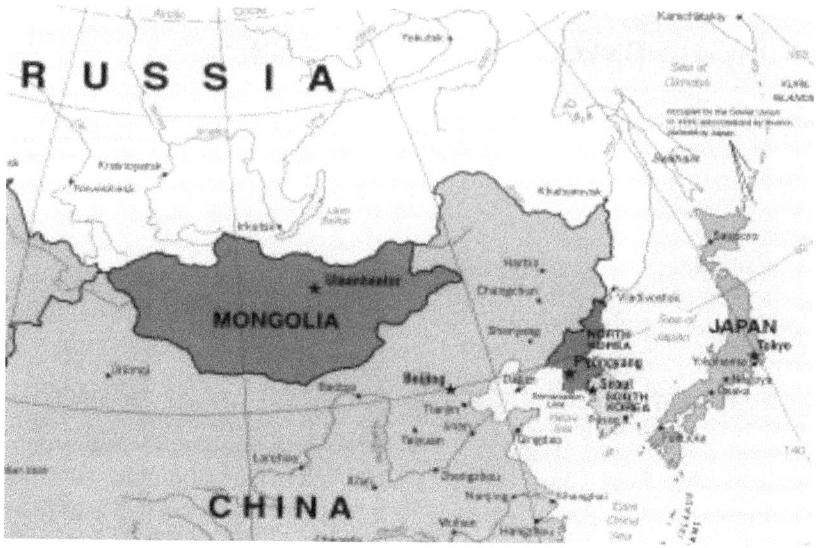

Figure 15.1 Korea is located in northeast Asia in the Korean penisula.

degrees. The percentage of people who received no formal education across the generation demonstrates how quickly Korea has evolved into a modern society. As Figure 15.2 illustrates that while 36% of the population in their seventies and 14% in their sixties did not attend school, less than 3% of the population younger than 60 received no formal education (Statistics Korea, 2005).

Brief history of neuropsychology

Several events preceded the birth of neuropsychology in Korea in the late 1980s and early 1990s. First and foremost, psychology as a field experienced major growth in Korea during the 1980s, like many sciences in the country, which partly can be accounted for by the steady growth of the South Korean economy. Psychology has demonstrated greater growth in the past 30 years than other scientific disciplines in Korea, probably due to increased awareness of the importance of psychology to human well-being. Clinical psychology grew the fastest. The number of Korean Psychological Association licensed clinical psychologists increased from 11 in 1977 to 507 in 2008 (see Figure 15.3).

Another significant event contributing to the growth of neuropsychology in Korea was the U.S. government's declaration of the decade of the brain for the 1990s, which was followed by similar pursuits in other countries. The nationwide support for brain research in the United States led to major advances in neurosciences, including neuropsychology, that underlined the importance of the brain mechanism and processes in human behavior and its disorders, and also promoted a clinical need for neuropsychology. Shortly before this initiative was implemented in the United States, a major influx of Korean students and clinicians began to

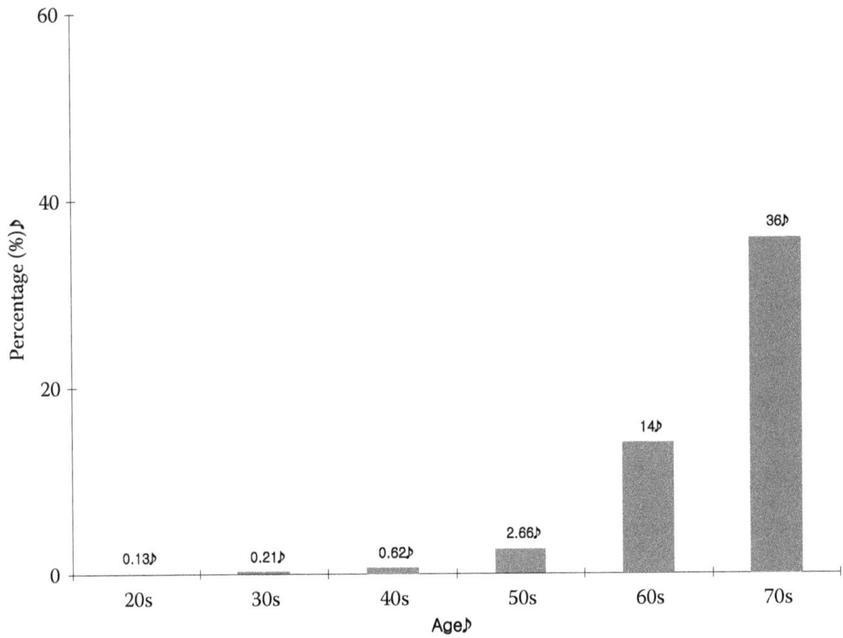

Figure 15.2 The percentage of people who received no formal education across generations. Note the drastic drop in rate in the populations who are less than sixty years old.

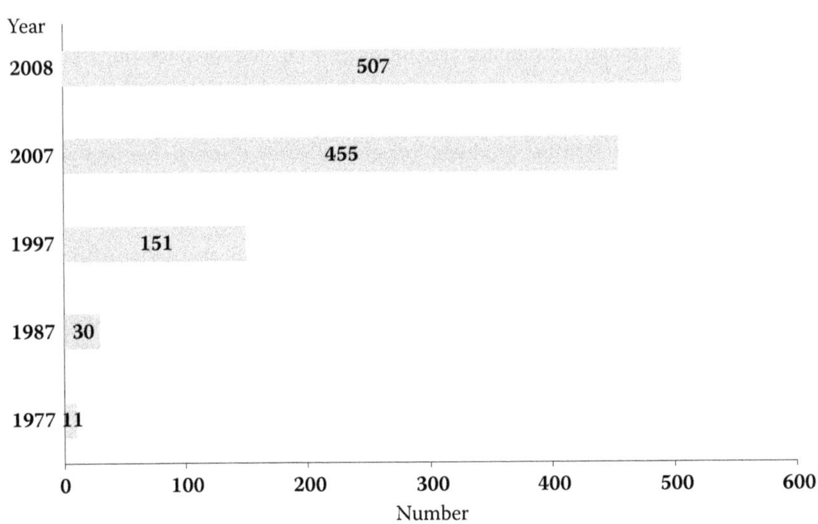

Figure 15.3 The cumulated number of Korean clinical psychologists. (*Source:* Korean Psychological Association, 2008.)

study and train abroad, especially in North America. Thus, the training of these students was heavily influenced by the *zeitgeist*. Upon completion of their study and training, many of these young scholars and clinicians returned to Korea, and introduced state-of-the-art science and technology to Korean psychology and other adjacent fields.

A third factor was the growing number of patients with brain disorders, such as head trauma, dementia, schizophrenia, and epilepsy, being evaluated in university hospitals, despite very few neuropsychological tools to be utilized. Thus, there existed a growing demand for neuropsychological services. The first official practice of clinical neuropsychology in Korea began in 1994, when a neuropsychology lab was instituted in the Neuroscience Center of Samsung Hospital. Neurologist Duk-Yeol Na and his colleagues invited Dr. Jeanyung Chey to open the nation's first clinical neuropsychology lab at the Department of Neurology.

Current practices

Korean neuropsychologists of the twenty-first century

The Society for Neuropsychology Research (SoNR) was founded in 1999 primarily by clinical neuropsychologists who have been at the frontier of Korean neuropsychology. Working as one of the research groups within the Korean Clinical Psychology Association, the goals of the Korean SoNR are to educate general clinical psychologists on current issues in neuropsychology, improve the practice of neuropsychology in Korean hospitals, and disseminate the latest knowledge from studies conducted on the Korean population. Dr. Yeon-Wook Kang at Hanlim University was the first president. She was succeeded by Dr. Jeanyung Chey at Seoul National University, Dr. Hyun-Soo Lee at Korea University Hospital, Dr. Hongkeun Kim at Daegu University Hospital, and Dr. Myunsun Kim at Sungshin Women's University. The society has successfully held quarterly workshops on various topics in neuropsychology.

Although three psychology graduate programs offer clinical neuropsychology, Hallym University, Seoul National University, and Sungshin Women's University, most clinical neuropsychology is practiced by clinical psychologists, and a handful of cognitive psychologists working with patients in hospitals. As in the United States, clinical psychologists are the only trained professionals who can evaluate patients' psychological functions comprehensively, including personality and emotional functions. Currently, there are no additional credentials to be earned in order to practice neuropsychology aside from the credentials of a clinical psychologist issued by the Korean Psychological Association, which requires a degree higher than the master's level in psychology and three years of clinical training.

Only a few sites offer formal neuropsychological training in Korea. Two neurology departments offer residency in Korea at this point, Samsung Seoul Hospital and Hallym University Sacred Heart Hospital, but a number of university hospitals are employing psychology graduates without a clinical psychology license to administer neuropsychological tests mostly as researchers. The vastly insufficient number of formal neuropsychological curricula and training, and the lack of advanced credentialing procedures are major challenges for Korean neuropsychology to overcome if it is to advance into a major professional field. A stronger professional relationship between the clinical neuropsychololgists and the medical community needs to be established in order to improve the quality of clinical practice. Further, systemic efforts from the Korean Clinical Psychological Association as well as the Korean SoNR are necessary in order for clinical neuropsychology to take a serious role in the clinical psychology community and Korean society in general.

Clinical populations of neuropsychology in Korea

Clinical populations in Korea are very similar to those found in the North American hospitals and clinics. In the 1970s and early 1980s, head trauma patients were one of the first populations to prompt clinical psychologists to search for neuropsychological tools to better assess existing cognition. It was, however, the increase in the dementia population due to aging of the society that really had a profound impact on how neuropsychology is practiced in Korea. A host of tests and assessment tools have been developed for the elderly population (see Tables 15.3 and 15.4), and major university hospitals employed clinical neuropsychologists or clinical psychologists to perform neuropsychological assessments on patients with dementia or age-related cognitive decline.

Neurosurgery patients, especially those suffering from intractable epilepsy, constitute another significant portion of the clinical population for neuropsychological evaluation, as well as patients with psychosis who might also undergo a traditional clinical psychological evaluation. The clinical need for the pediatric population is also growing rapidly in Korea. The main pediatric populations are children with attention-deficit hyperactivity disorder, learning disorder, and epilepsy. Patients with mental retardation, language disorder, and autism are also evaluated by clinical psychologists, and are often referred to special education professionals and speech-language therapists for further treatment and education.

Tests administered

Only a little more than a decade ago, clinical psychologists in Korea had to rely solely on intelligence tests, such as the Korean version of the Wechsler Adult Intelligence Scale–Revised, to assess patients with brain injury or diseases. Some informally translated versions of neuropsychological tests developed in North America were available, but few norms were established for the Korean population. Since then, however, a number of neuropsychological tools have been adapted and developed for the Korean populations, especially for the adult and elderly populations (see Figure 15.4 for the cumulative number of neuropsychological tests available for the Korean population). This change of events was propelled by the increasing number of clinical populations requiring neuropsychological assessment, and therefore a greater need for valid and efficient neuropsychological tools.

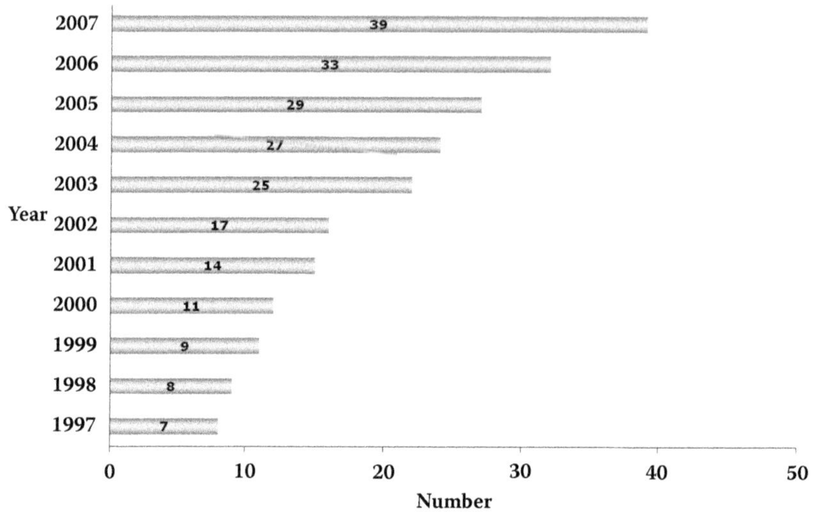

Figure 15.4 The cumulative number of neuropsychological tests published.

Adaptation and restandardization of the Western neuropsychological tools

The first phase of test development was mainly characterized by translation and adaptation of the Western neuropsychological tools and restandardization of the norms for the Korean population. During this period, Korean versions of the popular and user-friendly neuropsychological tools were developed, such as the Memory Assessment Scale (Lee, Ahn, & Jung, 1999; Williams, 1991), the Boston Naming Test (Kim & Na, 1997; Kaplan, Goodglass, & Weintraub, 1983), the Dementia Rating Scale (Chey, 1998; Mattis, 1973), and the CERAD (Woo et al., 2004; Morris et al., 1989). Similarly, it was common to compile a list of separate neuropsychological tools into a new battery that was appropriate for each clinical context. The Korean Benton Neuropsychological Assessment (Park, Kim, & Shin, 1996), the Rey-Kim Memory Test for Adults (Kim, 1999), and the Seoul Neuropsychological Screening Battery (Kang & Na, 2003) are popular examples. Since most Korean clinicians, including clinical psychologists, were new to neuropsychological assessment, the battery approach to neuropsychological assessment had instant appeal. Global cognitive function or memory indices given by these approaches were simpler for clinical psychologists to work with and provide interpretations.

As neuropsychology practice became more prevalent in Korea, a more process-oriented approach to neuropsychological assessment and tool development gained popularity. The process approach yielded more accurate and meaningful interpretations, as clinicians were able to parse out defective neuropsychological processes within a performance. The development of the Korean version of the California Verbal Learning Test (K-CVLT; Kim & Kang, 1997) and the children's version of the CVLT illustrate the newer trend of neuropsychological assessment in Korea (Table 15.2).

Indigenous test development

Korea, like many nations in Asia, has a unique language and cultural heritage that has had minimal interaction with the West until recently. Therefore, in order to understand and assess the Korean population accurately, clinicians need not only neuropsychological tools whose norms are based on the Korean population, but also those that are sensitive to the psychological differences in language, culture, and sociodemographics of Korea compared to Western countries. This is especially pertinent for the elderly population because the sociodemographics and culture are most discrepant in this age group as opposed to younger generations. Compared to the elderly population in North America and Europe, who grew up in the postindustrialized society, the elderly Koreans grew up in a predominantly agricultural society that valued Confucianism. During their childhood and adolescence, Westernized formal education was just beginning to take place in the communities, and a significant number of the elderly population did not attend school at all (Figure 15.2). Those with no formal education are mostly women, and some are illiterate. Considering the fact that Western neuropsychological tools were developed for elderly people who received a high school education, adaptation of Western neuropsychological tools proved to be insufficient in accurately evaluating this population. Frequently, normal elderly people with low educational background would perform so poorly that they met criteria for diagnoses of dementia or other brain disorders.

The Elderly Memory Disorder Scale (EMS; Chey, 2007) is one of the first efforts to develop neuropsychological tests to address the unique needs of a Korean population. More specifically, it was developed for the elderly Korean population, who are generally less educated. The tasks were made simpler and the materials consisted of familiar contents or themes for Koreans (e.g., Elderly Verbal Learning Test [EVLT], the Simple Rey Figure Test [SRFT], and the Story Recall Test [SRT]). Some tests included easier items (e.g., Digit Span and Spatial Span Tests [DSST]); other subtests utilized the testing-the-limits method of the Boston Process Approach (e.g., the EVLT, the SRT, the SRFT, the DSST, and the Clock Drawing Test). Not only do the subtests in EMS have smaller education effects than the Western tests, but test scores have been associated with volumes of the relevant brain regions in community-residing elderly Koreans (Chey, Na, Tae, Ryoo, & Hong, 2006.)

More recent efforts to develop novel paradigms to assess higher cognitive functions in the low-education population (Suk, Sa, & Chey, 2007) have been initiated. Since verbal conceptualization is an area in which persons with low education demonstrate significantly poorer performances than persons with at least a high school education, a test of nonverbal conceptualization, such as a proportional reasoning test, has been developed to assess conceptualization ability in this population, and has shown promise to actualize that goal.

Resource list

The tables mentioned below list published neuropsychological, intelligence, and achievement tests. A number of tests that have been developed, however, are not published, and thus this is not a comprehensive listing of the tests used in Korea today.

Tests of intelligence and general cognitive ability are presented in Table 15.1. These tests are administered to assess the overall cognitive functioning of an individual as well as serve as a database to infer premorbid intelligence (Lezak, Howieson, & Loring, 2004).

A summary of neuropsychological tests organized by function is presented in Table 15.2. Tests assessing memory and language have been developed more extensively than other functions, such as executive and higher-cognitive functions.

Many clinicians prefer screening tools or batteries that are developed for a particular population. Table 15.3 lists tests for special populations.

Questionnaires and rating scales used for gathering information on a client's everyday cognitive function and behavior are listed in Table 15.4.

Since brain disorders frequently affect the emotional functions and personality, the most widely used tests assessing these functions are presented in Table 15.5.

Overview of the literature

Adults

The earliest neuropsychological studies in Korea examined neuropsychological functions of psychiatric patients (Cho, 1982; Park, 1988; Moon, Oh, & Min, 1990). For example, studies examining schizophrenia found information processing deficits in attention (Moon et al., 1990; Pyo & Ahn, 1992a, 1992b), short-term memory (Cho, 1982; Jeong & Choi, 1987), and long-term memory (Kim, Jin, & Back, 1991; Park & Ahn, 1991) that were consistent with the findings at North American institutions. It is interesting that one of the first scientists in the United States to utilize cognitive psychology paradigms in schizophrenia research was the late Dr. Soon-Duk Koh, a University of Chicago psychopathologist who had previously been a professor at the Department of Psychology at Seoul National University (Koh, Kayton, & Schwartz, 1974; Koh, Kayton, & Berry, 1973; Koh, 1978).

The significant growth in neuropsychology during the mid-1990s is reflected in the contents of Korean psychology, psychiatry, and neurology journals. Neuropsychological studies on neurological patients, such as epilepsy patients (Jung & Choi, 1993; Jung, 1997), began to be published in the *Korean Journal of Clinical Psychology* and the *Journal of Korean Neurological Association* during this time. Reports on the validity and other issues concerning neuropsychological test development also appeared around this time (Kang, 1994; Kim & Kang, 1994, 1997; Jeun & Kang, 1994; Kim et al., 1995) as well. Since then, there has been a steady increase in the number of psychology journals publishing neuropsychological studies, such as the *Korean Journal of Clinical Psychology* and the *Korean Journal of Experimental and Cognitive Psychology*. Currently, more than 20 neuropsychological studies are published in

Table 15.1 Intelligence tests or tests that assess the general cognitive abilities

Name of the Test	*Authors*	*Characteristics*	*Publisher*	*Contact*
Korean Wechsler Adult Intelligence Scale (K-WAIS)	Tae ho Yum, Young Sook Park, Kyung Ja Oh, Jung Kyu Kim, Young Ho Lee	Korean version of WAIS-R	Korea Guidance	82-2-861-2161 www.guidance.co.kr
Korean Wechsler Intelligence Scale for Children-III (K-WISC-III)	Keum Joo Kwak, Hey Won Park, Cheong Tak Kim	Korean version of WISC-III	Special Education Publishing Co.	82-2-3280-0349 www.specialedu.co.kr
Korean-Wechsler Preschool and Primary Scale of Intelligence–Revised (K-WIPPI)	Hey Won Park, Keum Joo Kwak, Hey Won Park	Korean version of WPPSI-R	Special Education Publishing Co.	82-2-3280-0349 www.specialedu.co.kr
Korean Kaufman Assessment Battery for Children (K-ABC)	Su Baek Moon, Chang Jin Byun	Korean version of K-ABC (Kaufman & Kaufman, 1983)	Hakjisa	82-2-326-1500 www.hakjisa.co.kr
Korean-Leiter International Performance Scale–Revised (K-Leiter-R)	Soo Churl Cho, Min Sup Shin	Korean version of Leiter-R (in press)	Hakjisa	82-2-326-1500 www.hakjisa.co.kr
Korea Institute for Special Education–Korea Intelligence Test for Children (KISE-KIT)	Kyung Sook Park, Dong Young Chung, In Sook Jung	Korean intelligence test for children	Kyoyook-book	82-31-955-6956~8 www.kyoyookbook.co.kr
Multiple Intelligence Gardner School	Kyung Gwa Lee, Jin Yung Goh	Evaluate general intelligence of children	Mindpress	82-2-6221-0490 www.mindpress.co.kr
Korean Dementia Rating Scale (K-DRS)	Jeanyung Chey	Korean version of DRS (Mattis, 1988)	Hakjisa	82-2-326-1500 www.hakjisa.co.kr

Continued

Table 15.1 (Continued) Intelligence tests or tests that assess the general cognitive abilities

Name of the Test	*Authors*	*Characteristics*	*Publisher*	*Contact*
Korean Mini-Mental State Examination (K-MMSE)	Yeon Wook Kang, Duk L. Na, Hey Seung Han	Korean version of Mini-Mental State Examination (MMSE)		
Peabody Picture Vocabulary Test–Reedition (PPVT-R)	Young Tae Kim, Hye Sung Jang, Sun Sook Leem, Hyun Jung Baek	Korean version of PPVT-R	Seoul Community Rehabilitation Center	82-2-440-5700 www.seoulrehab.or.kr
Korean Coloured Progressive Matrices (K-CPM), Korean Standard Progressive Matrices (K-SPM)	Ho Chan Lim	Korean version of Raven's Progressive Matrices	Korea Guidance	82-2-861-2161 www.guidance.co.kr
Korean Cognitive Assessment System	Su Baek Moon, Young Jae Lee, Gwang Eung Yeo, Suck Hee Cho	Korean version of Cognitive Assessment System (Naglieri & Das, 1997)	Hakjisa	82-2-326-1500 www.hakjisa.co.kr

Table 15.2 The neuropsychological tests according to the functions assessed by the tools

Neuropsychological functions	*Name of the test*	*Authors*	*Publisher*	*Contact*
Multiple areas	Cognition Scale for Older Adults (CSOA)	Hong Keun Kim, Tae Yu Kim	Neuropsychology Publishing Co.	82-53-794-8138 www.neuropsy.co.kr
Multiple areas	Korean Benton Neuropsychological Assessment (K-BNA)	Bung Kyan Park, Jung Ho Kim, Dong Kyun Shin	Korea Guidance	82-2-861-2161 www.guidance.co.kr
Multiple areas	Korean-Leiter International Performance Scale–Revised (K-Leiter-R)	Soo Churl Cho, Min Sup Shin	Hakjisa (in press)	82-2-326-1500 www.hakjisa.co.kr
Multiple areas	Korean Luria-Nebraska Neuropsychological Battery for Children	Min Sup Shin	In press	shinms@snu.ac.kr
Sensation-perception	Korean Developmental Test of Visual Perception (K-DTVP-2)	Su Baek Moon, Gwang Eung Yeo, Tae Yong Cho	Hakjisa	82-2-326-1500 www.hakjisa.co.kr
Sensation-perception	Korean Test of Visual Perceptual Skills–Revised (K-TVPS-R)	Jung Min Kim	Special Education Publishing Co.	82-2-3280-0349 www.specialedu.co.kr
Attention	Korean Children's Color Trails Test (K-CCTT)	Min Sup Shin, Hun Jung Koo	Hakjisa	82-2-326-1500 www.hakjisa.co.kr
Attention	Korean Matching Familiar Figures Test (K-MFFT)	Nam Sung Kim, Hye Young Oh	Korea Guidance	82-2-861-2161 www.guidance.co.kr
Memory	Elderly Memory Disorder Scale (EMS)	Jeanyung Chey	Hakjisa	82-2-326-1500 www.hakjisa.co.kr

Continued

Table 15.2 (Continued) The neuropsychological tests according to the functions assessed by the tools

Neuropsychological functions	*Name of the test*	*Authors*	*Publisher*	*Contact*
Memory	Korean California Verbal Learning Test (K-CVLT)	Jung Ki Kim, Yeon Wook Kang	Special Education Publishing Co.	82-2-3280-0349 www.specialedu.co.kr
Memory	Korean Memory Assessment Scales (K-MAS)	Hyeon Soo Lee, Bung Kyan Park, Mi Ri Hae Kim, Chang Yil Ahn, In Kwa Jung	Korea Guidance	82-2-861-2161 www.guidance.co.kr
Memory	Rey-Kim Memory Test	Hong Keun Kim	Neuropsychology Publishing Co.	82-53-794-8138 www.neuropsy.co.kr
Memory	Rey-Kim Memory Test for Children	Hong Keun Kim	Neuropsychology Publishing Co.	82-53-794-8138 www.neuropsy.co.kr
Memory	Seoul Verbal Learning Test–Children version (SVLT-C)	Yeon Wook Kang	Human Brain Research & Consulting (in press)	82-2-6332-7447 www.humanbrainkorea.com
Memory	Seoul Verbal Learning Test–Elderly version (SVLT-E)	Yeon Wook Kang, Duk L. Na	Human Brain Research & Consulting (in press)	82-2-6332-7447 www.humanbrainkorea.com
Language	Korean version Boston Naming Test (K-BNT)	Hyang Hee Kim, Duk L. Na	Hakjisa	82-2-326-1500 www.hakjisa.co.kr
Language	Korean version Boston Naming Test for Children (K-BNT-C)	Hyang Hee Kim, Duk L. Na	Hakjisa	82-2-326-1500 www.hakjisa.co.kr

Language	Paradise-Fluency Assessment (P-FA)	Hyun Sup Sim, Moon Ja Sin, Eun Ju Lee	Paradise Institute for Children With Disabilities	82-2-2277-3296 www.paradise.or.kr
Language	Paradise · Korean version—The Western Aphasia Battery: (Paradise · K-WAB)	Hyang Hee Kim, Duk L. Na	Paradise Institute for Children With Disabilities	82-2-2277-3296 www.paradise.or.kr
Language	Peabody Picture Vocabulary Test–Reedition	Young Tae Kim, Hye Sung Jang, Sun Sook Leem, Hyun Jung Baek	Seoul Community Rehabilitation Center	82-2-440-5700 www.seoulrehab.or.kr
Executive function	Kim's Frontal-Executive Function Test	Hong Keun Kim	Neuropsychology Publishing Co.	82-53-794-8138 www.neuropsy.co.kr
Executive function	Kim's Frontal-Executive Function Test for Children	Hong Keun Kim	Neuropsychology Publishing Co.	82-53-794-8138 www.neuropsy.co.kr
Executive function	Korean STROOP/Color and Word Test–children's version	Min Sup Shin, Hun Jung Koo	Hakjisa	82-2-326-1500 www.hakjisa.co.kr
Reasoning	Korean Colored Progressive Matrices (K-CPM), Korean Standard Progressive Matrices (K-SPM)	Ho Chan Lim	Korea Guidance	82-2-861-2161 www.guidance.co.kr

Table 15.3 Screening tools or batteries for specific populations

Diagnostic group	*Name of the test*	*Authors*	*Publisher*	*Contact*
Dementia	7-Minute Screening Test–Korean version	Hyeong Mo Gu, Sun Gyu Go, Hye Jeong Go, Ui Jeong Kwon, Hyeong Seog Lee, Sang Yun Kim, Ji Hae Kim, Do Gwan Kim		khmpsy@hanmail.net
Dementia	Computerized Dementia Screening Test (CDST)	Sang-Yoon Kim, Jeanyung Chey, Belong Cho	Izentech	www. Izentech. com
Dementia	Korean Clinical Dementia Rating (CDR)	Korean Association for Geriatric Psychiatry		www.kagp.or.kr
Dementia	Korean Dementia Rating Scale (K-DRS)	Jeanyung Chey	Hakjisa	82-2-326-1500 www.hakjisa.cc.kr
Dementia	Seoul Neuropsychological Screening Battery (SNSB)	Yeon Wook Kang, Duk L. Na	Human Brain Research & Consulting	82-2-6332-7447 www.humanbrainkorea.com
Dementia	The Consortium to Establish a Registry for Alzheimer's Disease–Korean version (CERAD-K)	Ki Woon Kim, Sung Yun Kim, Ju Han Kim, Sung Il Woo, Jong In Woo, Jong Chul Yoon, Kang Wook Lee, Goon Hee Lee, Dong Youn Lee, Jung Hee Lee, Jin Hyung Ju, Sul Hee Han	Seoul National University Press	82-2-889-4424 www.snupress.com

Developmental disorders	ADHD Diagnostic System (ADS)	Kang Ui Hong, Min Sup Sin, Sung Jun Cho	IQBIG	82-2-552-1331 www.iqbig.co.kr
Developmental disorders	Korean Bayley Scales of Infant Development (K-BSID-II)	Bokhee Cho, Hyewon Park	KIDSPOP	82-2-3476-7004 www.i-lin.co.kr
Developmental disorders	Korean Developmental Indicators for the Assessment of Learning–3 (K-DIAL-3)	Byung Wun Jun, Gwang Soon Cho, Ki Hyun Lee, Eun Sang Lee, Jae Taek Leem	Special Education Publishing Co.	82-2-3280-0349 www.specialedu.co.kr
Developmental disorders	Korean version of Learning Disability Evaluation Scale	Min Sup Sin, Su Chul Cho, Gang Ui Hong	Hakjisa	82-2-326-1500 www.hakjisa.co.kr
Developmental disorders	Psychoeducational Profile–Revised (PEP-R)	Tae Lyun Kim, Lang Gyu Park	Special Education Publishing Co.	82-2-3280-0349 www.specialedu.co.kr
Developmental disorders	Sequenced Language Scale for Infants (SELSI)	Young Tae Kim, Kyung Hee Kim, Hye Lyun Yoon, Hwa Su Kim	Special Education Publishing Co.	82-2-3280-0349 www.specialedu.co.kr
Malingering	K-Malingering Diagnostic Test	Hong Keun Kim	Neuropsychology Publishing Co.	82-53-794-8138 www.neuropsy.co.kr

Table 15.4 Tests for evaluating emotion and personality

Name of the test	*Authors*	*Characteristics*	*Publisher*	*Contact*
Minnesota Multiphasic Personality Inventory–2 (Korean version)	Maumsarang	Korean version of MMPI-2	Maumsarang	82-2-511-1407 www.maumsarang.co.kr
Neuropsychiatric Inventory (Korean version)	Korean Association for Geriatric Psychiatry	Korean version of NPI	Korean Neuropsychiatric Association	www.knpa.or.kr
Symptom Checklist-90-R (Korean version)	Kwang Il Kim, Jae Hwan Kim, Ho Taek Won	Korean version of SCL-90-R		wonhotek@snu.ac.kr

Table 15.5 Miscellaneous neuropsychological tests or assessment tools

Name of the test	*Authors*	*Characteristics*	*Contact*
Seoul–Activities of Daily Living (S-ADL/S-IADL)	Doh Kwan Kim, Ji Hae Kim, Hyeong Mo Gu	Rating scales for elderly person's basic activities of daily living	khmpsy@nate.com
Literary Questionnaire	Jeanyung Chey	Evaluate level of literacy and classify functional illiteracy	jychey@snu.ac.kr
Handedness Inventory	Yeon Wook Kang	Assess lateral preference and cortical laterality	ykang@hallym.ac.kr
Elderly Cognition and Behavior Interview	Jeanyung Chey	Evaluate level of cognitive behavioral function by interviewing caretakers	jychey@snu.ac.kr
Samsung Dementia Questionnaire (SDQ)	Sung Hye Chey	Evaluate level of cognitive function and activities of daily living by interviewing caretakers	dukna@smc.samsung.co.kr
Korean Clinical Dementia Rating (CDR)	Korean Association for Geriatric Psychiatry	Korean version of CDR	www.kagp.or.kr

Korean Psychological Association journals annually, and many more neuropsychological studies on the Korean population are published in North American and international journals (e.g., *Neuropsychology, Neuropsychologia, Clinical Neuropsychologist, Brain Research, Journal of Neuroscience, Neurobiology of Aging*, etc.).

Geriatrics

Similar to many other countries, dementia is a prominent area of study in Korean geriatric neuropsychology. The first geriatric studies focused on test development for diagnosis and classification of the dementias, such as the Korean-Dementia Rating Scale (Chey & Lee, 1997; Chey, Na, Park, & Park, 1998) and the short forms of the Korean-Boston Naming Test (Kang, Kim, & Na, 1999; Park & Chey, 2000). Although many of the early Korean geriatric studies replicated findings from studies conducted in North America and Europe (Chey, Cho, & Kim, 2000), there have been unique findings that shed important implications on the development of dementia. The Cognitive Aging Study at Seoul National University, launched in 1998, examined risk factors for dementia in a nondemented community-residing Korean population for seven years. The study found that elderly with low cognitive performance (LCP) at baseline, who mostly had little education, demonstrated smaller brain volume at maximum maturity (Chey et al., 2006). Other lines of studies found that education effects on neuropsychological performance are much greater in Korean elderly than reported by North American studies (Chey, Na, Park, Park, & Lee, 1999; Kang, Na, & Han, 1997). It was concluded that neuropsychological evaluation of a person with low education, particularly for elderly suspected of having dementia, should involve age- and education-specific norms and also consider various issues associated with low education, such as illiteracy and socioeconomic status.

Children

The first pediatric populations studied with neuropsychological paradigms were children with attention-deficit hyperactivity disorder (ADHD) (Cheong & Oh, 1991; Koh, Shin, & Hong, 1996; Noh, Kim, Joung, & Hong, 1997; Chang & Shin, 1996; Song & Shin, 1998) and learning disorders (Chang & Shin, 1996; Lim, Kim, & Kim, 1997; Song & Shin, 1998). A study examining regional glucose metabolism and neuropsychological measures in ADHD patients illustrates collaborative efforts between clinical psychologists and medical staff (Kim, Lee, Shin, Cho, & Lee, 2002). Despite great interest in the pediatric population, only recently have children's versions of neuropsychological tests been developed and validated (Kang, 2003; Kim, 2006a, 2006b). These tools have empowered clinical psychologists to conduct rigorous studies in pediatric populations and further expand their service to other pediatric populations.

Summary

Neuropsychology is one of the fields in Korean psychology that has experienced dramatic accomplishment in recent years. In the early 1990s a small number of neuropsychologists initiated neuropsychological services to neurological and psychiatric patients, while universities began to offer neuropsychology courses in clinical psychology programs. No neuropsychological tools for the Korean population were available then, which was one of the many challenges facing the first generation of neuropsychologists in the country. Since then, almost 40 neuropsychological tools have been developed for the Korean population, and a number of universities offer neuropsychology classes or graduate programs. Further, many psychiatric and neurological patients receive neuropsychological services in hospitals and clinics around the country. This rapid and dynamic development of neuropsychology in Korea was largely propelled by the founding of the Society for Neuropsychology Research in 1999, which has been a major venue for educating in neuropsychology currently practicing clinical psychologists and trainees in hospitals and clinics. Despite many challenges facing Korean neuropsychologists today, the future of neuropsychology in Korea is promising in light of the increasing demand for neuropsychological services, the dedication of a number of neuropsychologists who have shared their knowledge with the Korean neuropsychological community, and the advancement of neuroscience in general.

References

Chang, E. J., & Shin, M. S. (1996). A comparative study on the cognitive deficits between the attention deficit/hyperactivity disordered children and learning disordered children. *Korean Journal of Psychopathology, 5*(1), 46–62.

Cheong, K. M., & Oh, K. J. (1991). Effects of task type and feedback on vigilance task performance of ADHD children. *Korean Journal of Clinical Psychology, 10*(1), 217–230.

Chey, J. (1998). *Korean-Dementia Rating Scale*. Seoul, Korea: Hakjisa.

Chey, J. (2007). *The Elderly Memory Disorder Scale*. Seoul, Korea: Hakjisa.

Chey, J., Cho, H., & Kim, J. (2000). Effects of apolipoprotein E phenotypes on the neuropsychological functions of community-dwelling elderly individuals without dementia. *Neuroscience Letters, 289*, 230–234.

Chey, J., & Lee, S. (1997). Development of the norms for the Korean-Dementia Rating Scale. *Korean Journal of Clinical Psychology, 16*(2), 423–433.

Chey, J., Na, D. G., Tae, W. S., Ryoo, J. W., & Hong, S. B. (2006). Medial temporal lobe volume of nondemented elderly individuals with poor cognitive functions. *Neurobiology of Aging, 27*, 1269–1279.

Chey, J., Na, D. L., Park, S., & Park, E. (1998). Validity and reliabilityof the Korean Dementia Rating Scale. *Korean Journal of Clinical Psychology, 17*(1), 247–258.

Chey, J., Na, D. L., Park, S., Park, E., & Lee, S. (1999). Effects of education in dementia assessment: Evidence from standardizing the Korean-Dementia Rating Scale. *The Clinical Neuropsychologist, 13*, 293–302.

Cho, S. W. (1982). A study on short-term memory in schizophrenics. *Korean Journal of Clinical Psychology, 3*(1), 65–74.

Jeong, J. B., & Choi, J. Y. (1987). The effects of ECT on visual reproduction and generic memory. *Korean Journal of Clinical Psychology, 6*(1), 42–47.

Jeun, D. I., & Kang, Y. (1994). A validity study on the Raven Progressive Matrices Test as an intelligence test. *Korean Journal of Clinical Psychology, 13*(1), 65–81.

Jung, A. J. (1997). Results on the neuropsychological test of temporal lobe epileptics. *Korean Journal of Clinical Psychology, 16*(1), 199–207.

Jung, J. B., & Choi, J. Y. (1993). Cognitive performances and psychiatric symptoms in epilepsy. *Korean Journal of Clinical Psychology, 12*(2), 105–112.

Kang, Y. (1994). Who is left-handed? Measurement of handedness in Koreans. *Korean Journal of Clinical Psychology, 13*(1), 97–113.

Kang, Y. (2003). A normative study of the Seoul Verbal Learning Test–Children's version (SVLT-C). *Korean Journal of Clinical Psychology, 22*(2), 435–448.

Kang, Y., Kim, H. H., & Na, D. L. (1999). A short form of the Korean-Boston Naming Test (K-BNT) for using in dementia patients. *Korean Journal of Clinical Psychology, 18*(2), 125–138.

Kang, Y., & Na, D.L. (2003). *Seoul Neuropsychological Screening Battery*. Incheon, Korea: Human Brain Research & Consulting.

Kang, Y., Na, D. L., & Han, S. (1997). A validity study on the Korean Mini-Mental State Examination (K-MMSE) in dementia patients. *Journal of the Korean Neurological Association, 15*(2), 300–308.

Kaplan, E., Goodglass, H., & Weintraub, S. (1983). *Boston Naming Test*. Philadelphia, PA: Lee & Febiger.

Kim, B. N., Lee, J. S., Shin, M. S., Cho, S. C., & Lee, D. S. (2002). Regional cerebral perfusion abnormalities in attention deficit/hyperactivity disorder. *European Archives of Psychiatry and Clinical Neuroscience, 252*(5), 219–225.

Kim, E. K., Park, B. K., Chung, Y. C., Shin, D. K., Bae, H. S., & Ko, B. H. (1995). The clinical application of Benton Neuropsychological Assessment: Focusing on qualitative analysis. *Korean Journal of Clinical Psychology, 14*(1), 219–235.

Kim, H. (1999). *Rey-Kim Memory Test, professional manual*. Taegu, Korea: Neuropsychology.

Kim, H. (2006a). *Children's Rey-Kim Memory Test*. Seoul, Korea: Neuropsychology.

Kim, H. (2006b). *Children's Kim's Frontal-Executive Function Neuropsychological Test*. Seoul, Korea: Neuropsychology.

Kim, H., & Na, D. L. (1997). *The Korean-Boston Naming Test (K-BNT)*. Seoul, Korea: Hakjisa.

Kim, J. K., & Kang, Y. (1994). A validity study on the Korean version of the California Verbal Learning Test (K-CVLT). *Korean Journal of Clinical Psychology, 13*(1), 82–96.

Kim, J. K., & Kang, Y. (1997). Korean-California Verbal Learning Test (K-CVLT): A normative study. *Korean Journal of Clinical Psychology, 16*(2), 379–395.

Kim, Y. H., Jin, Y. S., & Back, Y. M. (1991). A study on memory clustering and the effect of mnemonic strategy in schizophrenics. *Korean Journal of Clinical Psychology, 10*(1), 170–185.

Koh, S. D. (1978). Remembering of verbal materials by schizophrenic young adults. Language and cognition. In S. Schwartz (Ed.), *Schizophrenia* (pp. 59–69). Hillsdale, NJ: Erlbaum.

Koh, S. D., Kayton, L., & Berry, R. (1973). Mnemonic organization in young non-psychotic schizophrenics. *Journal of Abnormal Psychology, 81*, 299–310.

Koh, S. D., Kayton, L., & Schwartz, C. (1974). The structure of word-storage in the permanent memory of nonpsychotic schizophrenics. *Journal of Consulting and Clinical Psychology, 42*, 879–887.

Koh, S. H., Shin, M. S., & Hong K. E. (1996). A study of attention problems and cognitive characteristics on KEDI-WISC and TOVA in children with psychiatric disorders. *Korean Journal of Clinical Psychology, 15*(1), 165–178.

Lee, H. S., Ahn, C. Y., & Jung, I. K. (1999). A preliminary study on standardization of K-MAS (Korean version of Memory Assessment Scales). *Korean Journal of Clinical Psychology, 18*(1), 221–241.

Lezak, M. D., Howieson, D. B., & Loring, D. W. (2004). *Neuropsychological assessment* (4th ed.). New York, NY: Oxford University Press.

Lim, Y. R., Kim, J. H., & Kim, S. T. (1997). The Cognitive-neuropsychological characteristics of the learning disorder subtypes. *Korean Journal of Clinical Psychology, 16*(1), 53–73.

Mattis, S. (1973). *Dementia Rating Scale, professional manual.* Odessa, FL: Psychological Assessment Resources.

Moon, H. S., Oh, K. J., & Min, S. K. (1990). Attention deficit of schizophrenic patients on continuous performance tests. *Korean Journal of Clinical Psychology, 9*(1), 77–86.

Morris, J. C., Heyman, A., Mohs, R. C., et al. (1989). The consortium to establish a registry for Alzheimer's disease (CERAD): I. Clinical and neuropsychological assessment. *Neurology, 39,* 1159–1165.

Noh, J. S., Kim, J. H., Joung, Y. S., & Hong, S. D. (1997). A study for diagnostic discrimination of T.O.V.A. and GDS in attention-deficit/hyperactivity disorder. *Korean Journal of Clinical Psychology, 16*(2), 355–365.

OECD (2007). Country statistical profiles. Retrieved March 3, 2009 from http://stats.oecd.org/Index.aspx?DataSetCode=CSP2009

Park, B. K., Kim, J. H., & Shin, D. K. (1996). *Korean Benton neuropsychological assessment.* Seoul, Korea: Korea Guidance.

Park, E., & Chey, J. (2000). A normative study of the short-form Korean-Boston Naming Test. *Korean Journal of Cognitive Neuroscience, 18*(2), 102–108.

Park, K. (1988). Memory for scripts in positive and negative schizophrenia. *Korean Journal of Clinical Psychology, 7*(1), 53–61.

Park, K., & Ahn, C. Y. (1991). Prose memory and mental process of comprehension in positive and negative schizophrenia. *Korean Journal of Clinical Psychology, 10*(1), 186–205.

Pyo, G. Y., & Ahn, C. Y. (1992a). The impact of distractors on perceptual organization in schizophrenic patients. *Korean Journal of Clinical Psychology, 11*(1), 115–131.

Pyo, G. Y., & Ahn, C. Y. (1992b). Search asymmetry in schizophrenic patients. *Korean Journal of Clinical Psychology, 11*(1), 132–144.

Song, J. Y., & Shin, M. S. (1998). Differences between reading disabilities and ADHD on K-LDES. *Korean Journal of Clinical Psychology, 17*(1), 185–196.

Statistics Korea (2005). Statistical database. Retrieved March 3, 2009 from http://kosis.kr/eng.

Suk, J., Sa, S., & Chey, J. (2007). Proportional reasoning abilities: A potential neuropsychological function sensitive in detecting dementia in elderly populations with low educational background.

Williams, J. M. (1991). *Memory assessment scales. Professional manual.* Odessa, FL: Psychological Assessment Resources.

Woo, J. I., Kim, K. W., Kim, S. Y., Kim, J. H., Woo, S. I., Yoon, J. C., … Han, S. H. (2004). *The consortium to establish a registry for Alzheimer's disease—Korean version.* Seoul, Korea: Seoul National University Press.

16 Neuropsychology in Malaysia

Normah Che Din

Brief description of Malaysia

Malaysia is a tropical country located in the heart of Southeast Asia. It comprises the southern tip of peninsular Malaysia and the western and northern sections of Borneo, and covers approximately 330,000 km^2. This strategic position enticed traders from major powers that dominated the region throughout its history. Malaysia was described in both legend and literature of India, China, Greece, and Rome as a golden land of mineral and forest riches (*suvarnabumi* in Sanskrit and the Golden Chersonese in ancient Greek). In fact, Chinese, Indian, Dutch, Portuguese, and British communities have survived into the present and bear testimony to Malaysia's leading role as a trading center centuries ago (Deva, 2004).

Malaysia gained independence from British rule in 1957. The name *Malaysia* was adopted in 1963 when the Federation of Malaya (Malay: *Persekutuan Tanah Melayu*), Singapore, Sabah, and Sarawak formed a 14-state federation. Singapore was expelled from the federation in 1965 and subsequently became an independent country. Currently, Malaysia consists of 13 states and 2 federal territories. Nine of the states are ruled by nine sultanates, two states governors, and two federal territories.

Malaysia is currently embarking on an ambitious effort to become a developed country by 2020.

The economy has changed from one producing raw material to one manufacturing consumer goods and services. The per capita income, which was under US$1,000 at independence, has now surpassed US$4,000, and the gross national product is over US$100 billion. With the strengthening economy, the government has been able to overhaul the colonial health system and provide better services for its people. For example, improvements in health care have resulted in low infant mortality rates and an increased life expectancy that has recently crossed the 70-year mark (Deva, 2004). Increases in expenditures for education have improved the literacy rates in both adults (1980, 71.2%; 2003, 88.9%) and children (1980, 90%; 2004, 97.2%) (Globalis, 2008).

Demographics

Malaysia is a highly diverse society with a population of 24 million. Indigenous peoples, including Malays, Ibans, Dayaks, Kadazan-Dusun, and a variety of tribes in the east and west, comprise about 54% of the population. The remaining 46% are of immigrant Chinese, Indian, Pakistani, Sri Lankan, Thai, Filipino, Indonesian, and Eurasian (and others in small numbers) origin. Demographically, Malaysia is a young nation. More than 33% of the population are under 12 years of age, and a further 19% are aged 12–24. Over 60% of the population live in rural areas.

Neuropsychology in Malaysia

Clinical psychology is a nascent discipline in Malaysia, with postgraduate education beginning in 1994. Currently, only two universities, the Universiti Kebangsaan Malaysia and International Islamic University of Malaysia, offer programs in clinical psychology. Practice requirements include completion of a master's degree in psychology and a practicum supervised by a clinical psychologist. Clinical neuropsychology is a subspecialty of clinical psychology, with training only offered at Univeriti Kebansaan. There are no specific credentials for practicing neuropsychological services in Malaysia. Since 1994, the Universiti Kebangsaan Malaysia has produced 10 groups of clinical psychologists, with 30 clinical psychologists receiving training in neuropsychology.

Neuropsychological services have been provided primarily to adult and elderly populations and rarely to the children. Adult populations include persons suffering from epilepsy, head injury, stroke, HIV/AIDS, and memory impairments. Elderly patients are usually referred for neuropsychological assessments to rule out a dementia. Courts are another common referral source.

Tests administered

Thus far, Malaysian neuropsychological tests have generally been adaptations of Western tests. The most commonly administered tests include the Wechsler Adult Intelligence Scale–Revised and Third Edition (WAIS-R; Wechsler, 1981; Wechsler, 1997), Wechsler Memory Scale–Revised (Wechsler, 1987), Clock Drawing Test (Freedman et al., 1994), Elderly Cognitive Assessment Questionnaire (ECAQ; Kua & Ko, 1992), Mini-Mental Status Examination (MMSE; Folstein, Folstein, & McHugh, 1975), Benton Visual Retention (BVRT; Benton-Sivan & Spreen, 1996), Rey Auditory Verbal Learning Test (RAVLT; Rey, 1958), Dementia Rating Scale (Mattis, 1976), Wisconsin Card Sorting Test (WCST, Heaton, 1981), Rivermead Behavioral Memory Test (Cockburn & Smith, 1989), Blessed Functional Rating Scale (BFRS; Blessed, Tomlinson, & Roth, 1968), Raven's Progressive Matrices (Raven, 1938), and Trail Making Test (TMT; Reitan, 1992). These tests have been translated into Malay, normed on local samples, and evaluated for reliability and validity. The following are examples of test adaptations and psychometric studies.

The two most common neuropsychological tests administered in Malaysia are the WAIS-R and the WISC. The author and colleagues translated these tests into Malay. Several of the items were modified to increase the face validity and reduce content bias (see Table 16.1).

Table 16.1 The Malaysian substitute items for the information subtest of the WAIS-R

	Malaysian items	*Acceptable responses*
Information subtest		
1	What are the colors of the Malaysian flag?	White, red, yellow, blue
6	Name four men who have been the prime minister of Malaysia since 1957.	Tengku Abdul Rahman, Tun Razak, Tun Dr. Ismail, Dr. Mahadir Muhamad
8i	Who is P. Ramlee?	Singer, actor, musician, director
9	In what direction would you travel if you went from Malaysia to Australia?	Southwest
13	Who was the prime minister of Malaysia during the confrontation between Malaysia and Indonesia?	Tun Abdul Razak
14	Who is Ibu Zain?	Author
23	How far is it from Kuala Lumpur to Singapore?	400–500 km
27	What is the population of Malaysia?	24–26 million

The internal consistency of the WAIS-R in a sample of 47 epilepsy patients was very high (Cronbach's alpha = .91) (Normah, Saralla, Azlinawati, & Raymond, 2008). Construct validity for the Malay population was established by correlating WAIS-R scores to level of education (r = .48 to .67), years of formal education (r = .47 to .62), and neuropsychological tests such as the RAVLT (r = .18 to .64), BVRT (r = .37 to .46), TMT Part A (r = –.54 to –.57), and TMT Part B (r = –.55 to –.56) (Table 16.2).

The Rey Auditory Verbal Learning Test (RAVLT) is another widely used neuropsychological test in Malaysia. It was translated verbatim into Malay language despite

Table 16.2 The construct validity of the modified WAIS-R for Malaysian population

	Verbal IQ	*Performance IQ*	*Full-scale IQ*
Years of education	.62**	.47**	.60**
Level of education	.67**	.48**	.65**
RAVLT trial 1	.18	.19	.20
RAVLT trial 2	.44**	.48**	.50**
RAVLT trial 3	.58**	.58**	.62**
RAVLT trial 4	.57**	.53**	.59**
RAVLT trial 5	.59**	.60**	.64**
RAVLT trial 6	.46**	.46**	.52**
RAVLT trial 7	.49**	.43**	.50**
BVRT	.46**	.37*	.46**
TMTA	–.54**	–.55**	–.57**
TMTB	–.55**	–.56**	–.52**

* $p < .05$.
** $p < .01$.

Table 16.3 The original RAVLT (list I and list II) and two new Malay lists (list IA and IIA)

List I	*List IA*	*List II*	*List IIA*
Drum	Dram	Desk	Meja
Curtain	Langsir	Ranger	Askar
Bell	Loceng	Bird	Burung
Coffee	Kopi	Shoe	Kasut
School	Sekolah	Stove	Dapur
Parent	Ibu	Mountain	Gunung
Moon	Bulan	Glasses	Cermin
Garden	Taman	Towel	Tuala
Hat	Topi	Cloud	Awan
Farmer	Petani	Boat	Perahu
Nose	Hidung	Lamb	Kambing
Turkey	Ayam	Gun	Senapang
Color	Warna	Pencil	Pensil
House	Rumah	Church	Masjid
River	Sungai	Fish	Ikan

differences in word lengths, commonalities, and equivalencies across languages (Table 16.3).

Reliability was developed through determining the internal consistency of items in a group of adolescents (Cronbach's alpha = .88) (Normah, Nursan, & Mahadir, 2005) and adults (Cronbach's alpha = .91) (Normah, Saralla, et al., 2008) with epilepsy and in a study among 226 police officers at the Police Training Centre, Kuala Lumpur (Cronbach's alpha = .86). Validity was determined by correlating RAVLT Trials II to IV and the Immediate and Delayed Recall with Verbal Paired Associate I (Immediate Recall) (r = .14 to .37) and Verbal Paired Associate II (Delayed Recall) (r = .24 to .30) of the Wechsler Memory Scale–Revised (Normah, Khairiyah, et al., 2008) (Table 16.4).

The Trail Making Test (TMT) is widely employed for diagnosing brain damage, screening for cognitive impairment, and assessing simple cognitive processing speed

Table 16.4 Concurrent validity of RAVLT with the verbal paired associates I and II of WMS-R

RAVLT	*WMS-R immediate recall*	*WMS-R delayed recall*
Trial 1	.039	.037
Trial 2	.136*	.097
Trial 3	.301**	.274**
Trial 4	.365**	.290**
Trial 5	.280**	.241**
Trial 6 (distraction list)	.039	.079
Trial 7 (immediate recall)	.372**	.299**
Trial 8 (delayed recall)	.314**	.284**

and mental flexibility (Perianez et al., 2007; Groth-Marnat, 2000). A reliability and validity study was conducted among 227 police officers who attended a six-month training at the Police Training Centre, Kuala Lumpur. Six versions of the TMT were administered, Parts A, B, C, D, B_N, and A_{N+L}. The time to complete Trails A was the fastest, with an average of 32.86 ± 11.99 seconds, followed by the time to complete Trails A_{N+L} (52.06 ± 19.81 seconds), while Trails B took the longest time to complete (70.52 ± 27.31). An alternate form of reliability was analyzed by correlating Forms A and C ($r = .39$, $p < .01$) and TMT Parts B and D ($r = .49$, $p < .01$). Validity was determined by demonstrating that Parts A and B are measuring different constructs. Two characteristics of each test were measured for each trial. Trail lengths were determined by measuring the distances between targets in Parts A and B. Visual interference was quantified by counting the number of targets not in sequence within 3 cm of the path between each target. The result indicated significant differences between the speed of each Trial ($F = 166.28$, $p < .01$). The total number of visual interference for Trails B was found to be significantly greater than that for Trails A ($t = -2.52$, $p < .05$) (Normah, Khairiyah, et al., 2008a).

The Mini-Mental State Examination (MMSE) (Folstein et al., 1975) is the most widely used cognitive screening tool in Malaysia. The initial translation and validation study in Malaysia was conducted by Zarina and Zahiruddin (2004) on 185 elderly subjects recruited from various senior homes in Kota Bharu, Penang, Tanjung Rambutan, and Kuala Lumpur. The mean total score of MMSE was 17.78 ± 4.51 (score ranged from 7 to 27). The Pearson correlation with the Clock Drawing Test showed a positive relationship ($p < .000$). Other studies have provided further validity for the Malaysian MMSE. In a study with 67 stroke patients who attended their follow-up at the Neurology Outpatient Clinic and Stroke Rehabilitation Centre, the mean MMSE score was 24.33 ± 7.30. No differences were found between acute and chronic stroke patients. The MMSE was highly correlated with the Dementia Rating Scale ($r = .649$, $p < .01$) and negatively correlated with the Blessed Rating Scale ($r = -.29$, $p < .05$), General Health Questionaire–12 ($r = -.36$, $p < .01$), and Beck Depression Inventory ($r = -.30$, $p < .05$) (Normah et al., 2007). Normah, Khairiyah et al. (2008) administered the MMSE to 226 police officers at the Police Training Centre, Kuala Lumpur. The mean MMSE score was 29.19 ± .97, with almost zero variability among the subjects. MMSE was found to have low association with the test of verbal short-term memory (RAVLT) ($r = 0.03$ to 0.16), nonverbal short-term memory (BVRT) ($r = 0.08$), and the test of psychomotor speed (Trail Making Test) ($r = 0.06$ to 0.17).

Raven's Progressive Matrices (RPM) is a test of nonverbal reasoning and problem solving that is purported to be a culture-fair test (Raven, 1938). RPM was validated in Malaysia by Chiam (1994, 1995), who tested 5,384 subjects ranging from 7 to 12 years in age. The mean score obtained was 89 (mean = 100, *sd* = 15), which is lower in comparison to the British and U.S. norms (Raven, 2000). A subset of 1,459 Chinese Malaysians had a mean score of 99, which is higher than the total sample (Chiam, 1994). No differences were found between genders at each age level (Lynn & Irwing, 2004).

Indigenous test development

Many tests that have been developed in Malaysia are not related to neuropsychological evaluation. Two indigenous intelligence tests were developed by a group of researchers from the Faculty of Education, Universiti Kebangsaan Malaysia. One of the tests is the Malaysian Multiple Intelligence Test (MAMIT) (Ariffin et al., 2006), which is based upon Gardner's (1983) conceptualization of many autonomous intellectual competencies. The MAMIT measures nine domains of intelligence: naturalist, spatial, interpersonal, intrapersonal verbal linguistics, mathematical logic, music, bodily kinesthetic, and spiritual intelligence.

It consists of 165 items and is scored according to multiple measuring methods, such as symbol matching, open-ended questions, picture arrangements, mathematical questions, plan drawings, multiple-choice questions, map reading, calligraphy, weaving, and dichotomous questions. The MAMIT is available online at http://www.ukm.my/mamit with an automatic scoring system in a profile form. The candidate's individual profile will be compared with the Standard Malaysian Multiple Intelligences Profile. This profile will assist individuals to identify their strong and weak intelligences, and a therapist will be able to devise an intervention program. An important application of the MAMIT is assisting teachers to individualize their approaches to each student by recognizing individual study patterns and employing teaching styles to accommodate a student's talents and abilities.

Another nontraditional indigenous IQ test is the Malaysian Emotional Intelligence Inventory System (MEQI), which is based on the concept proposed by Salovey and Mayer (1990). It was developed by a team of eight researchers headed by Dr. Noriah Mohd Ishak, an associate professor from the Faculty of Education, Universiti Kebangsaan Malaysia. The MEQI measures four aspects of emotional intelligence: self-awareness, self-regulation, self-motivation, and social skills. It was validated on a sample of 4,000 persons and has three versions, targeting adults, students of higher learning institutes, and adolescents. Mohd Ishak et al. (2004) envisioned the MEQI as a useful tool for selection processes in business and institutes of higher learning by identifying individuals with strong interpersonal and leadership characteristics.

The MAMIT and MEQI differ from traditionally Western-developed intelligence tests that measure general intelligence, or *g*. It is believed that these Western tests are inadequate to measure the intelligence of Malaysia's ethnically diverse society. Indeed, there is some evidence that Malays think differently than Western societies. Western cultures are purported to be more individualistic, analytical, and context independent, the latter describing a tendency to focus on objects and their attributes. By contrast, collectivist cultures tend to think holistically and are more context dependent in the sense that attention is focused on the relations between objects and their entire fields (Kim & Markus, 1999; Kühnen, Hannover, & Schubert, 2000; Nisbett, Peng, Choi, & Norenzayan, 1999). Cognitive differences between cultures are supported in a study by Kühnen et al. (2001), who compared performances on the Embedded-Figure Test (EFT) (Witkin, 1950) between two individualist cultures (United States and Germany) and two collectivist cultures (Malaysia and Russia).

The EFT measures field dependence, which is the ability to detach simple geometrical figures from more complex geometrical patterns in which they are embedded. Results indicated that the Malaysian and Russian samples were more field dependent than the United States and German samples.

Resource lists

Universiti Kebangsaan Malaysia: http://www.ukm.my/mamit
Malaysian Journal of Psychiatry: http://www.psychiatry-malaysia.org
Jurnal Pendidikan Malaysia: http://www.penerbit.ukm.my/jpend.htm
Medical Journal of Malaysia: http://mma.org.my/medical-journal-of-malaysia
Malaysian Journal of Medical Sciences: http://www.medic.usm.my/publication/mjms/
Singapore Medical Journal: http://www.openj-gate.org/Articlelist
Malaysia: http://.en.wikipedia.org/wiki/Malaysia; www.gov.my/; https://cia.gov/library/publication/the-world-facthood/geos/my.html
Department of Statistics Malaysia: http://www.statistics.gov.my
Malaysian Institute of Road Safety Research: http://www.miros.gov.my/

Research: Children

Malaysian studies on children have generally been conducted on special education students in the school system. Studies are primarily descriptive in nature, focusing on epidemiology, diagnosis, interventions, and symptoms of populations with neurological disorders. A minority of the studies include neuropsychological testing. The majority of this research was conducted as part of the general requirement for the undergraduate and postgraduate theses requirements in special and general education programs. Populations receiving the most attention include general learning difficulties, dyslexia, and mental retardation.

Learning difficulties

Mohd Jelas (1990) defined learning difficulties as all behaviors that disturbed the functioning of a child in teaching and learning settings. The percentage of pupils perceived as experiencing learning problems in grades 1 and 2 are similar (35.3% and 35.5% respectively), while the percentage in grade 3 is lower (29.3%). Boys were perceived to have more learning problems (62.7%) than girls (37.3%). The majority of students with learning problems (73.8%) experience difficulties with language. There is a significant difference in the number of learning problems between pupils in the rural areas and pupils in the urban schools. The prevalence of learning problems in urban areas is 8.6% in Sarawak, 10% in Kelantan, and 6.0% in Johor. By contrast, the prevalence is much higher in rural areas, with 22.7% in Sarawak, 22.1% in Kelantan, and 16.85% in Johor demonstrating learning problems.

Dyslexia

The prevalence of a specific learning disability or dyslexia in Malaysia is 290,000 out of 4.9 million (5.9%) school children (Ministry of Education Malaysia, 2001). Dyslexic children have been identified as having the following problems: (1) difficulties in learning language, (2) disparities with intellectual abilities, (3) poor fluency in reading printed materials, (4) poor writing skills (difficulties in copying from the board or book), (5) eyes become easily fatigued after a few minutes of reading printed words, and (6) limited attention span (auditory or visual) (Zhagan, 1999). Dyslexic children are placed in both regular and special education classes (Abdul Wahab, 2001; Abdullah, 2001). A survey conducted by Kasim (2003) to determine the characteristics of dyslexic children in remedial classes indicated that dyslexics had high interest in skill subjects rather than language and mathematics, behavioral problems, and health problems. Girls were found to have more problems in academic achievement than boys, while boys demonstrated more behavioral problems than girls. About 17.5% of the remedial students were identified as having severe dyslexia (Kasim, 2003).

Children who are suspected of having learning problems are often referred for diagnostic neuropsychological testing. Of the 342 cases of children aged 6 to 16 years referred to the author (Normah, 1995–2007), 132 were diagnosed with a learning disorder. Among these children, 59% were diagnosed with learning disorders without comorbidity, while the rest include attention-deficit hyperactivity disorder (ADHD) with learning disorders (17%), specific learning disabilities or dyslexics (14%), and 19% were slow learners. Mean scores on the WISC-III were verbal IQ, 87 ± 19; performance IQ, 97 ± 13; and full-scale IQ, 92 ± 18. On the Child Behavior Checklist (CBCL), the sample demonstrated borderline level scores on total CBCL and internalizing problems (T-score = 67 and 65, respectively) and within normal range for externalizing problems (T-score = 60). Comparison between 33 dyslexic children and mainstream school children on the CBCL showed significant differences on all subscales except for the somatization subtest (Normah, Shalisah, & Nor'izam, 1999).

A significant problem in treating dyslexia is late diagnosis, as both parents and teachers lack awareness and knowledge in detecting the signs and symptoms of dyslexia. A survey by Chu (2006) examining knowledge of dyslexia in 60 special education teachers from the Kuala Lumpur Federal Territory revealed that teachers were "moderate" in their understanding of dyslexia. Educators were most familiar with the writing problems of dyslexics, followed by problems in reading, spelling, general achievement, behaviors, and arithmetic. Interestingly, years of experience in special education was not related to knowledge of dyslexia.

A study on dyslexic symptoms among preschool children was conducted among 40 preschoolers using the Dyslexia Early Screening Test, which includes tasks such as letter naming, rhyme detection, and phonological discrimination. Results indicated that 27.5% of the preschoolers had dyslexic symptoms, while 15% were identified as being high risk for dyslexia. More boys had dyslexic symptoms (10%) than girls (5%) (Mohd Noor & Mohd Majzub, 2003).

Table 16.5 The IQ level and adaptive skills of mentally retarded children

Scale	*Mean*	*SD*
Wechsler intelligence scale for children–third edition		
Verbal IQ	57.26	8.14
Performance IQ	62.66	11.47
Full-Scale IQ	56.53	8.79
Verbal Comprehension Index	58.86	6.26
Perceptual Organization Index	66.22	10.40
Freedom From Distractibility Index	64.60	11.30
Processing Speed Index	66.77	16.93
Vineland adaptive behavior scales		
Communication Skills	51.69	13.08
Daily Living Skills	76.19	22.35
Socialization Skills	71.62	19.68
Adaptive Behavior Composite	63.29	21.41

Mental retardation

The diagnosis of mental retardation is generally determined by child psychiatrists and clinical psychologists. Mental retardation was the diagnosis of about 32.8% of all cases referred to the author between 1997 and 2007 (Normah, 1995–2007). Routinely, the Wechsler Intelligence Scale for Children–Third Edition and the Vineland Adaptive Behavior Scale are administered when evaluating for mental retardation. Other assessments were used depending on the problems presented by the children. The IQ and adaptive skills of mentally retarded children are presented in Table 16.5.

A specific etiology of mental retardation studied in Malaysia is Down's syndrome. Down's syndrome is characterized by cognitive, social, speech, and language delays, as well as delays in reading and mathematical development. The intellectual level of these individuals is below average, and there are limitations in more than two adaptive functioning areas, such as communication skills, self-help skills, domestic skills, socialization skills, community adaptation, life goals, security and health, academic functioning, recreation, and job. Down's children have problems in mastering the academic skills and they are dependent on others (Tee & Boon, 1992). Cytogenetic analysis indicated that 9% of cases of mentally retarded children have Down's syndrome. Besides trisomy 21 (84%), other types of chromosomal abnormalities, such as mosaic Down's syndrome (15%) and a Robertsonian translocation case (1%), have been identified. About 45% of Down's syndrome babies were born to parents between the ages of 31 and 40 (Fatimah et al., 2003).

Self-help skills training is one of the primary interventions for improving functioning in mentally retarded children. Malie (1998) conducted an effectiveness study on 20 children diagnosed with mental retardation at two schools under the management of the Wisma Harapan, Kuala Lumpur. Among the self-help skills included in the training were dressing, eating, and toileting. Results indicated that the mentally retarded children were able to acquire 70% of the eating skills and 75% of the drinking skills, while 50% were able to use the toilet and dress without assistance. Overall, 50% of the mentally retarded children were able to acquire self-help skills.

Mental retardation as a chronic disability imposes a great deal of strain on the family or caregivers. The responsibility of raising a disabled child may be detrimental to the well-being of mothers. A cross-sectional study was conducted on the coping styles of 81 mothers of mentally disabled children who attended two rural Community Rehabilitation Centers (Noorzaidah, Normah, & Khairani, 2004). Overall, the mothers used a mixture of coping strategies. Task-oriented and emotion-oriented coping styles were the most frequently used strategies, while other coping styles, such as avoidance, distraction, and social diversion, were used less often. Divorced mothers, most with low educational level, were more inclined to use emotion-oriented coping strategies, while mothers with younger children (<5 years old) used more avoidance-coping strategies. Coping styles of mothers are similar in terms of their age, ethnicity, duration of marriage, number of siblings, child's birth order, and gender.

Research: Adults

Similar to research on children, Malaysian studies on adult neurological disorders are primarily descriptive in nature. The two most widely studied disorders are head injury and dementia.

Head Injury

Head injury secondary to road accidents is a significant health problem in Malaysia. Nearly 17 people are killed and over 120 others are injured daily as a result of road accidents. Motorcyclists accounted for more deaths than persons riding in automobiles. Road accidents accounted for 79.4% of preoperative deaths (Lim, 2003). The Economic and Social Committee of Asia Pacific (ESCAP) reported that Malaysia had the third highest rate of road accidents (248.3 per 10,000 vehicles), behind Germany (471.8) and Finland (338.9).

A study on psychosocial and neuropsychological outcomes of head injury was conducted on 30 chronic head injury patients treated at the Neurological Outpatient Clinic of Hospital Kuala Lumpur, Malaysia (Normah & Norhuzaifah, 2006). The sample consisted of 19 males (63%) and 11 females (37%). Demographics are presented in Table 16.6. According to Glasgow Coma Scale (GCS) scores upon admission, 43% sustained mild injuries, 40% sustained moderate injuries, while 17% had a severe head injury. The majority of subjects experienced loss of consciousness lasting less than a day (57%), while 73% experienced retrograde amnesia and 60% anterograde amnesia. Cognitive functioning was assessed with the Mini-Mental Status Examination (MMSE), Rey Auditory Verbal Learning Test (RAVLT), and

Table 16.6 Demographic data of the head injury subjects

Demographic data	*Frequency*		*Percentage*
Age groups	15–29 years	16	53%
	30–45 years	14	47%
Marital status	Single	15	50%
	Married	15	50%
Gender	Male	19	63%
	Female	11	37%
Ethnic groups	Malay	13	43%
	Chinese	10	33%
	Indian and others	7	24%
Occupation	Working	19	63%
	Not working	11	37%
Glasgow Coma Scale	Minor (12–15)	13	43%
	Moderate (9–11)	12	40%
	Severe (3–8)	5	17%
Types of cognitive impairment	Localized	17	57%
	Globalized	13	43%
Duration of LOC	Minor (less than 1 day)	17	57%
	Moderate to severe	13	43%
Retrograde amnesia	Yes	22	73%
Anterograde amnesia	Yes	18	60%

Brain Injury Checklist. Psychosocial outcomes following head injury were assessed using the Beck Depression Inventory (BDI) and General Health Questionnaire–12 (GHQ-12). Age, education, ethnicity, and severity of head injury were selected as independent variables, while the psychosocial and cognitive outcomes of head injury were the dependent variables.

Results indicated no significant differences between younger and older patients on cognitive and psychosocial outcomes with the exception of the RAVLT Trial V. Educational differences were demonstrated on subtests of the Brain Injury Checklist. No differences were found between ethnic groups on head injury outcomes. Significant differences between head injury severity were demonstrated on the MMSE ($p < 0.01$) and all subtests of the Brain Injury Checklist ($p < 0.001$). Correlations between psychosocial and cognitive outcomes of head injury showed negative relationships between MMSE and GHQ-12 ($r = -.268$) and BDI ($r = -.380$), while Trial VI of the RAVLT was slightly correlated with the GHQ-12 and BDI. The results indicated that cognitive impairment affects the mental health and well-being of head injury victims.

Geriatrics

Similar to countries around the world, Malaysia is experiencing rapid growth in its aging population. According to United Nations estimates, the world population of elderly aged

60 years and older will reach 1.2 billion by 2025, the majority of whom will be from developing countries. In Malaysia, the number of persons aged 65 and over was around 1 million in 2000, but is estimated to almost triple to 2.7 million by the year 2025. Among the elderly, 833,000 will be age 75 and older by 2025 (Arokiasamy, 1997).

Cognitive impairment and dementia are major problems of the elderly. Two studies with both suburban and rural populations estimated about 24% and 22.2% of elderly experience cognitive deficits, respectively (Krishnaswamy, 1995; Sherina, Rampal, & Mustaqim, 2004). In rural areas, cognitive impairment in the elderly was significantly associated with age, gender, ethnicity, marital status, and level of education (Sherina et al., 2004). Rates of dementia are 6% for persons aged 65 and above, and increase to 14% for those over age 75. Depression (13%) and anxiety disorders (12%) are also common among the elderly (Krishnaswamy, 1997).

References

Abdul Wahab, M. (2001). *The characteristics of dyslexia among remedial class students at Pudu Zone of Federal Territory.* Unpublished master's thesis, Universiti Kebangsaan Malaysia.

Abdullah, M. A. (2001). *A survey on the knowledge of special education teachers on dyslexia at Hilir District of Perak.* Practical training, Universiti Kebangsaan Malaysia, Bangi.

Ariffin, S. R., Mohd Ishak, N., Ahmad, A. G., Majid, R., Mustapha, R., & Salleh, N. (2006). *Malaysian Multiple Intelligence Test.* Universiti Kebangsaan Malaysia.

Arokiasamy, J. T. (1997). Malaysia's ageing issues [Editorial]. *Medical Journal of Malaysia, 52*, 197–201.

Benton-Sivan, A. B., & Spreen, O. (1996). *Der Benton Test* (7th ed.). Bern, Switzerland: Huber.

Blessed, G., Tomlinson, B., & Roth. M. (1968). The association between quantitative measure of dementia and of senile change in the cerebral grey matter of elderly subjects. *British Journal of Psychiatry, 114*, 797–811.

Chiam, H. K. (1994). *Is the Raven Progressive Matrices valid for Malaysians?* Paper presented at the 23rd International Congress of Applied Psychology, Madrid, Spain.

Chiam, H. K. (1995). *The standardisation of several tests in Malaysia.* Unpublished manuscript, School of Education, University of Malaya, Kuala Lumpur.

Chu, C. L. (2006). *The level of knowledge of special education teachers toward dyslexia: A survey of secondary schools of Kuala Lumpur Federal Territory.* Unpublished practicum training report, Faculty of Education, Universiti Kebangsaan Malaysia.

Cockburn, J., & Smith, P. T. (1989). *The Rivermead Behavioral Memory Test.* Suffolk, England: Thames Valley Test Company.

Deva, M. P. (2004). Malaysia mental health country profile. *International Review of Psychiatry, 16*(1–2), 167–176.

Fatimah, R. S., Suhaida, M. A., Aqsoriah, K., Mariam, I. S., Ros Sidek, M., Mokhtar, K. I., … Isa, M. N. (2003, May). *Cytogenetic analysis in Husm (8 years review): Incidence of Down's syndrome associated with paternal and maternal ages.* Eighth National Conference on Medical Sciences, Universiti Sains Malaysia.

Folstein, M. F., Folstein, S. E., & McHugh, P. R. (1975). "Mini-mental state." A practical method for grading the cognitive state of patients for the clinician. *Journal of Psychiatric Research, 12*, 189–198.

Freedman, M., Leach, L., Kaplan, E., Winocur, G., Shulman, K. I., & Delis, D. C. (1994). *Clock Drawing: A neuropsychological analysis*. New York, NY: Oxford University Press.

Gardner, H. (1983). *Frames of mind: The theory of multiple intelligences*. New York, NY: Basic Books.

Globalis. (2008). *Malaysia*. Retrieved March 3, 2008, from http://globalis.gvu.unu.edu/indicator_detail.cfm?country=MY

Groth-Marnart, G. (2000). *Neuropsychological assessment in clinical practice: A guide to test interpretation and integration*. New York, NY: John Wiley & Sons, Inc.

Heaton, R. K. (1981). *Wisconsin Card Sorting Test* [Manual]. Odessa, FL: Psychological Assessment Resources, Inc.

Kasim, M. (2003). *A survey for the characteristic of dyslexia among the remedial children*. Unpublished undergraduate in special education thesis, Faculty of Education, Universiti Kebangsaan Malaysia.

Kim, H., & Markus, H. R. (1999). Deviance or uniqueness, harmony or conformity? A cultural analysis. *Journal of Personality and Social Psychology, 77,* 785–800.

Krishnaswamy, S. (1995). Screening for dementia among elderly Malays in urban settlements in Kuala Lumpur. *Malaysia Journal of Psychiatry, 3,* 654–658.

Krishnaswamy, S. (1997). Psychiatric problems among the elderly in Malaysia. *Medical Journal of Malaysia, 52,* 222–224.

Kua, E. H., & Ko, S. M. (1992). A questionnaire to screen for cognitive impairment among elderly people in developing countries. *Acta Psychiatrica Scandinavica, 85,* 119–122.

Kühnen, U., Hannover, B., Roeder, U., Shah, A. A., Schubert, B., Upmeyer, A., & Zakaria, S. (2001). Cross-cultural variations in identifying embedded figures: Comparisons from the United States, Germany, Russia, and Malaysia. *Journal of Cross-Cultural Psychology, 32,* 366–372.

Kühnen, U., Hannover, B., & Schubert, B. (2000). *A semantic-procedural interface model of the self: The role of self-knowledge for context-dependent versus context-independent modes of thinking*. Manuscript submitted for publication, University of Michigan.

Lim, K. G. (2003). Traumatic deaths. *Malaysian Journal of Medical Sciences, 10,* 100–117.

Lynn, R., & Irwing, P. (2004). Sex differences on the progressive matrices: A meta-analysis. *Intelligence, 32,* 481–498.

Malie, Y. (1998). *Examining the achievement of self-management skills among mentally retarded children at the Wisma Harapan*. Unpublished undergraduate thesis, Faculty of Education, Universiti Kebangsaan Malaysia.

Mattis, S. (1976). *Dementia Rating Scale: Professional manual*. Odessa, FL: Psychological Assessment Resources.

Ministry of Education Malaysia. (2001). *Working paper on long-term and short-term planning for the special education programme*. Department of Special Education, Ministry of Education Malaysia.

Mohd Ishak, N., Mustapha, R., Mahmud, Z., & Ariffin, S. R. (2004). *Malaysian Emotional Intelligence Inventory System*. Universiti Kebangsaan Malaysia.

Mohd Jelas, Z. (1990). *Current remedial teaching: Implementation and challenges*. Paper presented at the Remedial Teaching Seminar, Pasir Panjang Teacher's College, Kuala Terengganu.

Mohd Noor, S., & Mohd Majzub, R. (2003). *A study of dyslexic symptoms among preschool children*. Unpublished undergraduate thesis, Faculty of Education, Universiti Kebangsaan Malaysia.

Mohd Yunus, K. R., & Mohd Jelas, Z. (1994). A prevalence study on learning disabled among grade one students based on the teacher's perception. *Jurnal Pendidikan, 19,* 9–26.

Nisbett, R. E., Peng, K., Choi, I., & Norenzayan, A. (1999). *Culture and systems of thought: Holistic versus analytic cognition*. Manuscript submitted for publication, University of Michigan.

Normah, C. D. (1995–2007). Child cases referred for psychological assessment at the Health Psychology Unit, Faculty of Allied Health Sciences, Universiti Kebangsaan Malaysia.

Normah, C. D., Khairiyah, M., Nadzirah, A. B., Nur Farhana, H., Nurrul Hidayah, M. T., Shairah, A. W., … Ng, L. O. (2008). *Cognitive and psychosocial profiles of the police at the Police Training Centre, Kuala Lumpur*. Health Psychology Unit, Faculty of Allied Health Sciences, Universiti Kebangsaan Malaysia.

Normah, C. D., Mahadir, A., Shazli E. G., Ponnusamy, S., Siti Hazlina, A., Siti Aminah, O., & Maryam Thoraya, A. (2007). *The Influence of personality types, activities of daily living, and cognitive functions toward mental health of stroke patients*. UKM Grant NN-005-2003.

Normah, C. D., & Norhuzaifah, Z. (2006). *Psychosocial and cognitive outcomes of minor head injury*. Unpublished degree thesis, Universiti Kebangsaan Malaysia.

Normah, C. D., Nursan J. S., & Mahadir, A. (2005). *Predictors of memory in adolescents with epilepsy*. Abstract of the Mid-Year International Neuropsychological Society Meeting, Dublin, Ireland.

Normah, C. D., Saralla, M. C., Azlinawati, N. M., & Raymond, A. A. (2008). *Neuropsychological profiles of epilepsy patients referred for presurgical evaluation*. Abstract of the 4th Malaysian Indonesia Brunei Medical Sciences Conference, Faculty of Medicine, Universiti Kebangsaan Malaysia.

Normah, C. D., Shalisah, S., & Nor'izam, M. A. (1999). Behavior profiles of specific learning disabilities and normal children. *Malaysian Journal of Psychiatry*, *7*, 35–44.

Noorzaidah, A. H., Normah, C. D., & Khairani, O. (2004). Coping styles of mothers with disabled children at rural community rehabilitation centres in Muar, Malaysia. *Medical Journal of Malaysia, 59*, 384–390.

Perianez, J. A., Rios-Lago, M., Rodriguez-Sanchez, J. M., Adrover-Roig, D., Sanchez-Cubillo, I., Crespo-Facorro, B., … Barcelo, F. (2007). Trail Making Test in traumatic brain injury, schizophrenia, and normal aging: Sample comparisons and normative data. *Archives of Clinical Neuropsychology, 22*, 433–447.

Raven, J. (2000). The Raven's Progressive Matrices: Change and stability over culture and time. *Cognitive Psychology, 41*, 1–48.

Raven, J. C. (1938). *Progressive Matrices: A perceptual test of intelligence*. London, UK: H.K. Lewis.

Reitan, R. M. (1992). *Trail Making Test. Manual for administration and scoring*. South Tucson, AZ: Reitan Neuropsychology Laboratory.

Rey, A. (1958). Memorisation d'une serie de 15 mots en 5 repetitions. In A. Rey (Ed.), *L'examen clinique en psychologie*. Paris, France: Presses Universitaires de France.

Salovey, P., & Mayer, J. D. (1990). Emotional intelligence. *Imagination, Cognition and Personality, 9*, 185–211.

Sherina, M. S., Rampal, L., & Mustaqim, A. (2004). Cognitive impairment among the elderly in a rural community in Malaysia. *Medical Journal of Malaysia, 59*, 252–257.

Tee, C. T., & Boon, K. B. (1992). *Special education and remediation of basic reading*. Kuala Lumpur, Malaysia: Dewan Bahasa dan Pustaka.

Wechsler, D. (1981). *WAIS-R manual*. New York, NY: Psychological Corporation.

Wechsler, D. (1987). *Wechsler Memory Scale—Revised manual*. New York, NY: Psychological Corporation.

Wechsler, D. (1991). *Manual for the Wechsler Intelligence Scale for Children* (3rd ed.). San Antonio, TX: The Psychological Corporation.

Wechsler, D. (1997). *Wechsler Adult Intelligence Scale* (3rd ed.). San Antonio, TX: Harcourt Assessment.

Witkin, H. A. (1950). Individual differences in the case of perception of embedded figures. *Journal of Personality, 19*, 1–15.

Zhagan, M. (1999). *The effect of Malay Language Teaching Approach towards the understanding and word output among dyslexic children aged 8 to 9 years at transition class.* Unpublished practicum report, Faculty of Education, Universiti Kebangsaan Malaysia.

Zarina, Z. A., & Zahiruddin, O. (2004.) *Validation of Malay version of Mini-Mental State Examination and its correlation with Clock Drawing Test in dementia.* Abstract of the University Sains Malaysia Medical Alumni Society National Scientific Meeting, Kota Bharu, Kelantan, Malaysia.

17 Neuropsychology in the Philippines

Maria Raquel Lopa-Ramos and Lourdes Ledesma

Description of the country

The Republic of the Philippines is an archipelago of 7,107 islands located in Southeast Asia. The islands are divided into three major areas: Luzon, Visayas, and Mindanao. The capital city of Metro Manila is found in Luzon. The Philippines is a developing country with an agricultural base, light industry, and service sector economy (Toh & Cawagas, 2005).

The Philippines is considered the 12th most populous country in the world, with the population estimate for 2007 at 89 million (National Statistics Office, Republic of the Philippines, n.d.). The Filipino is basically of Malay heritage, but many are partly of Spanish, Chinese, American, or Arab ancestry and are sometimes called *mestizo* for their mixed heritage (Abigan, 1998). Eighty percent of the population is Roman Catholic, the Spanish colonization's lasting legacy (Republic of the Philippines Official Web Site, n.d.).

More than 170 languages and dialects are spoken in the country, almost all of them belonging to the Malayo-Polynesian language family (Tope, 1994). However, Filipino and English are the two official languages of the country, the latter primarily due to five decades of American occupation. Filipino is predominantly based on Tagalog, one of the country's major languages, and it also incorporates elements of other Philippine languages as well as borrowings from English and Spanish. Many Filipinos understand, write, and speak Filipino, English, and their respective regional languages. The Philippines has one of the highest literacy rates in the East Asian and Pacific area, with about 92% of the population 10 years of age and older considered literate (Toh & Cawagas, 2005).

The country's history can be divided into distinct phases (Republic of the Philippines Official Web Site, n.d.). In the pre-Spanish period, Indonesian, Chinese, and Malayan peoples settled in the Philippines and established trade with nearby countries. Spanish colonial rule began after Ferdinand Magellan arrived in 1521 and lasted until 1898. The Spaniards introduced Christianity and ruled over three centuries, a period marked by sporadic uprisings (Abigan, 1998). In 1898, the Philippine revolution against Spain resulted in the proclamation of the first Philippine Republic. But in that same year, the United States acquired the Philippines through the Treaty of Paris by virtue of Spain's defeat in the Spanish American War. The Americans governed the country until the Japanese occupation during World War II. After the war, the United States granted the Philippines its independence in 1946. Democratic institutions were established until martial law was imposed by Ferdinand E. Marcos in 1972. A peaceful "people power" revolution overthrew his dictatorship in 1986 and installed Corazon C. Aquino as president. An emergent democracy continues to characterize the country's sociopolitical situation.

History of neuropsychology

The early roots of neuropsychology in the Philippines can be traced back to the mid-1970s when the Philippine General Hospital, through a bilateral agreement between the Philippine government and the French government, sent a neurosurgeon to train in neuropsychology under Dr. Francois Lhermitte at the Hospital Pitie-Salpetriere, University of Paris 7. Under the same program, a nurse with a specialization in neurology and a doctorate degree in counseling was also sent for a year-long fellowship in the early 1980s. During this period, an adult neurologist received a grant from the University of Bergen in Norway to train in neuropsychology, specifically in the use of the Halstead-Reitan battery. These medical professionals eventually returned to the Philippines but did not formally pursue neuropsychology. Their training and experiences nonetheless influenced their subsequent practice. Informally, they applied assessment techniques they learned to gain further insight into their patients' impaired functioning. They generally acknowledged that their neuropsychology training was beneficial, as it provided them with an additional perspective from which to view the various cases in their practice.

It was in 1980 that the first formally trained neuropsychologist began practicing in the Philippines. Unlike the others, Dr. Lourdes K. Ledesma was a psychologist by training who earned her doctorate in counseling psychology at Boston College, Massachusetts. She was then granted a fellowship at the Department of Psychiatry, Harvard Medical School, and was the first intern in the pediatric neuropsychology training program headed by Dr. Natalie Sollee. This program included an adult rotation at the Boston Veteran's Administration Hospital, where she was mentored by Dr. Edith Kaplan. When she returned to the Philippines, she initially established a private clinical practice for neuropsychological assessments. Shortly after, she was invited to join the neurology section at the Philippine General Hospital, a government-run tertiary care facility that services indigent patients. Over the succeeding years, Dr. Ledesma helped establish and eventually headed an adult memory clinic at the Philippine General Hospital and at a private medical facility. She likewise started the neuropsychology section at two neurodevelopmental centers, one at a government pediatric hospital and another at a private medical facility. The branching out of her practice signaled the recognition of neuropsychology as a valuable subspecialty in the neurosciences.

Current practices

Inspired by Dr. Ledesma's success, several other psychologists trained abroad in neuropsychology. These professionals obtained their doctorates from Georgia State

University, Temple University, Fordham University, State University of New York at Stony Brook, and McGill University in Canada. Of these, only one has returned to practice in the Philippines, while the rest have opted to practice or seek more advanced training abroad. One psychologist obtained a master's degree in education and neuroscience at Columbia University and established a practice in the Philippines, but has recently migrated to Canada. Another psychologist is currently completing her doctorate at Fuller Theological Seminary. Dr. Ledesma also supervises psychologists who assist in her neuropsychological assessments through the centers in which she is affiliated. These psychologists hold master's degrees in psychology, and many are working on their doctorate degrees.

In response to the great need for more neuropsychologists in the country, the University of the Philippines (UP) in Diliman is establishing a clinical neuropsychology track within the developmental psychology doctoral program. A joint initiative between the UP School of Medicine at the Philippine General Hospital and the UP Department of Psychology has also resulted in plans to offer a master's of science degree in the neurosciences, with clinical neuropsychology as one of its tracks. In addition, there have been informal discussions among various psychology department heads of colleges and universities in Manila, spearheaded by the Dementia Council of the Philippine Neurological Association, to establish training programs in neuropsychology. These efforts underscore the growing awareness in the academy of the important contributions of neuropsychology in helping those with neurological-based conditions, and the need to train specialists in this field.

There are primarily four centers where neuropsychological evaluations are conducted. Two cater to adult patients: The Center for Memory and Cognition is located at the Philippine General Hospital and focuses on memory screenings and evaluations for the elderly. The Neurocognitive and Neurobehavioral Clinic is located at the Medical City, a private medical facility, and administers neuropsychological evaluations for patients 16 years and older who present with cognitive and behavioral changes attributed to neurologic or other medical conditions. These centers are part of the neurology department of the facilities in which they are located. Pediatric patients are seen at two neurodevelopmental centers, one at Philippine Children's Medical Center, a government-run tertiary care facility for indigent patients, and another at St. Luke's Medical Center, a private medical facility. The neuropsychologists at these multidisciplinary units work closely with pediatric neurologists, developmental pediatricians, child psychiatrists, speech pathologists, occupational therapists, reading specialists, and special educators.

The centers are all located in the country's capital city, Metro Manila, and patients from all over the country as well as those from other countries in the region, including Hong Kong, Indonesia, Singapore, and Brunei, come to these centers for neuropsychological services. Adult patients typically present with conditions such as dementia and mild cognitive impairment, cerebrovascular disease and strokes, transient global amnesia, seizures, head trauma and brain injury, and viral encephalopathies. Pediatric patients include children with neurological conditions such as seizure disorder, history of central nervous system (CNS) infections, or congenital malformations, and those with neurodevelopmental problems, such as mental retardation, learning disabilities, pervasive developmental disorders, and attention-deficit/hyperactivity disorder. A neuropsychological evaluation is also included in the protocol of procedures, such as deep brain stimulation (DBS), in epilepsy surgery (which includes the Wada test), and in neuro-oncology involving brain tumors. A wide spectrum of patients from various socioeconomic backgrounds are seen, from those in urban areas who are highly educated to those from rural settings with limited educational opportunities.

Neuropsychological tests

Test batteries used in neuropsychological assessment are mainly Western-developed tools. Local norms for such tests are still unavailable; hence, test scores are always interpreted with caution. Testing of clinical limits is undertaken as well to further explore the possible underlying reasons for a patient's performance on a test. In addition, emphasis is placed on qualitative descriptions, observations, and analyses in order to arrive at diagnostically sound conclusions.

Informal adaptations of Western instruments are also made to assist in the evaluation process. For instance, questions may be translated into the vernacular, or culturally rooted themes may be substituted with similar but more locally relevant ones (e.g., a question about seasons in a temperate climate is substituted with one related to the tropical climate of the country). When English language proficiency is limited, informal tests in Filipino are usually given to supplement the English battery. These tests are commonly clinically designed tools whose objective is to provide the neuropsychologist with additional information about the patient's functioning vis-à-vis his or her performance on a Western test (e.g., Story Memory using Filipino in comparison to Story Memory on the Wide Range Assessment of Memory and Learning–Second Edition). Literacy skills are likewise informally assessed in the patient's dominant language, such as by making him or her read and answer questions about a story in a graded Filipino textbook used in the local schools.

Over the past years, there have been several attempts to formally develop local instruments that incorporate more applicable methods and materials. One is the "de-Westernization" of a dementia screening scale. This project was undertaken in recognition of the fact that a patient's poor performance on a Western dementia scale may actually be due to educational and sociocultural factors. Specifically, elderly patients from rural areas from low-income brackets with less educated backgrounds tend to do poorly on such Western scales. The De-Westernized Dementia Screening Scale was developed for such a population (Ledesma, Diputado, Orteza, & Santillan, 1993). Similar to other dementia screening scales, the instrument included subtests such as behavior and activities of daily living, memory, orientation, mental tracking, praxis, calculation, language, abstract thinking, and judgment. However, to de-Westernize the instrument, changes were incorporated, which included making the testing setting more comfortable for the patient by allowing a family member or caregiver to be present during the assessment, using the patient's native tongue as the medium of testing, using familiar objects, and employing indigenous constructs (e.g., asking a patient to give directions to a place using landmarks like trees, mountains, etc., rather than in miles or kilometers since this is how Filipinos usually provide directions). Taking illiteracy into consideration, no reading or writing skills were required, and items relied mostly on verbal-auditory and visuographic skills. The result was a diagnostic tool that was more relevant and meaningful for the target population.

Another tool is the Manila Motor-Perceptual Screening Test (MaMPS; Javier, Luna-Reyes, Walter, Ledesma, & Reyes, 1988). The MaMPS is a screening test for preschool children (ages 4 to 6 years), which was created to aid in the early identification of children at risk for learning disabilities. Specifically, the test was developed to evaluate the motor, sensory, and perceptual skills of these young children. It was made to resemble an indigenous child's game, *piko*, which is similar to hopscotch, and was designed to be easily administered and interpreted so that schoolteachers can conduct the evaluation. Children are assessed by evaluating activities that occur naturally within the game, such as gross motor coordination, eye-hand coordination, balance, spatial awareness, laterality, color perception, fine finger dexterity, and understanding of instructions. These activities included connect the dots, throwing a "marker" to specified color boxes in the game diagram, hopping and skipping, and balancing while placing a specified hand or foot on the game diagram. Visual shape identification, tactile shape identification, and color recognition activities were also incorporated using simple materials (e.g., picture cards, wooden blocks). The field investigation included 1,071 boys and girls, ages 4 to 6 years, from both public and private schools in Metro Manila. It was hoped that the screening would eventually be used in schools nationwide to help identify children who could benefit from early intervention, or at least to raise the index of suspicion of the teachers to seek further consultation. However, limitations in resources as well as shifting priorities and policies at the government level have been an obstacle.

There is undeniably a great need to develop more indigenous tests with local norms, but lack of resources, primarily funding, remains a major difficulty. Such a situation often compels and challenges Filipino neuropsychologists to be creative and resourceful in their work, without sacrificing the integrity of their findings.

Research

Research is another area that needs further development in the Philippines. Limitations in resources similarly have impacted this pursuit. There is currently one primary psychological journal in the country, the *Philippine Journal of Psychology*. A review of the issues from its inception in 1968 to the present reflects a dearth of studies in neuropsychology. Nonetheless, in recent years, there appears to be a growing interest in neuropsychology in that affiliated specialists (e.g., neurodevelopmental pediatricians) have begun to incorporate neuropsychological topics in their research. Most of the research, however, remains unpublished.

The majority of the studies conducted in the Philippines have focused on children. A few examine the use of Western tests on Filipino children. Alianan (2004), for instance, studied the validity of the Mental Processing scale of the Kaufman Assessment Battery for Children (K-ABC) when administered to Filipino school-age children (ages 6 to 11 years) in Metro Manila. Analyses showed that the latent structure of the various subtests based on the performance of the participants conformed to the theoretical constructs defined by the scale. The conclusion was that the scale was deemed appropriate for use with Filipino urban school children, pending the development of local norms and instruments.

To date, there are no epidemiological studies of neurological or developmental disorders that affect children, but there have been a number of hospital-based studies that present the clinical profiles of Filipino children with speech and language delay, global developmental delay, attention-deficit/hyperactivity disorder, and learning disabilities (e.g., Ledesma et al., 1991; Conducto, Avendaño, Reyes, Ortiz, & Tañega, 2000; Prudencio, Ledesma, & Reyes, 2002).

One emerging focus of research recognizes the important role of the Filipino's bilingual background. There have been investigations into how language proficiency in Filipino and English influences the development of literacy skills in normal children and in those with dyslexia (e.g., Ocampo, 2002; Ledesma, 2002). Ocampo (2002) investigated the literacy development and the cognitive and linguistic factors that were related to reading difficulties among bilingual children. The study involved 479 bilingual-biliterate children aged 6 to 13 years (grades 1 to 6). A group of children from grades 3 to 6 with poor single-word reading skills was identified as the dyslexic group. One conclusion made from this study is that literacy development among bilinguals is different from that of monolinguals. The transparent orthography of Filipino appears to provide earlier development of phonological abilities in this language that consequently facilitate the development of the same processes underlying literacy development in English. It was also found that literacy difficulties manifest differently in the two languages due to differences in their orthographic depth.

Ledesma's study (2002) investigated early reading development among 81 bilingual boys in kindergarten (pre–grade 1) attending two schools in Metro Manila, with one school using Filipino as the medium of instruction and the other using English. Aside from language of instruction, she examined the relationship of language preference, orthography, and other reading-related skills (e.g., phonological awareness, rapid naming) to reading decoding and reading comprehension. Results indicated that language preference may facilitate reading performance in the preferred language. However, more basic and universal skills (e.g., phonological awareness, rapid naming) underlie reading decoding skills in the two languages. These underlying skills appear to develop independently of language preference or language of instruction. In contrast, reading comprehension (especially English cloze passage comprehension) seems to be more influenced by language use, vocabulary knowledge, and proficiency. Filipino instruction predicted better performance on all Filipino reading measures, while English instruction predicted better English reading comprehension but not English decoding. Similar to Ocampo, Ledesma's findings underscore the complex interplay of factors involved when dealing with bilingual populations, and more research in this area is merited.

The studies on adults have examined dementia, stroke, epilepsy, and memory. As with the studies on children, some studies with adults have looked at the use of Western instruments with Filipinos. Orteza (1999) examined the use of the Fuld Object Memory Evaluation on Filipino adults and elderly. She cites inherent characteristics of the measure that make it amenable to this population; in particular, the use of 10 common stimulus objects was felt to circumvent cultural, socioeconomic, and educational differences. A sample of 100 aging and adult participants was tested to establish normal values based on age, years of education, and gender, factors that were found to affect performance on the test. Using this test was recommended as an adjunct to the Mini-Mental State Exam and other screening procedures for elderly patients presenting with memory complaints.

Neuropsychology in a developing country such as the Philippines certainly faces many challenges. Yet the field continues to grow, encouraged by the increasing appreciation of its significant contribution in the neurosciences and by the support of the medical practitioners, educators, and family members in need of its services.

References

Abigan, E. R. (1998). *The Philippine Atlas.* Manila, Philippines: Philippine Guides, Inc.

Alianan, A., Jr. (2004). *A validation of the Kaufman-Assessment Battery for Children in Metro Manila.* Unpublished doctoral dissertation, Ateneo de Manila University, Philippines.

Conducto, C. C., Avendaño, E., Reyes, A., Ortiz, M. H., & Tañega, A. (2000). Clinical profile of attention-deficit/hyperactivity disorder among Filipino children in a tertiary referral center [Abstract]. *Philippine Medical Children's Center Book of Abstracts (1995–2006)*, 129.

Javier, S. B., Luna-Reyes, O. B., Walter, R. T., Ledesma, L. K., & Reyes, T. M. (1988). The Manila motor-perceptual screening test: Its development and field investigation. *Santo Tomas Journal of Medicine, 37,* 126–169.

Ledesma, H. M. (2002). *Language factors influencing early reading development in bilingual (Filipino-English) boys.* Unpublished doctoral dissertation, Georgia State University, Georgia, USA.

Ledesma, L. K., Diputado, B. V., Orteza, G. O., & Santillan, C. E. (1993). De-Westernization of a dementia screening scale: The Philippine experience. *Philippine Journal of Psychology, 26,* 30–38.

Ledesma, L. K., Ortiz, M. H., Gonzaga, F., Lee, L. V., Palines, E. V., Panlilio, J. R., & Tuazon, M. N. (1991). Speech delay in Filipino children: A clinical profile. *Philippine Journal of Psychology, 24*, 20–25.

National Statistics Office, Republic of the Philippines. (n.d.). *Philippines in figures*. Retrieved September 8, 2007, from http://www.census.gov.ph

Ocampo, D. (2002). *Effects of bilingualism on literacy development.* Unpublished doctoral dissertation, University of Surrey, England.

Orteza, G. O. (1999). Testing for memory in the Filipino elderly. *Philippine Journal of Psychology, 32*, 60–85.

Prudencio, M. A., Ledesma, L. K., & Reyes, A. (2002). Profile of Filipino children with learning disabilities at the Philippine Medical Children's Center for the past 3 years [Abstract]. *Philippine Medical Children's Center Book of Abstracts (1995–2006)*, 125.

Republic of the Philippines Official Web Site. (n.d.). *General information.* Retrieved September 8, 2007, from http://www.gov.ph/aboutphil/general.asp

Toh, S. H., & Cawagas, V. F. (2005). *Our nation, our world.* Quezon City, Philippines: Sibs Publishing House.

Tope, L. R. (1994). *Cultures of the world: Philippines.* New York, NY: Marshall Cavendish.

18 Neuropsychology in Singapore

Simon L. Collinson and Donald Yeo

Singapore is a prosperous and vibrant multicultural society of 4.5 million people consisting of a mixture of Chinese (77%), indigenous Malay (14%), Indian (8%), and other ethnic minorities (1%). The majority of Singaporeans speak English, which is taught in school as the national language, although a variety of other languages and dialects may be the first or second language spoken at home, including Mandarin, Malay, Hokkien, Cantonese, Teochew, and Tamil. Whereas older generations of Singaporeans may have experienced low levels of prosperity and education, in recent decades Singapore has developed a buoyant economy with a high standard of living and education. On average, students attend 12 years of formal education prior to a 3- to 4-year undergraduate university degree. Singapore has a high standard of literacy. Global statistics estimate the adult literacy rate for Singapore was 93% for ages 15 and older during the period 2000 to 2004 (World Bank, 2006).

The leading causes of morbidity and mortality in Singapore are the major noncommunicable diseases, and with an aging population, dementia is emerging as a major public health concern. Despite high-quality medical services, with active promotion of preventive medicine and the presence of established psychology departments in local universities, the development of clinical psychology and neuropsychology in Singapore has lagged behind that of comparable economies in the Western world. In recent years, there has been significant development of clinical neuropsychology research, test development, and training in several institutions in Singapore. The many local languages, dialects, and cultures impose unique challenges for neuropsychologists in Singapore, but as the country seeks to establish itself as a regional leader in the clinical neurosciences, these challenges are taking on growing significance.

Neuropsychology, as a separate discipline, has evolved organically in Singapore as an offshoot of general clinical psychology. The first formal clinical service in psychology in Singapore grew from a single clinical appointment at Woodbridge Hospital, now known as the Institute of Mental Health. In 1956, V. W. Wilson, an Australian, was appointed to develop a full psychological service providing for medical, social welfare, and educational applications as well as government advisory. In the late 1950s and 1960s several key figures, including M. K. Wong and F. Y. Long, who trained at the Institute of Psychiatry London and Sydney University, respectively, developed the assessment component of the service beyond IQ testing to include personality testing and projective techniques. The 1960s and 1970s saw an expansion in Woodbridge Hospital's psychology services to include a range of consultancy services to other hospitals and government bodies in Singapore.

Formal clinical neuropsychological assessment, along the lines of the British assessment approach, was introduced to Woodbridge Hospital in 1981. Short batteries of tests or subtests (e.g., Nelson's Short Wisconsin Card Sorting Test, Reitan Trail Making Test, Wechsler Memory Scale subtests, Benton Visual Retention Test, Wechsler Adult Intelligence Scale subtests, Rey-Osterreith Complex Figure, Token Test, short version of Minnesota Aphasia Test, Graham-Kendall Memory for Designs, etc.) were used for detection and diagnosis as well as lateralization and lesion localization. This approach has remained the dominant method of assessment. With the influence of greater numbers of Singaporeans trained in Australia, Britain, and the United States in the 1980s and 1990s, psychology departments began to emerge in the major public hospitals around Singapore.

In 1998, Singapore's first dedicated neuropsychology unit opened at Singapore General Hospital. Staffed by research psychologists, clinical psychologists, and clinical neuropsychologists, the unit provides clinical services to patients from the departments of neurology, neurosurgery, behavioral medicine, geriatric medicine, and rehabilitation medicine. Its primary roles include diagnostic clarification, cognitive characterization and monitoring, and therapeutic intervention. The unit also provides research support in psychometric testing for clinical trials in hospitals and community-based research projects.

Singapore's advanced medical system and high standards of medical care contribute to the country's reputation as a regional hub for medical services. There are several large public hospitals in Singapore, including Singapore General Hospital, Changi General Hospital, National University Hospital, and Tan Tock Seng Hospital, which have established departments of neurology, neurosurgery, geriatrics, rehabilitation, and psychological medicine, and many with subdepartments of clinical psychology that perform the majority of neuropsychological assessments. The largest public employer of clinical psychologists in Singapore remains the Institute of Mental Health, a large psychiatric facility with over 2,500 inpatient beds that is entirely dedicated to psychiatric patients, and those with developmental and neurodegenerative disorders. Research in neuroscience and neuropsychology is also conducted at the National Neuroscience Institute, a center of clinical neuroscience training and research in Singapore, as well as the various universities in Singapore.

In Singapore, there is currently no formal registration of clinical psychologists. However, voluntary registration has been introduced via the Singapore Psychological Society (SPS)—the main professional body for local psychologists. Of the approximately 110 psychologists registered with the SPS, only a small proportion have postgraduate clinical training. Similarly, the Singapore Ministry of Health (MOH) estimates that only 30 clinical psychologists working within the public sector in Singapore have postgraduate qualifications in clinical psychology, with an unspecified number working in the private sector. A significant number of practitioners are Singapore-educated psychologists with applied master's working in public hospitals. These data indicate that independent practitioners vary in their level of clinical training from no postgraduate professional training up to PhD level–trained clinical psychologists with pre- and postdoctoral specializations. Due to the lack of trained psychologists, some forms of screening and computerized cognitive assessment have been undertaken by parallel professions, such as speech and language pathology or occupational therapy, although formal neuropsychological assessment remains in the domain of psychology.

The relatively low percentage of post–graduate level clinical psychologists is largely due to the absence of homegrown clinical professional training programs. For example, up until recently, the National University of Singapore, the island's largest university, had a relatively small joint department of social work and psychology. Only in 2005 was an independent department of psychology formed, which has been growing steadily, with 20 faculty as well as adjunct and visiting staff. There are now academic departments of psychology in two local universities.

Notwithstanding the current small number of professional clinical psychologists currently working in Singapore, the number of clinically trained psychologists is set to increase substantially with the National Mental Health Blueprint, which prioritizes the development of mental health manpower as a key focus area for Singapore from 2007 to 2011.

The absence of a clinical program in Singapore has resulted in the need for students to seek clinical training abroad. Of the range of clinically trained psychologists currently working in Singapore, the majority have trained in Australia, with master's level qualifications in clinical psychology. A significant percentage of them practice some clinical neuropsychology as part of their overall remit as clinical psychologists. Those who have trained in Australia have training in psychometry and IQ assessment. In comparison, U.S.- and UK-trained clinical psychologists may have subspecialty training in clinical neuropsychology during their postgraduate studies, or as a postdoctoral specialization. In Singapore, there are only a handful of postgraduate-trained clinical neuropsychologists. All have been trained in Australia, where neuropsychology is a separate postgraduate training specialization to clinical psychology. These clinicians are involved in a range of activities, including clinical work, research, and teaching.

The major difference between the Australian and British clinical psychology programs and their North American counterparts is the length of training. As a consequence of earlier specialization in psychology at the undergraduate level, British Commonwealth clinical training tends to be shorter and requires proportionally more clinical contact in a shorter amount of time. However, increasingly students are opting for DPsych and professional PhD programs, and Singapore is beginning to see greater numbers of doctoral level clinicians in the health services. The MOH has indicated a need to upgrade the qualifications of clinical psychologists in Singapore, and has intentions to implement formal regulation of clinical psychology with minimum standards of training.

The high standards of infrastructure, safety, and accountability in Singapore distinguish it from other, less wealthy regional countries with respect to rates of injury and disability. In many respects, Singapore is no different from other developed economies in terms of health care concerns and priorities. The leading causes of morbidity and mortality in Singapore are the major noncommunicable diseases, such as cancer, coronary heart disease, stroke, diabetes, and hypertension, and head injuries, with the recent emergence of dementia as a growing public health concern due to an aging population. In 2006, cancer, cardiovascular diseases, and stroke together accounted for approximately 60% of the total causes of death.

With growing recognition of the value of clinical neuropsychology among the medical community, there is support for the application of neuropsychological services beyond tertiary hospitals to other health care settings. In the private sector there is a high demand for educationally related psychometric assessment, typically performed by educational psychologists, and medicolegal assessment following head injury, usually performed by clinical neuropsychologists or clinical psychologists within hospitals. Singapore employs workers from a range of regional nations on short-term employment visas, many of whom work as construction workers and incur head injuries from workplace accidents.

There are currently few local adaptations of clinical tests commonly used in the West. This problem is significantly mitigated by the strong English language skills of many Singaporeans, but it remains one of the major challenges to best practice. A recent survey of Singapore Psychological Society registered clinically practicing psychologists (unpublished data) indicated that the overwhelming majority (+90%) of respondents used the Wechsler tests almost exclusively, including the WAIS-III, WISC-III, WIAT-II, and WIPPSI-III. The Peabody Individual Achievement Test–R and Connors Continuous Performance Test II are also widely used. In all, few of the respondents used more than the Wechsler tests on a routine basis, and the majority administered tests in all local languages, including English, Mandarin, Tamil, and Malay. It is noteworthy that these psychologists are relying upon their own individual translation of these tests, as none of these proprietary tests have been validated in local languages. Unfortunately, the absence of local norms has made it necessary for Singaporean psychologists to use UK, Australian, or U.S. norms for comparison, and these norms are made less reliable by cultural references that are inappropriate to the local population. As Singapore was formerly a British colony until 1963, UK versions may have greater applicability to the local population than U.S versions. Presently, the development of local tests and normative studies remains in its infancy in Singapore. Data on comparative norms between Singapore and other countries, and issues of cross-cultural cognitive testing in Singapore have not been systematically investigated at present, but this could potentially be valuable as a research focus in future studies.

Despite the dearth of locally normed tests, there is a growing number of studies in Singapore in both psychology and the clinical neurosciences that have used or examined locally validated tests. Few published studies with local norms exist in the pediatric literature, although particular government agencies have developed local norms for commonly used psychometric tests. In separate studies, Lim and colleagues (Lim, Chan, & Yoong, 1994; Lim et al., 1996) validated a Singapore version of the Denver II Developmental Screening Test (DDST) on 2,459 children, in five ages: 3 months, 9 months, 17 months, 37 months, and 60 months. Children with "questionable," "abnormal," and "untestable" scores were screened out, equating to a screened-out rate of 12.6%. Among these cases, the DDST had a high false positive rate of

83.5% and a lower false negative rate of 3.7%, compared to the full developmental assessment. However, it was suggested that the high false positive rate could be significantly reduced by doing repeat screening on the questionable cases and having all cases assessed by trained physicians. Nonetheless, DDST was viewed as a useful tool in identifying children who would otherwise be missed without formal screening.

In adults, there have been no major validation studies of neuropsychological tests undertaken in Singapore. However, a small but growing rehabilitation literature has developed, thanks in part to the existence of the Tan Tock Seng Rehabilitation Center, a centralized facility for the management and rehabilitation of neurological disorders. Among the disorders of relevance to neuropsychology, stroke has been examined in relation to short-term (Auchus, Chen, Sodagar, Thong, & Sng, 2002) and medium-term (Tham et al., 2002) outcome, as well as primary subarachnoid hemorrhage (Yap & Chua, 2002) and pediatric head injury (Yen & Wong, 2007). A series of studies have examined neuropsychological deficits caused by a range of encephalopathies, including Nipah virus (Ng, Lim, Yeoh, & Lee, 2004) inorganic chemical exposure in occupational spray painters (Ng, Lim, & Win, 1992), video tape manufacturing workers (Chia, Ong, Phoon, Tan, & Jeyaratnam 1993), workers exposed to Toulene (Boey, Foo, & Jeyaratnam, 1997), and those susceptible to inorganic lead exposure (Chia, Huijun, Theng, & Yap, 2007).

In recent years, there has been ongoing development of a local validation of the Brief Assessment of Cognition in Schizophrenia (BACS) (Keefe et al., 2004). As the title suggests, this brief measure is designed with schizophrenic patients in mind and assesses five different domains of cognitive function with six tests (verbal memory, working memory, verbal fluency, attention, and speed of information processing and executive functions) and takes about 35 minutes to administer.

The aging population of Singapore has raised the important issue of early detection of mild cognitive impairment (MCI) and conversion to dementia (Lim et al., 2003). Sahadevan and colleagues (Sahadevan, Tan, Tan, & Tan, 1997a, 1997b; Sahadevan, Lim, Tan, & Chan, 2000) embarked on a series of studies to validate a neuropsychological assessment battery to identify early Alzheimer's disease (AD) in elderly community-dwelling Chinese in Singapore, taking into account the age and education of the local elderly population. Sahadevan et al. (1997a) reported education-stratified normative data on a localized 10-item Word List Recall, Animal Fluency, 15-item Boston Naming, Block Design, and Object Assembly. Although difficult to statistically compare these norms with Western norms due to differences in age ranges and educational ranges, upon visual examination means and standard deviations on the Sahadevan-developed tests appear very similar to norms from the West. Later, Sahadevan et al. (2000) validated their battery on 55 cognitively healthy elderly Chinese and 72 predominantly mild AD patients. Their results showed that the majority of tests validly identified early AD in the aged Chinese subjects. Verbal memory, verbal fluency, and aspects of visuospatial functioning were the best diagnostic predictors in line with findings from Western populations. A more recent study by Yap, Ng, Niti, Yeo, and Henderson (2007) examined the CLOX (Royall, Cordes, & Polk, 1998), a drawing test that is sensitive to executive dysfunction, in 73 subjects with mixed-etiology AD, compared with 75 healthy controls, and found diagnostic accuracy of 84% to 85% for CLOX1 and CLOX2 and sensitivities and specificities in the 75% to 80% range in differentiating vascular-related dementia from AD.

Kua and Ko (1992) examined the validity of the 10-item Elderly Cognitive Assessment Questionnaire (ECAQ) and compared it with the Mental Status Questionnaire (MSQ). The ECAQ and the MSQ were administered to 105 elderly subjects (aged 65 years and above) from two day centers and a psychiatric outpatient clinic in Singapore. The sensitivities of the scales were similar. The ECAQ demonstrated properties similar to those of Western normed tests, with a sensitivity of 85.3%, specificity of 91.5%, and positive predictive value of 82.8%. More recently, Li, Ng, Kua, and Ko (2006) examined combinations of instruments to improve screening accuracy MCI and early AD. They compared the Mini-Mental State Examination (MMSE), Immediate and Delayed Recall (Logical Memory I and II), informant reports, and an activities of daily living (ADL) scale with the Clinical Dementia Rating (CDR) in 88 cognitively intact, 37 MCI, and 19 early AD patients. Screening accuracy was lowest for MMSE, whereas combinations of informant report, ADL, and cognitive measures of memory were better at predicting MCI.

The same research group examined ethnic differences in MMSE in discriminating between demented and nondemented elderly Asians (Ng, Niti, Chiam, & Kua, 2007). The subjects of this large-scale study of 1,092 community-living elderly, comprising Chinese, Malays, and Indians in Singapore, were given MMSE, Geriatric Mental State, and other demographic and health questionnaires, and significant ethnic differences in mean MMSE scores were found among noneducated but not educated Chinese, Indians, and Malays. Overall, the MMSE scores discriminated well between subjects with and without dementia, and scores were superior in higher-educated subjects. Lower education had a significant effect on specificity, which persisted after adjusting for differences in sociodemographic, health, and behavioral variables. Cutoff scores for determining dementia were very similar to those for Western studies (e.g., 23/24 for subjects with a sixth-grade education and above). Analysis of a comprehensive neuropsychological battery administered to these same subjects is currently under way.

In summary, while it is apparent that the development of clinical neuropsychology in Singapore has been somewhat slower than in some Western nations, it remains that Singapore, with its dynamic economy and many similarities to Western countries, faces many of the same challenges that have led to the development of clinical neuropsychology in the Western world. With the advent of neuroimaging, the subsequent decade of the brain in the 1990s, and increasing recognition of neuropsychology as a clinical profession abroad, many Singaporeans have sought training overseas in neuropsychology and the clinical neurosciences, and some are beginning to return and utilize their overseas experience to the betterment of the profession within Singapore. With rapid expansion of neuroscientific knowledge, the growth of psychology departments within the major hospitals, and an increasing number of Singaporeans wishing to pursue clinical psychology and clinical neuropsychology as a career, neuropsychology as a clinical profession is gaining a stronger presence. This growth will increase further with the planned introduction of the first home-grown clinical psychology program at the National University of Singapore in 2008, and the potential for the development of postgraduate clinical programs at other local universities. With these developments, Singapore is well placed to become a regional hub for training, research, and practice in clinical neuropsychology in years to come.

Acknowledgments

The authors particularly thank Associate Professor Fred Long from Nanyang Technological University, and acknowledge the help of Miss Quah Soo Li and Dr. Catherine Hayes in the preparation of this review.

References

Auchus, A. P., Chen, C. P., Sodagar, S. N., Thong, M., & Sng E. C. (2002). Single stroke dementia: Insights from 12 cases in Singapore. *Journal of Neurological Science, 15,* 203–204.

Boey, K. W., Foo, S. C., & Jeyaratnam, J. (1997). Effects of occupational exposure to toluene: A neuropsychological study on workers in Singapore. *Annals of the Academy of Medicine Singapore, 26,* 184–187.

Chia, S. E., Huijun, Z., Theng, T. M., & Yap, E. (2007). Possibilities of newer ALAD polymorphism influencing human susceptibility to effects of inorganic lead on the neurobehavioral functions. *Neurotoxicology, 28,* 312–317.

Chia, S. E., Ong, C. N., Phoon, W. H., Tan, K. T., & Jeyaratnam, J. (1993). Neurobehavioural effects on workers in a video tape manufacturing factory in Singapore. *Neurotoxicology, 14,* 51–56.

Keefe, R. S., Goldberg, T. E., Harvey, P. D., Gold, J. M., Poe, M. P., & Coughenour, L. (2004). The brief assessment of cognition in schizophrenia: Reliability, sensitivity, and comparison with a standard neurocognitive battery. *Schizophrenia Research, 68,* 283–297.

Kua, E. H., & Ko, S. M. (1992). A questionnaire to screen for cognitive impairment among elderly people in developing countries. *Acta Psychiatrica Scandinavica, 85,* 119–122.

Li, M., Ng, T. P., Kua, E. H., & Ko, S. M. (2006). Brief informant screening test for mild cognitive impairment and early Alzheimer's disease. *Dementia Geriatric Cognitive Disorders, 21,* 392–402.

Lim, H. C., Chan, T., & Yoong, T. (1994). Standardisation and adaptation of the Denver Developmental Screening Test (DDST) and Denver II for use in Singapore children. *Singapore Medical Journal, 35,* 156–160.

Lim, H. C., Ho, L. Y., Goh, L. H., Ling, S. L., Heng, R., & Po, G. L. (1996). The field testing of Denver Developmental Screening Test Singapore: A Singapore version of Denver II Developmental Screening Test. *Annals of the Academy of Medicine Singapore, 25,* 200–209.

Lim, H. J., Lim, J. P., Anthony, P., Yeo, D. H., & Sahadevan, S. (2003). Prevalence of cognitive impairment amongst Singapore's elderly Chinese: A community-based study using the ECAQ and the IQCODE. *International Journal of Geriatric Psychiatry, 18,* 142–148.

Ng, B. Y., Lim, C. C., Yeoh, A., & Lee, W. L. (2004). Neuropsychiatric sequelae of Nipah virus encephalitis. *Journal of Neuropsychiatry and the Clinical Neurosciences, 16,* 500–504.

Ng, T. P., Lim, L. C., & Win, K. K. (1992). An investigation of solvent-induced neuro-psychiatric disorders in spray painters. *Annals of the Academy of Medicine Singapore, 21,* 797–803.

Ng, T. P., Niti, M., Chiam, P. C., & Kua, E. H. (2007). Ethnic and educational differences in cognitive test performance on Mini-Mental State Examination in Asians. *American Journal of Geriatric Psychiatry, 15,* 130–139.

Royall, D. R., Cordes, J. A., & Polk, M. (1998). CLOX: An executive clock drawing task. *Journal of Neurology, Neurosurgery and Psychiatry, 64,* 588–594.

Sahadevan, S., Lim, P. P., Tan, N. J., & Chan, S. P. (2000). Diagnostic performance of two mental status tests in the older Chinese: Influence of education and age on cut-off values. *International Journal of Geriatric Psychiatry, 15,* 234–241.

Sahadevan, S., Tan, N. J., Tan, T., & Tan, S. (1997a). Cognitive testing of elderly Chinese people in Singapore: Influence of education and age on normative scores. *Age and Ageing, 26,* 481–486.

Sahadevan, S., Tan, N. J., Tan, T.C., & Tan, S. (1997b). Cognitive testing of elderly Chinese from selected community clubs in Singapore. *Annals of the Academy of Medicine Singapore, 26,* 271–277.

Tham, W., Auchus, A. P., Thong, M., Goh, M. L., Chang, H. M., Wong, M. C., & Chen, C. P. (2002). Progression of cognitive impairment after stroke: One year results from a longitudinal study of Singaporean stroke patients. *Journal of Neurological Science, 15,* 49–52.

World Bank. (2006). *World development report 2007: Development and the next generation.* Washington, DC: World Bank Publications.

Yap, E. C., & Chua, K. S. (2002). Rehabilitation outcome after primary subarachnoid haemorrhage. *Brain Injury, 16,* 491–499.

Yap, P. L., Ng, T. P., Niti, M., Yeo, D., & Henderson, L. (2007). Diagnostic performance of Clock Drawing Test by CLOX in an Asian Chinese population. *Dementia Geriatric Cognitive Disorders, 24,* 193–200.

Yen, H. L., & Wong, J. T. (2007). Rehabilitation for traumatic brain injury in children and adolescents. *Annals of the Academy of Medicine Singapore, 36,* 62–66.

19 Neuropsychology in Thailand

Kattiya Ratanadilok

Thailand is a Southeast Asian nation bordered by Laos, Mynamar, Cambodia, and Malaysia. It is subdivided into 76 provinces, which constitute four natural regions: the North; the Central Plain, or Chao Phraya River Basin, which includes the capital city Bangkok; the Northeast, or the Korat Plateau; and the South, or Southern Peninsula, which borders on Malaysia. The population of Thailand is estimated to be just over 65 million (2007) and is distributed throughout the country as follows: central Thai (36%), Thai-Lao (32%), northern Thai (8%), and southern Thai (8%) (Thailand Board of Investment (BOI), 2008). About 75% of the people are ethnically Thai. Chinese make up 14% of the population, while Malays, Cambodians, Vietnamese, and Indians account for the remaining 11%. Approximately 25% are under the age of 15 (Thailand BOI, 2008).

The government of Thailand is a constitutional monarchy. His Majesty King Bhumipol Adulyadej ascended to the throne in 1946 at age 19, and is the longest reigning monarch in the world. As head of state, the king has the authority to exercise sovereign power through the national assembly, the council of ministers, and the courts. The government is run by the prime minister, who functions in the name of the king and is responsible for all royal commands regarding the affairs of the state. His majesty the King and Her Majesty Queen Sirikit are the cultural and spiritual leaders for all Thai people. Buddhism is the national religion, which is practiced by 95% of the population (Thailand BOI, 2008).

Thailand has the second largest economy in Southeast Asia, following Indonesia. Although still a major agricultural economy, Thailand has experienced significant growth in its industrial sector, including automotive and electronics exports. Tourism is another growth industry. The currency is the Thai Baht.

The official language of Thailand is Thai, which is a tonal language. In other words, meaning is dictated by the tones or inflections in which the word is spoken. There are also numerous dialects of Thai spoken in regional areas that are influenced by the languages of border countries. For example, in the Northeast, dialects are heavily influenced by Laotian. Bahasa Melayu influences the dialects in the South and in some provinces closer to Malaysia. Dialects can differ to the point that Thais living in different regions have difficulty communicating. In fact, some Thais living in border areas are considered to speak a different language. Thai also has its own written language.

The Thai government places a strong emphasis on education, resulting in a high literacy rate (93%) (Thailand BOI, 2008). English is a compulsory subject in public schools; however, it is not yet a second language for most Thais. English is only spoken and understood in major cities such as Bangkok and is primarily used in the business community and tourism industries.

The life expectancy for Thais is 72.6 years (male, 70.2 years; female, 75 years) (Thailand BOI, 2008). The top five causes of mortality include HIV/AIDS (14%), ischaemic heart disease (7%), cerebrovascular disease (6%), diabetes mellitus (5%), and road traffic accidents (5%) (WHO, 2006). According to the National Statistical Office (NSO), Thailand's population growth rate is declining.

Psychology in Thailand

Although not a new discipline, psychology has taken long to develop in Thailand, partially due to cultural interpretation and biases toward mental illness. This section describes a brief history of psychology in Thailand as well as current practice patterns of clinical psychologists.

In 1953, the Thailand Department of Public Health established the first mental health clinic in Thailand. The Sukhawittayajit Clinic, currently known as the Rachanakarin Children and Adolescent Mental Health Institute, was opened with assistance from the World Health Organization (WHO) after Margaret Stepan, MD, helped train medical doctors in the field of psychiatry. At that time, mental health services were the purview of psychiatry.

The discipline of psychology emerged a decade later. In 1963, Somsong Suwannalert became the first Thai clinical psychologist after she completed her training at the University of Toronto (Suwannalert, 2006). In Thailand the first undergraduate program in clinical psychology was offered at Chiang Mai University under the Faculty of Humanity in 1964. Slowly, more Thai universities developed psychology departments, including Thammasat Unversity (1965), Kasetsart University (1975), Ramkhamhang University (1994), and Narasuan University (2000). In 1979, a master's degree program in clinical psychology was established in the Mahidol University Department of Psychiatry at Siriraj Hospital. This program is still the only institution offering a graduate level degree in clinical psychology in Thailand.

The Thai Clinical Psychologist Association (TCPA), the first and only Thai organization of clinical psychologists, was established in 1976. Membership includes both academic and clinical psychologists. One of the TCPA's missions is to improve standards of practice throughout the country. The efforts of the organization culminated in the passing of a psychology licensure requirement law in 2003.

To be eligible for licensure, a candidate must have a bachelor's degree in clinical psychology and complete a six-month internship. The licensing process consists of a written examination and an interview with the Thai licensing board. Statistics from 2006 indicate that 344 psychologists have been granted licenses.

The TCPA is aware that Thailand is behind most of the world in providing education and training for psychologists. To address the needs for higher standards of training, the TCPA has invited clinical psychologists and psychiatrists from countries such as America, Sweden, and the Netherlands to provide workshops and short courses on treatment and assessment techniques. Training programs usually last for a few days to a few weeks. Other psychologists have sought training abroad, enrolling in master's and doctoral programs in psychology from other countries. Currently, the author is the only Thai psychologist attaining a doctorate in clinical psychology with a concentration in neuropsychology. The lack of well-trained and educated personnel has led to slow progress in the development of the field.

Historically, clinical psychologists have worked almost exclusively in psychiatric departments of medical hospitals. Psychologists are included in interdisciplinary teams, alongside nurses, social workers, and psychiatrists. The psychiatrist is typically regarded as the team leader. Primary duties include psychological assessments and psychotherapy. Freestanding counseling centers or private psychotherapy services are generally nonexistent. No specific mental health law permits clinical psychologists to open a clinic by themselves without the supervision of a psychiatrist. In addition, there are some cultural reasons for this limited practice. First, many Thais perceive all ailments as medical problems, and thus seek medical treatment when experiencing stressors or emotional problems. Second, due to the tendency toward somatization, many Thais do not recognize mental problems in family members and may not know where to go for treatment, or that mental health problems are curable. Third, Thais are a collectivist culture, yet many Thais are very private. They tend to keep problems within the family and resort to religion, such as Buddhist teachings, to reduce their mental discomfort. Finally, the stigma of mental illness is very strong in Thai culture. Thus, many Thais feel uncomfortable seeking counseling from a mental health clinic for fear of being labeled "crazy," and typically seek treatment only when their condition becomes intolerable and requires immediate medical attention. As a result, mental health services are generally found within the medical setting.

Given these limitations, it will be many years before clinical psychology is commonly practiced outside of medical settings and the umbrella of psychiatry. Still, a few opportunities have emerged. For example, the Department of Juvenile Observation and Protection (DJOP) under the Ministry of Justice (MOJ) has significantly expanded juvenile training schools. Nearly 50% of Thai psychologists are working in this setting. Other psychologists have pursued careers in related fields, such as AIDS counseling, community mental health prevention (Tapanya, 2001), and crisis intervention, the latter for people suffering from posttraumatic stress disorders due to natural disasters such as tsunamis and terrorist attacks.

Neuropsychology

Neuropsychology is a subspecialty of clinical psychology in which a growing number of Thai psychologists are beginning to practice. An informal survey on clinical and neuropsychological practice was conducted by the author at the 2007 annual conference sponsored by the Thai Clinical Psychologist Association (TCPA) ($N = 35$). Subjects of the survey were registrants in the author's lecture on neuropsychology of attention-deficit/hyperactivity disorder (ADHD) and learning disability (LD). The majority of participants worked in the psychiatry department of a medical hospital, while a few worked in the neurology department. A small number reported working in children's psychiatric care, regional health clinics, and juvenile training schools.

Job duties included psychological evaluation and intervention with a few neuropsychological evaluations and treatments. The largest population serviced were children and adolescents with the following diagnoses: learning problems, attention-deficit/hyperactivity disorder, substance abuse, autistic disorder, and Asperger's syndrome. The second most common population consisted of geriatric patients with dementia, stroke, Alzheimer's disease, and other systemic diseases, such as diabetes. The three most common referral sources were psychiatrists, physicians, and schoolteachers.

Neuropsychological tests used by Thai psychologists are primarily adaptations of Western tests. The most common intelligence tests include the Wechsler Adult Intelligence Scale (WAIS), the Wechsler Intelligence Scale for Children (WISC), Raven's Progressive Matrices (RPM), and the Stanford-Binet Intelligence Scale. The most popular neuropsychological tests used were the Bender Gestalt Test and the Mini-Mental Status Exam (MMSE)–Thai version. A few psychologists reported using the Wechsler Memory Scale (WMS-III), the Wisconsin Card Sorting Test (WCST), the Boston Naming Test, the Rey Complex Figures Test, and the Trail Making Test, and one reported using the Halstead-Reitan. Test selection appears heavily dependent upon availability to the psychologist. Tests are translated into Thai via nonstandardized processes by a small group of psychologists. For example, back translations are typically not done. Thai psychologists generally use the original Western norms when interpreting test results. Because of the growing interest in neuropsychology, an increasing number of tests are being imported from other countries.

Currently, there are many challenges in neuropsychological practice in Thailand. As illustrated above, a significant problem is the validity of the tests that are being used. The vast majority of neuropsychological instruments are translated versions of Western tests. Translation processes are not standardized, and tests are usually older versions. In addition, there are no local norms and few local validation studies; thus, test interpretation is subject to sampling biases. Both limitations question the validity of the testing for the Thai population.

Attempts have been made to standardize Western tests on the Thai population. These projects have been sponsored by Western countries studying the HIV epidemic in Thailand. For example, Maj et al. (1993) evaluated two neuropsychological tests, the WHO/UCLA Auditory Verbal Learning Test (AVLT) and Color Trails 1 and 2, which were designed to minimize cultural bias. Tests were administered to subjects in developed countries (Germany and Italy) and developing countries (Thailand and Zaire). Results showed that the new testing instruments measured the same functional domains. The researchers also found that the instruments were sensitive to HIV-21-related cognitive impairment across different cultures (Maj et al., 1993). More recently, the South East Asian Research Collaboration with Hawaii (SEARCH), an international HIV study headed by Victor Valcour at the University of Hawaii, collected norms on a number of neuropsychological tests, including Finger Tapping, EIWA digit symbol, Grooved Pegboard, Verbal Fluency—names and animals, Trail Making A, EIWA Block Design, and the two aforementioned WHO measures.

Local norm collection or studies examining test validity are rare; however, a few attempts have been made. For example, Kaewpornsawan and Ariyanuchitkul (2000) collected norms on a sample of 127 Thai children ages 6 to 11 for an adapted version of the computerized Continuous Performance Test (CPT). Their modified version of the CPT used simple pictures instead of letters.

Tantilipikorn (2003) attempted to validate the Reitan-Indiana Aphasia Screening Test on a Thai population by comparing scores in samples of 75 neurologically normal subjects, 22 epilepsy patients, and 55 patients with either right or left hemisphere lesions. Results indicated that the test was able to discriminate between the left and right brain lesion subjects and the normal and epilepsy subjects; however, no significant differences were found between the left and right brain lesion subjects. Tantilipikorn suggested that the lack of differences between these groups may have been due to educational level. Alternatively, because of the tonal nature of the Thai language, it is possible that language skills in Thais may be less lateralized than the language skills of persons in Western countries.

Another challenge is that Thai psychologists do not receive adequate training in neuropsychology. None of the Thai university psychology programs offer courses in neuropsychology. Many Thai psychologists learn how to administer and interpret tests simply from reading the test manuals. Accurate test interpretation is also affected, as many Thai psychologists hold false assumptions about neuropsychological testing. For example, they often use negative findings from a visual motor integration test to rule out organic brain injury, they believe that the intellectual functioning test can be used to diagnose learning disability, and they assume that nonverbal tests are culture free. Thus, similar to psychology, there are limitations in training and practice that need to be addressed to develop the discipline.

Research in neuropsychology

There have only been a handful of studies examining neuropsychology in Thailand. Studies have generally been descriptive in nature, examining test performance or differential diagnoses with child, adolescent, psychiatric, and geriatric populations.

For example, Phattharayuttawat (1999) examined IQ test scores and scatter profiles on the Wechsler Intelligence Scale for Children (WISC) to differentiate children with mental retardation (MR) from those with a learning disability (LD). Tubmanee (2001) studied the relationship between depression and dementia using the Thai Geriatric Depression Scale (TGDS) and the Thai Mental State Examination (TMSE) in a random sample of 270 elderly individuals. The prevalence of depression was approximately 35% and 27%, respectively, for dementia. Another study using the same instruments compared dementia in stroke survivors and patients with Parkinson's disease (Poungvarin, 1996). Results indicated that 33% of stroke patients and 26% of Parkinson's disease patients scored below the 23-point cutoff scores for dementia.

Other studies have examined the prevalence of, or individual cases of, misdiagnoses. Arayawichanont (2000) believed that dementia was underdiagnosed by treating physicians. To examine this hypothesis, he determined the cognitive status of 150 inpatients through clinical evaluation, neurological examination, and mental state examination. Arayawichanont identified 49 of the sample as having a dementia. Of these cases, only two had been diagnosed with a dementia by attending physicians, and both of those patients had previously been diagnosed with dementia before admission to the hospital.

Puttipornopas (2006) reported the case study of a 30-year-old Thai man diagnosed with paranoid schizophrenia for 7 years who demonstrated poor response to treatment. After a systemic evaluation by an interdisciplinary team, which included physical, mental, and laboratory tests, the patient was diagnosed with frontal lobe atrophy and hydrocephalus. His treatment regimen was changed and included ventriculoperitoneal shunting, the administration of an antidementic drug, and life skills training to increase his quality of life.

As mentioned previously, international researchers have collaborated with Thai researchers in studying HIV populations in Thailand. Specifically, studies have examined neuropsychological abnormalities in patients with HIV/AIDS (Valcour et al., 2007), neuropsychological differences between patients treated with antiretroviral therapy medication and control groups (Koekkoek et al., 2006), and HIV-related neuropsychological abnormalities in patients living in different cultures (Maj et al., 1991).

In summary, despite a lack of knowledge and appropriate training, Thailand's need for qualified practitioners in neuropsychology increases each year as a result of the development of medical science and an ever-increasing acknowledgment of neurological disorders in Thai people. However, the current knowledge base among psychologists and the paucity of training opportunities pose significant challenges to the field. Ultimately, better education and training for practitioners, standardized test translation procedures, collection of local norms for neuropsychological tests, and research on clinical populations, test validity, and clinical interventions are needed to develop the field of neuropsychology in Thailand.

Acknowledgments

The author expresses her gratitude to Mr. Thomas E. Smith for his kind suggestions and editorial assistance in the preparation of this review.

References

Arayawichanont, A. (2000). Do physicians recognise dementia? *Siriraj Hospital Gazette, 52*, 528–532.

Kaewpornsawan, T., & Ariyanuchitkul, S. (2000). Normal values of computerized continuous performance test for measuring the sustained attention in Thai students. *Siriraj Hospital Gazette, 52*, 180–185.

Koekkoek, S., Eggermont, L., De Sonneville, L., Jupimai, T., Wicharuk, S., Apateerapong, W., et al. (2006). Effects of highly active antiretroviral therapy (HAART) on psychomotor performance in children with HIV disease. *Journal of Neurology, 253*, 1615–1624.

Maj, M., D'Elia, L., Satz, P., Janssen, R., Zaudig, M., Uchiyama, C., et al. (1993). Evaluation of two new neuropsychological tests designed to minimize cultural bias in the assessment of HIV-1 seropositive persons: A WHO study. *Archives of Clinical Neuropsychology, 8*, 123–135.

Maj, M., Janssen, R., Satz, P., Zaudig, M., Starace, F., Boor, D., et al. (1991). The World Health Organization's cross-cultural study on neuropsychiatric aspects of infection with the human immunodeficiency virus 1 (HIV-1): Preparation and pilot phase. *British Journal of Psychiatry, 159*, 351–356.

Phattharayuttawat, S. (1999). IQ discriminance analysis between mental retardation and learning disabilities in children. *Siriraj Hospital Gazette, 51*, 92–97.

Poungvarin, N. (1996). Comparison of dementia in stroke survivors and patients with Parkinson's disease in Thai subjects. *Siriraj Hospital Gazette, 48*, 291–301.

Puttipornopas, P. (2006, July). *Report of patients with frontal lobe dementia with eating disorder and the interdisciplinary intervention program.* Abstract of the 5th International Mental Health Conference, Prince Palace Hotel, Bangkok, Thailand.

Suwannalert, S. (2006). Thirty years of Thai clinical psychology. *Journal of Clinical Psychology, 37*, 1–8. (Original work published in Thai)

Tantilipikorn, C. (2003). A study of aphasia screening test: A subtest of Halstead-Reitan Neuropsychological Test Battery in brain lesion patients as compared to normal subjects. *Journal of Clinical Psychology, 34*, 44–57.

Tapanya, S. (2001). Psychology in medical settings in Thailand. *Journal of Clinical Psychology in Medical Settings, 8*, 69–72.

Thailand Board of Investment (BOI). (2008). *Thailand in brief: Demographic.* Retrieved February 29, 2008, from http://www.boi.go.th/english/how/demographic.asp

Tubmanee, M. (2001). Depression and dementia in Thai community dwelling elderly in Bangkok. *Journal of Clinical Psychology, 32*, 43–57.

Valcour, V. G., Sithinamsuwan, P., Nidhinandana, S., Thitivichianlert, S., Ratto-Kim, S., Apateerapong, W., et al. (2007). Neuropsychological abnormalities in patients with dementia in CRF 01_AE HIV-1 infection. *Neurology, 68*, 525–527.

World Health Organization. (2006). *Mortality country fact sheet 2006—Thailand.* Retrieved February 29, 2008, from http://www.who.int/whosis/mort/profiles/mort_searo_tha_thailand.pdf

Index

www.ingramcontent.com/pod-product-compliance
Ingram Content Group UK Ltd.
Pitfield, Milton Keynes, MK11 3LW, UK
UKHW022003180926
475701UK00003B/179
* 9 7 8 1 1 3 8 8 8 2 9 6 6 *